Human Resources Management for Health Care Organizations

A Strategic Approach

JOAN E. PYNES

DONALD N. LOMBARDI

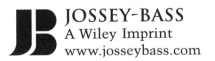

JOSSEY-BASS
A Wiley Imprint
www.josseybass.com

Library of Congress Cataloging-in-Publication Data

Pynes, Joan.

  Human resources management for health care organizations : a strategic approach / Joan E. Pynes, Donald N. Lombardi.—1st ed.

        p. cm.

  Includes bibliographical references and index.

  ISBN 978-0-470-87355-7 (pbk.); 978-1-118-15273-7 (ebk.); 978-1-118-15274-4 (ebk.); 978-1-118-15275-1 (ebk.)

  1. Health services administration.   2. Health facilities—Personnel management.   I. Lombardi, Donald N., 1956- II. Title.

  RA971.35.P96 2012

  362.1068—dc23

2011038828

Printed in the United States of America

FIRST EDITION

PB Printing 10 9 8 7 6 5 4 3 2 1

CONTENTS

Preface   xv

The Authors   xxi

PART ONE

Human Resources Management in the Health Care Business Arena

4/4 Chapter 1: Introduction to Health Care Human
               Resources Management   3

       Defining Elements of Progressive Health Care
          Organizations   4

       Current Perceptions of Health Care Organizations   7

       Spheres of Influence Model   9

Five Significant Change Dynamics of Modern
   Health Care   12

Profile of a Progressive Health Care Organization   22

Composition of a Progressive Health Care Human
   Resources Management Department   27

Chapter 2: Strategic Health Care Human Resources
            Management and Planning   31

The Changing Role of Human Resources Management   32

Human Resources Outsourcing   35

Strategic Human Resources Management and Human
   Resources Planning   36

Anticipating Future Needs   38

Evaluating the Effectiveness of Strategic Human
   Resources Management   42

Problems and Implications of Strategic Human
   Resources Management   44

Chapter 3: Organizational Culture Standards for Health
            Care Human Resources   49

Performance Matrix of Superstars, Steadies, and
   Nonplayers   50

PACT Formula   54

Strategic Requirements for a Progressive Health Care
   Human Resources Management Department   74

Chapter 4: Equal Employment Opportunity Laws
            and Health Care Human Resources
            Management   83

Federal Equal Employment Opportunity Laws   84

Proving Employment Discrimination   96

Affirmative Action: Executive Orders and Other
    Federal Laws   98

Constitutional Rights   102

Additional Protections for Employees   109

Chapter 5: Managing the Unique Health Care
                Workforce   115

Cultural Factors Relevant to Health Care Human
    Resources   122

Practical Application: A Tale of Two Jersey
    Cultures   129

Chapter 6: The Importance of Volunteers in Health
                Care Organizations   135

Selection and Placement Strategy Considerations for
    Volunteers   136

Maximizing Health Care Volunteer Performance   143

Agenda Topics for Volunteer Summits   148

Ten Essential Rules for Volunteer Placement   150

PART TWO

Methods and Accountabilities of Health Care Human Resources

Chapter 7: Critical Job Analysis and Design   155

Legal Significance of Job Analysis   157

Job Analysis Information   158

Designing a Job Analysis Program   163

Job Descriptions and Job Specifications   164

Competency Modeling   168

Job Analysis Techniques   170

4/18

4/18

4/11

Chapter 8: Recruitment, Interviewing, and Selection
                  Strategies   177

    Preselection Process   178

    Critical Dimensions of External Recruitment   195

    Preparing and Planning for the Interview   198

    Conducting the Interview   199

    Evaluating the Interview   204

Chapter 9:   Maximizing Performance Management
             and Evaluation   209

    Developing an Evaluation Program   210

    Using Defusers—the Return to Objectivity Formula   241

Chapter 10: Compensation Strategies   247

    Motivation   248

    Equity   253

    Executive Compensation and Benefits   265

    Federal Laws Governing Compensation   267

Chapter 11: Benefits   271

    Government Required Benefits   272

    Discretionary Benefits   276

    Quality-of-Work and Quality-of-Life Issues   282

PART THREE

Maximizing Health Care Human Resources

Chapter 12: Training and Development   289

    Needs Assessment   291

    Developing Training Objectives   293

Developing the Curriculum   294

Delivering Training   302

Evaluating Training   303

Career Development   306

Health Care Training and Development in
    Application   308

Relevant and Resonant Health Care Organizational
    Training and Development   310

Chapter 13: Organizational Development Strategies   319

Essential Objectives of Health Care Organizational
    Development   319

Organizational Development Strategies for Building
    Pride   329

Organizational Development Strategies for Escalating
    Accountability   338

Organizational Development Strategies for Team
    Building   344

Chapter 14: Labor-Management Relations   353

Collective Bargaining in the Private Sector   354

Collective Bargaining in Health Care Organizations   355

Collective Bargaining in Federal Government Agencies   358

Collective Bargaining in State and Local Government
    Agencies   359

Concepts and Practices of Collective Bargaining   360

Chapter 15: Strategic Health Care Human Resources
    Technology   377

Information Systems Technology   378

Organizational Change   380

Types of Information Systems   381
Human Resources Information Systems   384

Bibliography   393

Index   409

TABLES AND FIGURES

Tables

3.1	Performance Matrix	51
4.1	Federal Statutes Related to Equal Employment Opportunity	103
5.1	Cultural Dynamics of the Hoboken Gen X Crew	130
5.2	Cultural Dynamics of New Jersey Retirees	131
6.1	Progressive Placement of Medical Center Volunteers	146
10.1	Typical Compensable Factors	256
10.2	Salary Table 2010-GS Incorporating the 1.50 Percent General Schedule Increase (Annual Rates by Grade and Step)	259
11.1	Employee Benefits	277
13.1	Organizational Development Themes from Great American Innovators	326
14.1	National Labor Relations Board Jurisdictional Standards for Nonprofit Health Care Organizations (in Effect July 1990)	356

Figures

1.1	Spheres of Influence Model	10
1.2	Organizational Chart—Midsize Community Hospital	23
1.3	Organizational Chronology of a Health Care Professional	25
1.4	Organizational Chart—Health Care Human Resources Management Department	27
3.1	PACT Formula	55
3.2	Time Line Review of the Huntington VA Medical Center, West Virginia	60
3.3	Defined Values of a Progressive Health Care Leader	66
3.4	Decision-Making Criteria and Process	77
5.1	Unique Facets of the Health Care Workforce	116
5.2	Cultural Composition Foundations	123
6.1	Identifying Background Strengths of Health Care Volunteers	137
7.1	Example Job Analysis Questionnaire	160
7.2	Example Structured Checklist	161
7.3	Example Job Description	166
8.1	Recruitment Sources	182
8.2	Candidate Evaluation	194
8.3	Interview Dyad Dynamics	202
9.1	Example Trait Rating Scale	213
9.2	Example Critical Incident Report	214
9.3	Example Behaviorally Anchored Rating Scale	216
9.4	Example Behavioral Observation Scale	217
9.5	Example 360-Degree Evaluation	218
12.1	Critical Dimensions of Health Care Training and Development	308
12.2	The "I" Formula	314

13.1   Essential Tenets of Health Care Organizational
       Development   320

13.2   Majuro Medical Center Credo of Nursing   330

13.3   Example Criteria Page for an Organizational Handbook
       of Values   332

13.4   Huntington VA Medical Center (VAMC) Fact Sheet   348

I N AN ERA in which health care organizations are contending with ever-escalating expectations, increased demands for services, and critical scrutiny from all constituencies, the need to maximize the performance of human resources at every level and in every regard is the most significant component of a health care organization's essential charter. Strategic human resources management (SHRM) is the integration of human resources management (HRM) with the strategic mission of the organization that innovates human resources policies and practices to meet the challenges health care agencies face today, as well as those they will face in the future. Human resources management departments must take a proactive role in guiding and supporting health care organizational efforts to meet the changing demands of the customer-patient community and the challenges confronting every member of the health care organization.

With these daunting challenges, there has been a renewed emphasis on human capital and human resources management as a responsibility of all health care leaders, as health care organizations face the realization that the combined strength of their employees is undoubtedly their most important organizational asset. Workers define the organization's character, affect its capacity to perform, and represent its knowledge base—a confluence that results in the provision of the best possible health care to the community. To be true strategic partners, human resources management departments must possess high levels of professional and business knowledge and must establish viable foundations and vivid links to enhancing organizational performance that offer a fundamental, measurable basis for the continued success and recognized excellence of the organization.

Health care organizations must stay dynamically attuned to the needs of society and seek to improve the quality of their services by engaging in strategic human resources management. Recruitment and selection strategies must be innovative, career development opportunities must be provided progressively, work assignments must be thoughtfully designed, and policies must reward superior performers while resolving performance problems posed by marginal employees. These policies must be developed and administered according to the principles of equity, efficiency, and effectiveness; performance standards must be designed to promote the stated goals and resonant values of the progressive health care agency so that it truly evolves into an accountable care organization.

PURPOSE AND AUDIENCE

This book works as a comprehensive guide to the essential areas of health care human resources management by defining what each aspect of human resources addresses, why it is specifically essential to a health care organization, and then how it can be incorporated strategically using best practices and vanguard programs. This book particularly emphasizes the importance of HRM functions and SHRM planning balanced with the current and emergent dynamics apparent in the most important resource of a health care organization—its people.

This book was written to be an immediately useful practical handbook for practitioners as well as a textbook for use as part of health care management undergraduate and graduate programs. By infusing academic discourse with current proven strategies, the book is intended to be relevant, resonant, and realistic in its scope and viability in both the classroom and the health care workplace.

OVERVIEW OF THE CONTENTS

Part One introduces the context of human resources management in the unique health care business arena, and moves in a "general to specific" progression by examining the critical dimensions of the customer-patient environment, the composition of a progressive health care organization, and the human resources management needs of a health care professional. Chapter One provides an introduction to the health care human resources business setting, replete with methods for strategic analysis and examples from a triad of community health care organizations powered by strong human resources management departments. Chapter Two explains how SHRM and human resources planning are imperative if health care agencies are to remain competitive and be able to accomplish their mission. Chapter Three presents organizational culture standards for progressive health care human resources management using an organizational assessment tool as a focal point. Chapter Four presents the legal environment of human resources management, incorporating practical perspectives and validated guidance. Chapter Five explores the methods for managing the unique health care workforce and moves from the overarching subject of organizational culture to practical perspectives and pertinent application. Then, the importance of managing volunteers and how SHRM practices can assist in making the volunteer experience both productive for the agency and satisfying to volunteers and board members is discussed in Chapter Six.

Part Two presents the techniques and functional areas of human resources management, supported by methods and accountability programs for health care organizations. Each chapter provides ample practical examples. Chapter Seven explains the importance of job analysis before executing HRM policies or developing job descriptions, performance appraisal instruments, training and development programs, and recruitment and selection criteria. A variety of job analysis techniques are discussed. Chapter Eight addresses recruitment, selection, and hiring techniques. Drug testing, physical ability testing, psychological examinations, and other essential selection programs are also summarized.

Performance management and evaluation of employee performance are the focus of Chapter Nine. The chapter explains different performance appraisal techniques, identifying their strengths and weaknesses, noting the importance of rater training and thorough documentation. Ethical issues in performance appraisal are discussed, as are critical dynamics of merit pay and 360-degree evaluations relative to health care organizations. Chapter Ten identifies the internal and external factors that influence compensation policies and practices. The chapter discusses fully the techniques used to develop pay systems, provides examples of job evaluation systems, and explains nontraditional pay systems. Chapter Eleven's discussion addresses employer-provided benefits and pensions with the objective of providing not only an overview but a critical examination of benefits strategies and programs for health care organizations.

Part Three provides a spectral view of strategies for maximizing health care human resources progressively, positively, and purposefully in an accountable care organization. The focus of Chapter Twelve is training and development activities, as changes in technology and demographics and the development of new responsibilities and expectations have made training and career development more important than ever. Identifying training needs, developing the training objectives and curriculum, and evaluating training are explored, and different training formats are summarized. The chapter concludes with examples of management training and career development programs.

Chapter Thirteen articulates the vibrant role of organizational development in health care as a leading factor in the growth and development of the organization itself. Basic strategies, case exemplars, and a wealth of field-proven programs are illustrated comprehensively and in context. Chapter Fourteen discusses collective bargaining in health care settings, and explores the legal environment of labor-management relations for health care agencies. Definitions and explanations are provided for such concepts as unit determination, union security, unfair labor practices, management rights, impasse resolution, and grievance arbitration. Chapter Fifteen discusses strategic human resources management and information technology.

ACKNOWLEDGMENTS

The authors would like to thank Andy Pasternack and Seth Schwartz from Jossey-Bass/Wiley for their insightful guidance and steadfast support, as well as the following individuals for their many thoughtful and helpful comments on the completed manuscript: Jane Nelson Bolin and David Hernandez. In addition, Ben Choe, USMC(R), was stellar in his innovation and effectiveness working with all of the diagrams and visual materials that enrich this book.

We are also very grateful to all of the great health care leaders—at every level and across the national health care business arena—whose insights contributed to the practical strategies in this text. Moreover, we appreciate all of the good work they do every day to take good care of all of us, and hope that this book assists in a small way in their extraordinary mission.

Joan would like to acknowledge her husband, Mike, and her sister, Robyn, for their support; Don would like to thank his wife, Debbie, and all fourteen of his godchildren.

THE AUTHORS

JOAN E. PYNES PhD, is a professor of public administration at the University of South Florida. She is the author or coauthor of four books, most recently the third edition of *Human Resources Management for Public and Nonprofit Organizations: A Strategic Approach* (Jossey-Bass, 2009) and *Effective Nonprofit Management: Context and Environment* (M. E. Sharpe, 2011). She is the author or coauthor of more than fifty academic articles, book chapters, technical reports, and encyclopedia entries about public and nonprofit human resources management.

DONALD N. LOMBARDI PhD, USMC(R), is the Industry Professor and director of the Stevens Healthcare Educational Partnership and the academic director of the Veterans Program at Stevens Institute of Technology. He has consulted for over 170 health care organizations in all fifty states and ten foreign countries; has developed seven accreditation programs for the American College of Healthcare Executives since 1986; and has written eleven books, including *The Handbook for the New Healthcare Manager* (Jossey-Bass, 2001). He holds more than fifty U.S. copyrights on strategic planning, human resources management, and organizational development systems for text, on-site, and online delivery.

Human Resources Management for Health Care Organizations

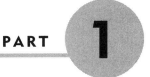

Human Resources Management in the Health Care Business Arena

1

Introduction to Health Care Human Resources Management

LEARNING OBJECTIVES

- Identify the components of the unique health care business arena
- Delineate the five critical change factors in the health care business environment
- Understand the basic leadership roles and functions of the emergent health care organization
- Recognize the context for progressive human resources management in a health care organization

HEALTH CARE IN the United States is provided by organizations that are singularly unique in nature and construction, and that have few comparative models across American industry. Many health care organizations are among the best-known institutions in their geographic area, yet they typically operate as nonprofit entities. Although they employ a large number of local citizens, their pay scale and compensation levels are normally below those of many of the much smaller for-profit organizations in their service community. Very few community hospitals are truly public institutions, yet because they provide emergency care for absolutely everyone coming through their doors, they are widely perceived as public institutions supported largely and directly by federal, state, and local tax revenue.

This chapter explores in a general way the composition of American health care organizations as it relates to human resources management to set a working context for specific organizational development and human resources strategies. Although these organizations can range in size from a small neighborhood or rural clinic to a large metropolitan hospital employing thousands of professionals, there are many instructive similarities, which will be examined first broadly, and then with a specific focus on human resources management. This chapter details the roles and responsibilities of the executive cadre and respective operational ranks of the administrative and patient care sectors of a health care organization, and then describes the causal relationship between a progressive health care organization and its customer-patient community. In addition, this chapter begins to introduce the components of a progressive, successful health care organization by establishing the mainstay foundation—strong human resources management that extends from the human resources office to the executive suite, through the medical ranks onto the patient floors, and across the entire organization. Finally, the chapter concludes with a practical discussion of the critical and significant role that human resources management plays in the daily operations and ongoing success of a progressive health care organization.

DEFINING ELEMENTS OF PROGRESSIVE HEALTH CARE ORGANIZATIONS

Most health care organizations are among the largest employers in their service community and are nonprofit institutions that rely on a very complicated labyrinth of reimbursement funds, charitable contributions, physician fees, and an assortment of other revenue sources to meet their budgetary requirements. Because federal law dictates that no American can be denied health care services from any community medical center's emergency room, for example, health care organizations are perceived to be community bedrocks in the same manner as public schools. Such organizations as the U.S.

Department of Veterans Affairs, which includes nearly 120 large medical centers employing an average of three thousand people as well as nearly four hundred community-based outpatient clinics, are indeed formidable community players, especially in current times.

Many health care organizations also share a laudable history with their respective communities. Urban New Jersey provides three excellent examples of health care organizations that share a wonderful legacy, lore, and legend with their community. In Hoboken, New Jersey, commonly known as the birthplace of Frank Sinatra and the centerpiece of the classic movie *On the Waterfront,* Hoboken University Medical Center (HUMC) has served its diverse community—which features constituencies ranging from Wall Street stockbrokers to newly arrived immigrants living within two miles of the Statue of Liberty—since 1863. In that year, the medical center opened its doors, as did many organizations that were founded during the nineteenth century, as a de facto hospice in which doctors sent severely ill patients to receive terminal care or critical services. Through the years Hoboken University Medical Center, in a city featuring waterfront, education-based, technology-based, and tourist businesses, evolved into both a major community employer and a health care organization that can lay claim to having the most sophisticated technology tracking and assessment system in the state of New Jersey.

Furthermore, HUMC is a community-driven health care organization that seriously embraces the charter of providing its community with stellar "cradle to grave" services—everything from childbirth to pediatric services to emergency care, and across the spectrum of critical and elective surgery care. Health care organizations maintaining this charter are the ones that the majority of experts believe will be most likely to thrive in an era in which American health care constituents are more exacting, demanding, and educated, because they represent the first defining element of a progressive health care organization:

We do everything here.

Newark Beth Israel Medical Center (NBIMC) opened its doors in 1898 in the state's largest city. By 2009 it had become one of the flagship organizations of Barnabas Health, the second-largest employer of any kind in the state of New Jersey—particularly noteworthy when one considers that New Jersey is the most densely populated state in the United States—with nearly 24,000 employees, six major medical centers, and over forty clinics and ambulatory care centers. Despite the religious resonance of the system's name (based on its flagship medical center, which coincidentally is also the state's oldest), Barnabas Health is secular and nonprofit, and rates second only to the state of New Jersey itself as major employer, human services provider, and educational center in terms of employee populace. Since its opening as a prototypical general hospital, Newark Beth Israel Medical Center, now 3,585 employees strong, also includes the Children's Hospital of New Jersey and one of the highest-rated cardiology centers in the United States, and is the major provider of virtually every type of health care service needed in the state's largest urban center. As an organization that prides itself on "growing its own and hiring from within the community," it is not uncommon to find employees at NBIMC who are third-generation "Beth employees." Further, one of the current vanguard initiatives of NBIMC is the Start On Success (SOS) Program, which is the epitome of a community employee development program. This program provides selected high school seniors in the City of Newark public school system with an opportunity to complete their education in the morning on the campus at The Beth (as NBIMC is commonly known across the organization and in its service community). In the afternoon the students undertake responsibilities in part-time jobs that provide training in such areas as patient transport, entry-level nursing, security, food services, and other critical vocational areas that are always in demand in a health care organization. With this everyday, resonant charter, proven over a hundred years now, The Beth personifies the second defining element of a progressive health care organization:

Quality care begins with quality people.

Across town, in Belleville, New Jersey, made famous as the home neighborhood of pop icons Frankie Valli and the Four Seasons and Connie Francis, Clara Maass Medical Center (CMMC) has been in business since 1888. Originally named German Hospital because it tended at its inception to the majority community population of recent American immigrants from Germany, CMMC—still with its original, formidable brick facade—became the local provider of choice, establishing a reputation as a training center for medical and nursing personnel. In fact, a cohort of physicians and nurses not only provided research and direct patient care in the areas of general medicine in the late 1880s but also became pioneers of critical medical research. Specifically, a group of physicians and nurses from German Hospital worked assiduously for a cure of yellow fever. One of the nurses—Clara Maass herself, a young German American nurse from the neighborhood—not only participated in the research but also offered her life in volunteering to be the first human subject for the vaccine that eventually cured the malady of yellow fever. The hospital was rightfully rechristened in her honor and to this day exemplifies the third defining standard of a progressive American health care organization:

What we did yesterday might be good enough for today, but we constantly have to learn anew and face the challenge of being better tomorrow.

Health care organizations such as these three have survived the conundrum of how to provide quality health care by adhering to these principles, which, as we will see, take root in strong health care human resources management.

CURRENT PERCEPTIONS OF HEALTH CARE ORGANIZATIONS

At present many **customer-patients** consider themselves to be educated about health care and, thanks to mass advertising through traditional media sources and on the Internet, often pride themselves on being informed consumers. As already mentioned, many American health care organizations possess a reputation, sometimes good and sometimes not so good, in their community based on history and past performance. However, with the recent spotlighting of health care by politicians and legislators, among other factors to be discussed later in this chapter, health care organizations today endure more scrutiny than ever before.

This scrutiny begins at the physician's office, the time-honored entry point of health care in the United States. Starting with this interaction, the health care consumer believes the *what* of health care—that is, the actual product of health care, augmented and supported by cutting-edge technology and the latest medical devices—is likely to provide a sure cure at the highest possible level of care. However, what is being more closely assessed now than at any other point in health care history is the *how* of health care—that is, the "human touch" that is afforded to customer-patients by all employees, volunteers, medical professionals, and administrative leaders that they encounter through their healing experience. Because health care customer-patients pay more, and believe that they are better educated than health care consumers of previous generations and are aware of more dimensions of care, the element of health care that we define as the human touch—and that traditionally has been referred to as bedside manner—often supersedes the actual product when patients evaluate care. This reality demands a strong human resources management department that can help maximize the organization's human capital on a daily and progressive basis.

On a related note, a consumer and a customer, as per the traditional thinking in marketing, can be two different people in health care. The consumer, for example, in an equation involving services for the aging, could be an aging parent. The customer—that is, the person making the decision— could be the son-in-law or daughter-in-law of the aging parent, because he or she is most likely to be objective in the decision making and the most demanding, wanting to achieve the highest possible level of satisfaction with the outcome. However, the customer patient's overall perception of the quality of care, which is always founded on the quality of his or her interaction with staff members, is still the primary consideration in the customer-patient's decision making.

The fact that health care nationally represents one-sixth of the U.S. economy by most government estimates, comprises organizations ranging from physicians' offices with a dozen employees to organizations like the Barnabas Health system that employ tens of thousands of employees, and offers a distinctive "high-demand, essential need" product only complicates the calculus when assessing the unique health care environment. Further-more, 18 percent of the national workforce works in the traditional delivery of health care, with another 9 percent estimated to work in ancillary organi-zations that provide products directly to health care organizations, such as food services organizations; uniform distributors; technology management firms; and others that help support these organizations, many of them with massive physical plant facilities. In numerous cities health care organizations are among the largest employers; in fact, in every one of the thirty largest U.S. and Canadian cities, health care organizations represent at least three spots on all lists of the top twenty employers. In the early 1960s any of those lists would have been replete with manufacturing organizations—service organizations now dominate those lists, and the largest organizations, both in terms of physical plant size and number of employees in the service sector, are part of health care.

SPHERES OF INFLUENCE MODEL

Figure 1.1 demonstrates the **Spheres of Influence Model,** which is a very useful tool in charting the various impact factors that influence the health care organization in general and the human resources management department in particular, which is the primary catalyst in a successful health care organization.

As pictured in the diagram, there are three sectors that make up the Spheres of Influence Model of health care. The first sector and the widest impact area is the customer-patient constituent community, which presents an array of risks and challenges on a daily basis to the modern health care organization. The community persistently puts a significant amount of pressure on the organization, based on customer-patient expectations centered on the naturally prominent role that a health care facility plays within its given operating environment. In addition, the ever-demanding customer-patient community's desire for new services and innovations must be sated by the health care organization. Demands for **nontraditional services,** such as preventive medicine and health education, must also be factored in when considering the expanding demands on a health care organization.

The second concentric circle in Figure 1.1 represents the primary recipient of the stress and pressures from the customer-patient community and external competitive environment—the health care organization. However, there are internal demands within every health care organization that also present a cacophony of challenges. To begin with, health care organizations are repeatedly confronted with major fiscal and financial pressures, and most nonprofit health care organizations struggle daily to "come out even" at the end of the given fiscal year. Health care organizations also wrestle with the difficulties involved in having a limited amount of skilled personnel in the face of customer-patients' increasing demands for new services and personal attention. Adding to this conundrum is the consistently high turnover even in well-managed and well-financed health care organizations operating in metropolitan areas in which there is a dearth of health care

Figure 1.1   Spheres of Influence Model

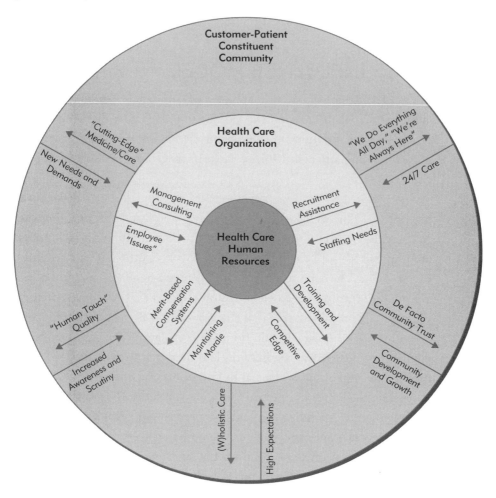

human capital talent. Turnover of personnel is even more perilous in areas in which consistency of performance can be threatened as staff members go from one organization to another for slightly better financial compensation.

Stress is also evident within a health care organization on the part of employees who live in the community—and approximately 90 percent of health care employees usually reside in their organization's service area—and contend with questions and comments about their employer constantly, even when going to a grocery store or attending a child's school activities.

Unlike their fellow citizens who work at a private corporation or somewhere outside of the community, health care workers are commonly known to their neighbors and friends, and are seen as a source of information and expertise. Finally, the stress caused by nonperformance on the part of nonplayers—an organization's employees who do not meet performance expectations but still manage to stay employed—can greatly affect the daily action of a health care organization and indeed can cause the implosion of significant work objectives.

The innermost sector of the Spheres of Influence Model is the human resources team, representing a nuclear department within a health care organization. As pressure for great performance moves from the customer-patient community through the organization to individual work groups, all members of a given department are challenged with the mantra "We must do more with less." The reality in health care human resources today is that many staff members are doing "everything with practically nothing" as they seek to meet the demands of the organization. In smaller departments, a turnover situation in which a vacant position is not filled immediately can create additional pressure on the other members of the group to work even harder and dedicate even more time to attending to the business of the department. In all cases, members of the human resources management department must have a strong working knowledge of their department's objectives in relation to the overall mission and vision of the health care organization to fully dedicate their efforts and talents to the accomplishment of organizational objectives.

The role of human resources in a health care organization cannot be understated. Given that human resources professionals are the prime agents, in concert with line managers, in recruiting, training, and developing employees, the charter of health care human resources is indeed challenging and demanding. Every health care employee is potentially the first point of contact for the customer-patient, and can create the all-important initial perception of the health care organization in the eyes of that individual. All health care employees are leaders, and are asked on a daily basis to "lead the action" relative to their technical expertise, which is the essential product of the health care organization. Furthermore, recall that most customer-patients are interested not only in the *what* of a health care organization but also more vitally in the *how*—the manner in which health care is delivered.

In fact, most customer-patients assume that they will get effective health care—what they are assessing is the human touch provided by each employee they encounter. Every employee therefore acts as an exemplar—good, bad, or marginal—of the entire organization's ethos. Together with their peers, employees collectively form an "organizational personality" that becomes the most formative aspect of the customer-patient's perception.

Considering the demands starting with the customer-patient and extending to each employee at the nucleus of the spheres of influence, it is important for an organization to constantly strive for a human resources composition that represents a majority of steadies and superstars. The application of a Performance Matrix (see Chapter Three), first in concept and then in daily practice, is vital in maintaining sound customer-patient services as well as in developing the organization to a maximum performance level.

Most people don't want to pay more taxes or higher bills. Moreover, all people want to have their money's worth, so as people pay more exponentially for health care services either through insurance premiums, indirect taxes, or a vexing combination of both, it is logical to assume that the customer-patient will be more demanding than ever for "perfect outcomes" in all of their personal experiences with health care. Accordingly, all health care organizations must provide the "latest and greatest" at the lowest cost ratio for the customer-patient; members of the human resources management department must, working with line managers, ensure that they hire individuals who not only demonstrate a mastery of the *what* of health care but also, and perhaps more important, perform at a high level in regard to the *how* of health care, best exemplified in the goal of providing an outstanding human touch in all interactions with all customer-patients.

FIVE SIGNIFICANT CHANGE DYNAMICS OF MODERN HEALTH CARE

The health care business arena is one that is teeming with change dynamics and daily challenges that affect each and every staff member of an organization. The antecedents of many of these changes are actually traditional demands on health care that have intensified over the past ten years due to a number of catalysts. In fact, most health care professionals would agree that there has been more change than ever over the past ten years of health care and, moreover, that there will be even more pressure and stress related to change forthcoming in the next five years. This section examines the five major change dynamics of health care, all of which have an impact on both the employee profile in all jobs in a health care organization and the organizational role that human resources plays in a health care organization.

The starting point for understanding the intensity of pressure on a health care organization is learning more about customer-patients' prevalent perceptions. In current American society, perception has become more important than reality. As a basic component of human nature, individuals develop strong beliefs, based on subjective observations, that ultimately result in an adopted perception and conviction. For example, if a customer-patient recently has had one negative experience with a member of a nursing staff at a given health care facility, a conviction takes root that the entire facility is bad news. In the perception of that customer-patient, the validation is "Hey, who hired that bad nurse to begin with?"

Subsequently and consequently, with a little negative word of mouth, a community perception could then be easily established that all of the nurses working at that health care facility are not particularly skilled—a perception that becomes more important than any facts or data presented in defense of the nurses' abilities. In this manner, perceptions are formed daily and almost instantaneously in our fast-paced society that demands quick satisfaction, immediately accessible data, and perfect results.

Therefore, it is vital to consider the most important "factual perception"—that customer-patients are perhaps more "customers" then "patients." This is the result of American consumers' understanding that they have a choice when selecting a health care provider. Not only will their insurance company inform them of their various choices and options through enrollment guides, 800-number help lines, and physician network listings, but also the attending physician will often provide an array of choices if they hold privileges at more than one hospital. As another example, such Web sites as WebMD provide information that is presented factually but can in fact can be more general than specific. However, customer-patients who believe that all information on the Internet is valid can form an erroneous "factual perception" (which indeed is a perilous oxymoron) before even visiting the doctor's office or a health care facility. At that point it becomes even more problematic and difficult for caregivers to gain the trust of their constituents, who have become apprehensive and fearful while forearmed with the "latest Internet facts" relative to their condition or malady.

With the terms *customer-patient* and *perceptual reality* in mind, it is time to explore five major impact factors that place ever greater demands both on health care facilities and on each employee trying to deliver sound health care during times of change, chaos, competition, and confusion.

Life-or-Death Outcomes

Customer-patients often believe that almost everything involving a health care facility can result in an outcome with a potentially drastic impact on their health care and quality of life. For example, if a six-year-old child attempting to ride his new two-wheeler bicycle falls on the pavement and opens a gash on his hands while bracing his fall, the parents' first move will be to rush the child to the emergency room. Try as we might to educate health care consumers on not abusing the emergency room with minor injuries, we must conclude that when the shocked parents of a young child see blood, they are going to make a dash, child in tow, to the nearest trauma center. Assuming that stellar health care is provided—that is, there are no problems with the attendant paperwork or with processing the insurance card, and a physician sutures the wound quickly and effectively—the prevailing question from the parents concerning this somewhat routine episode would be "Wow, my child received stitches! Will he have a scar *for life*?" It is also a fair assumption that the parents might even make an initial inquiry about the availability of plastic surgery at the facility in the future to remedy any scar resulting from the injury.

Another example of the "life-or-death" perception prevalent in the collective mind of American health care customer-patients is in full evidence every time you attend a birthday party. Whether the birthday boy or girl is four years old, fourteen years old, or forty years old, at a certain point during the celebration the parents of the honoree will recount for all of the attendees the adventure of the birthday celebrant's birth. If you listen carefully, you will hear not only an assortment of details about the *what* of the birth, such as the physiological details of the delivery, but also many of the *how* facets of the delivery, such as in the assistance provided by a security guard, the compassion of a nurse or doctor at a critical juncture, or even the extra effort put forth by a housekeeper or environmental services worker to make the new mom's room more accommodating for visitors. When the *how* factors are rated well, the perception of the parents and family—especially the mom—will undoubtedly be positive. However, even if the *what* factors are positive, if the *how* factors are negative the entire experience will be judged as negative, and the parents will probably seek another health care facility for their next medical need.

Escalating Expectations

In a general sense, it is somewhat easy to define the prevalent expectation of today's customer-patients. In essence, "they want everything at once without waiting in line with perfect outcomes, while great, skilled, intelligent staff employs the best equipment with the latest innovations in medicine and treatment while obtaining perfect outcomes while treating the customer-patient like royalty and without the customer-patient paying a dime for anything," to directly quote an emergency room nurse at a Philadelphia hospital. It is important to understand why this confounding expectation is evoked at present from coast to coast, regardless of the type of insurance or health care coverage an individual maintains.

To begin with, all of us pay exponentially more for our health care now than we did even a mere decade ago. Insurance costs have skyrocketed, and many large employers have passed the cost down to their employees. Even many major corporations with a reputation for being "best companies to work for," such as Wegman's, and strong state teachers' unions in Wisconsin and New Jersey have received constituent backlash and negative press coverage for asking their employees to incur the cost for a fractional part of their health care coverage. In the 1960s most American workers received full "hospitalization" as part of their employment package; in the early part of the twenty-first century, however, many American workers are becoming all too familiar with such terms as *health maintenance organization, physician organization,* and *copayer,* with the last term almost taking the semblance of an obscenity. The American way is to expect more when one pays more for services of any kind. Accordingly, it is at least logical to assume that customer-patients paying more for health care services from their own pockets expect more.

Furthermore, the American health care customer-patient believes that he or she has significant knowledge about health care. In the words of a nursing home director in Washington DC, "They either know more, think that they know more, or know that they better learn more about their coverage and the type of health care in their area." As individuals learn more about health care, whether or not their information is correct, they naturally expect more, as Web sites, the media, and even advertising from health care facilities present paragons of health care delivery that the customer-patient then expects as part of the routine delivery of health care. As a result, a pharmaceutical advertised on television, such as Claritin, becomes the "drug of demand," and the suggestion of a generic substitute is perceived—and remember, perception *is* reality—as an attempt of the caregiver to give the customer-patient second-rate care. As another example, the customer-patient who is familiar with the ubiquitous television commercial featuring open-air MRIs is likely to subsequently be less willing to endure an examination in a closed-air MRI. This type of commercial not only heightens the expectations of the customer-patient but also puts additional pressure and stress on the caregiver, who must break the customer-patient's adherence to a media-driven misconception of the relative efficacy of contrasting medical equipment and replace it with a truly realistic, effective treatment plan.

Health Care as a Media Target

Along with education, health care is a prominent sociological issue and a favorite target of the media. Because virtually every American has had experience with health care, any story dealing with health care will find resonance with an audience that is increasingly interested in the performance of local health care institutions. The media thus approaches health care from three different vantage points—the journalistic media, the advertising media, and, perhaps the most powerful, the popular media.

Today, in any part of the United States or Canada, there is bound to be a newspaper article about health care in some form, which is usually written from a negative point of view and often relates a "horror story" of negative circumstances. Reflecting the maxim that "bad news always sells," articles of this genre can be found both in tabloids and in more serious, respected newspapers and on news programs. With the emergence over the past fifteen years of such "twenty-four hours a day" news stations as CNN and MSNBC as well as a multitude of news-laden Web sites across the Internet, there are more news outlets than ever to bombard the sensibilities of the North American customer-patient. Major medical breakthroughs are reported misleadingly or are presented sensationally, such as through stories of the separation of Siamese twins or the repair of three-armed babies. Health care policy pieces that help inform and shape public opinion can often run alongside these "medical miracle" stories in the printed, broadcast, and Web-based outlets of today's daily news.

For example, *USA Today* recently displayed on its front page a "scientific survey" sponsored by a leading pharmaceutical company that listed the five most prominent fears of one thousand respondents who were facing surgery. Whereas fear of not recovering from the surgery was the "number one concern," an apprehension that the patient would be mistreated, misinformed, and mishandled by hospital staff was the "number three concern." Although it is disconcerting that this ranking was substantiated by the majority of the one thousand survey respondents who hold both fears to be valid, the fact that nearly four million people read *USA Today* on a daily basis and would be influenced negatively by this "scientific survey"—after all, it was on the front page of the paper!—is indeed troubling to any health care staff member attempting to settle the fears of a community member facing surgery.

The advertising media also contributes mightily to the creation of perceptions relative to health care. As mentioned previously, advertisements that feature "groundbreaking" new drugs, new equipment, and breakthrough procedures serve to heighten the expectations of customer-patients and create popular demand for the "newest and latest" medical innovations. According to one senior executive at a Connecticut medical center, "We do disservice to ourselves when we promise miracles." In every competitive health care market, there is at least one noted health care provider that spends an inordinate amount of money advertising a cutting-edge department, such as oncology; the ability to provide a new procedure, such as sophisticated eye surgery; or an affiliation that provides partner services with a nationally recognized "name" institution, such as Sloan Kettering Cancer Services or the world-renowned Mayo Clinic. Without question, the provision of new, sterling services is great for the community; however, in an unintentional but implicit manner it also creates higher expectations on the part of the customer-patient and the community.

Even investment firms have gotten into the act relative to the advertising media. For example, a major Wall Street financial management firm recently ran a print advertisement in such national magazines as *Time* and *Newsweek.*

The ad featured a patient who obviously just emerged from surgery, as evidenced by bandages around his head and his wearing of a surgical gown, who had to wash dishes to pay off his hospital bill. The caption under the ad read, "How do *you* plan to pay for unexpected medical bills?" Needless to say, such advertisements serve only to create fear, not only of the caregiving process but indeed of the entire business continuum of care from insurance coverage to payment of outstanding bills.

Even when positive health care images are presented in the advertising media, a "backfiring" effect can occur. For instance, if a potential customer-patient sees perfect outcomes, pleasant staff, and immaculate "guest" rooms in advertisements for a health care facility, she will expect absolutely nothing less to be the reality when she checks into that local hospital. If the conditions do not match the ideal situation featured in the ad, the customer-patient is certain to feel that the hospital was disingenuous from the outset. This quandary is similar to that of a hungry consumer who passes a billboard featuring a perfect hamburger from one of the many fast-food providers in his community. When he orders the hamburger featured on the billboard an hour later and it does not match the opulent appearance and tantalizing glow of the billboard version, disappointment and perhaps even anger form a negative consumer perception. In a similar but more important way, the natural inability of a community hospital to match the perfect conditions featured in its resplendent advertisements can also create initial distrust in the customer-patient service cycle.

Finally, the popular media is overflowing with characters and images that do not bode well for positive consumer perceptions of modern health care facilities. Consider the media icons of the 1960s and 1970s television world. Such physician heroes as Ben Casey were able to do three surgeries, set the administrator straight, conduct a very busy personal life, and perform laudable community service—all within an hour, including commercials. Marcus Welby, MD, never even left his house—he would send his young intern, played by a pluperfect James Brolin, off on a motorcycle to gather patients—and then would regularly save the day, week in and week out, through a series of house calls, office visits, and the strength of his august, patriarchal personality.

Today viewers are assaulted with a series of negative images and unsavory characters associated with health care that naturally create negative perceptions. The doctors on the erstwhile but syndicated hit show *ER* seem to spend more time delving into personal angst than attending to their patients in any purposeful manner. The thankfully canceled psychodrama *Chicago Hope* once aired an episode in which open-heart surgery resulted in the patient's heart's being dropped, kicked, rinsed off in a sink, and then stuck back into the unconscious patient's chest cavity. It would seem that media depictions of health care scenarios do little to assuage the fears and apprehensions already inherent in an always skeptical and often frightened customer-patient populace.

A good insight into the strategy of the popular media in regard to depicting health care was discernable in an interview for this book with an actress who plays a leading role on ABC's premier soap opera, *All My Children.* When discussing the script meetings for planning medical and health care sagas on the show, she said that the first consideration is always "What would be the best opportunity to inject drama into the mix?" Some recent scenarios resulting from these objective-based meetings include doctors blowing operations because they were thinking about their romantic lives and nurses failing to answer trauma calls because they were arguing on their cell phones with their most current paramour. When asked if any consideration was given to the fact that some viewers might think that those representations are "what really goes on in a hospital," our leading lady offered a pointed reminder that "that's not important in planning a *real* dramatic scene in my business."

Public Trust

We live in an era in which more people cast a vote for the best singer on *American Idol* than vote for the leader of the Free World in the U.S. presidential elections. The popularity and credibility of politicians have reached an all-time nadir as stories of corruption, higher taxes, and fiscal mismanagement appear daily throughout all forms of the media. Unfortunately, the delivery of health care is often perceived as a facet of public services. Although it is a fact that a number of municipal hospitals and the entire Department of Veterans Affairs medical system are true public trust entities directly supported by tax dollars, a number of academic surveys indicate that an overwhelming majority of American citizens believe that *all* health care facilities are supported by both property taxes and local sales taxes in the same manner that public schools receive financial support.

Accordingly, a comparison of public schools and local health care facilities is useful to understand how this perception abets the escalation of demands for constant improvement and new innovations in health care facilities. To begin with, when a child is registered at a local public school, the parents are not the least bit concerned about a tuition payment, as they inherently know that tax dollars will support the child's education, and, moreover, they hold close the patriotic belief that access to education is a given right for all American citizens. In a similar vein, any American citizen can receive health care at his or her local emergency room, where payment for services is often not a primary concern of the patient-customer yet is paramount to the hospital's survival. As a matter of law, no one can be refused treatment at an emergency room in any one of the fifty states, as evidenced in a landmark case in New England several years ago in which a civil judgment was made in favor of a patient who was refused treatment in an emergency room. This well-known case stands as a reminder that access to emergency room care is in actuality an unalienable right beyond just perception. From another perspective, when property taxes are raised in the community a common ploy of both politicians and real estate agents is to cite the excellence of both health care and education within the community as the reasons why property tax revenue must be increased. Also, consider how many of our local hospitals include in their nameplate the words *community, memorial,* and other appellations that suggest a connotation of public trust.

As a last point concerning this customer-patient perception, many Americans would agree that both health care and education could use vast improvement in many regards. However, the idea of "nationalizing" either entity is an anathema to any taxpayer who has worked hard to make a good income so that he or she can live in a community with solid schools and sound health care. In neither case will the taxpayer be willing to accept "nationalization leading to marginalization." This latter perception reflects the old adage of the late U.S. congressional leader Thomas (Tip) O'Neill that "all politics are local," and individuals are more interested in circumstances within their local community than in the entire national realm of health care and education. Accordingly, it is apparent that any nationally driven legislation attempting to "fix the broken American health care system" will meet popular resistance. In addition, a national opinion that health care and education are well funded but often lackluster in regard to quality will continue to have a deleterious impact on customer-patients' perceptions well into the future.

"People Intensity"

The number of people who work in health care facilities is also worth noting. In the 1960s the American economy was based on a reliance on manufacturing entities; now, with many manufacturing jobs exported overseas and with a centric focus on service industries, health care has emerged as a leading employer in every American community, as already discussed. Health care organizations are therefore perceived not only as agents of the delivery of services related to life and death but also as the "major employers in town," receiving increasing scrutiny across the country for their organizational ethics, hiring patterns, and competitive status relative to other organizations.

Also, the biggest daily challenge confronting health care leaders at every level—and an ongoing subject throughout this book—is maximizing the performance of their staff. However, the amount of time that a health care facility will spend interviewing and selecting a computer or information technology specialist, for example, is miniscule compared to the amount of time that the facility will spend in selecting the type of computer system. The problem here is that if a computer fails, a service contract includes a warranty to ensure its performance; if the computer specialist fails to meet organizational expectations, the organization will have to expend a significant amount of time, energy, and money in attempting to redirect performance and, often, subsequently terminating and replacing this unsatisfactory employee.

It is difficult to imagine that the impact on health care of any of these five significant change dynamics will lessen in the near future. It is therefore an imperative of every health care leader to select, develop, and retain stellar employees who will meet the ever-escalating expectations resulting from these five prevailing dynamics.

PROFILE OF A PROGRESSIVE HEALTH CARE ORGANIZATION

Given all of these realities, a successful health care organization must be structured to maintain timely response capabilities proactive planning, and sustained growth to meet the needs of a demanding constituency of customer-patients.

Figure 1.2 illustrates the functional composition of a progressive health care organization. Consider as an example the most common form of health care organization, which is a local, community-driven medical center. This representation not only is typical of the organizational dynamics at the majority of health care organizations but also contains components that can easily be extracted, reduced, or expanded to represent all health care organizations. This example will also provide a construct for an efficacious health care human resources component, which will be examined in detail later on in this chapter and indeed throughout the entire text.

The governance structure of a typical community-driven health care organization begins with the board of directors. Most health care organizations have a board of directors consisting of ten to twenty-five members drawn from the community, including business experts, local legislative and political leaders, medical and health care experts from other organizations, and educators and social leaders. The role of the board is to provide governance and guidance on such significant issues as growth and development plans, strategic direction, and relations with local and state governments. Most successful health care boards of directors have at least a committee or subcommittee that provides counsel on education, human resources, and organizational development issues.

The titular leader of a health care organization is typically the chief executive officer (CEO), or the president. As is the case in most industries, the CEO is the key decision maker who has the vision of the organization, the trust of the community, and the growth of the health care enterprise as his or her functional charter. At most health care organizations the CEO has ascended to the executive suite after an impressive career in either administrative management or medical leadership (usually the former). Although the CEO might only have seven to twelve direct reports, every member of the organization is in the CEO's chain of command. In any successful

Figure 1.2 Organizational Chart—Midsize Community Hospital

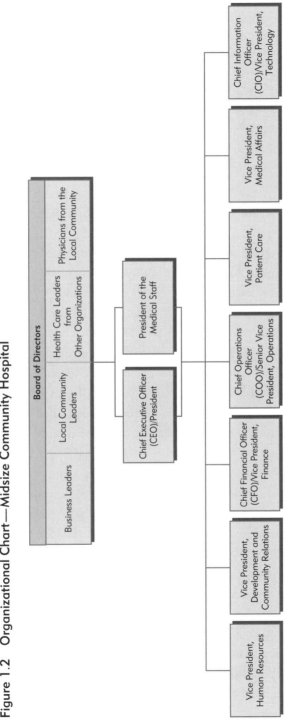

health care organization the CEO will take a fervent interest in human resources and be an active and appropriate participant in key recruiting decisions, training and education initiatives, and other high-priority human resources endeavors. The CEO's importance in the organization cannot be understated, as many health care organizations that have enjoyed the benefits of favorable demographics and potential high revenue have failed because of poor leadership at the top and decision making that was less than responsive to the emerging needs of their constituent community.

The next layer, as indicated in Figure 1.2, is commonly called the second tier of health care leadership. Most health care organizations have a chief operating officer (COO) who is often the second-in-command of the organization and is in charge of all of the physical plant operations, support operations, and other major facets of the health care organization. This individual usually has a set of directors, such as a chief of security, a director of food services, a manager of plant engineering, and other professionals who lead skilled staff in the daily operations of the health care organization. **Technical training** (often called in-service education in health care) is very important in health care operations, and that becomes a joint endeavor with the human resources management department in successful health care organizations in which a variety of perspectives are synergized into smart decisions. Naturally, recruiting for skilled positions is also a major concern for the COO, or the senior vice president of operations, as is the identification of competitive salaries, wages, and benefits needed to attract the highest possible level of professionals in the health care arena.

Another key leader in the second tier of a health care organization is the vice president of patient care, who normally is the executive leader for the largest employee population, as patient services encompasses nursing and other direct patient care departments. Because shortages abound in many patient care specialty areas, including nursing, pharmacy, physical therapy, dietary services, and other direct patient care sectors, the entire chronology of employee acquisition and development, as detailed in Figure 1.3, becomes critically important to the vice president of patient services. Often this individual has ascended to his or her position through a nursing career pathway and thus understands intrinsically that although many customer-patients might not remember the name of their operation or the specifics of their aftercare, they will *always* remember the name of the nurse and

Figure 1.3   Organizational Chronology of a Health Care Professional

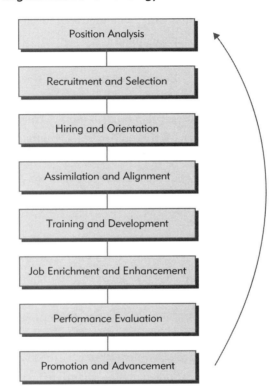

the other direct patient care providers who assisted them in a time of need. Therefore, by working in concert with the human resources management department, the strong nursing corps and augmenting team of diagnostic and therapeutic professionals that make up the patient services corps can become the flagship human capital component in a progressive health care organization.

An oft-recited mantra in health care is "No margin, no margin mission," alluding to the fact that financial revenue must be healthy if the health care organization is going to succeed in making its community healthy. This makes the role of the chief financial officer (CFO) at the second tier of the health care organization a pivotal one. With direct reports including personnel in internal auditing, accounts payable, and the all-important department of accounts receivable, the CFO might have one of the smallest staffs in a health care organization but obviously one of the most important. The CFO's critical role in health care human resources management can be seen in the establishment of merit-based compensation systems related to a criteria-based performance evaluation system. Fair, equitable, and incentive-driven compensation systems, when implemented effectively, help the progressive health care organization reward good performance, thus ensuring its overall and long-term success.

Most health care organizations also have at the second tier a chief information officer (CIO). With the emergence of technology driving everything from how medical records are kept to the work of the financial audit team to Internet-based training and development, the CIO plays a pivotal role in the success of the health care organization, although he or she usually does not have a particularly large staff. However, with the growing demand for more information and the reliance of all staff members on reliable and accurate data, the CIO's expertise and the acumen of his or her staff can spell the difference between the organization's ability or inability to maintain a competitive edge. Accordingly, top talent must be attracted to the organization through the efforts of the organization's human resources professionals, and expertise must be afforded to the CIO's staff quickly when an employee relations problem emerges, for example, so that an equitable and efficient resolution can help maintain a vibrant flow of technology support across the organization.

Finally, the second tier of the executive cadre of a progressive health care organization must include the vice president of human resources. As you will see in the next section of this chapter, the vice president of human resources should have a complete complement of specialists and generalists that can provide counsel and leadership on the human capital issues that are the heartbeat of any successful health care organization. Furthermore, the vice president of human resources should play a critical role in the strategic planning of the health care organization, and he or she should have a keen sense of demographics and psychographics of the community because upwards of 85 percent of a health care organization's staff members live within the organization's stated service area. Accordingly, many of the employees of a health care organization are also possible patients and constituents, and certainly become ambassadors to the community in regard to new initiatives and ongoing imperatives of the organization. And, given the unique nature of the health care organization, the human resources leader fills a community role that is as vitally important as that of a public school administrator or any elected representative within the local community, involving a wide array of civic responsibilities and accountabilities.

COMPOSITION OF A PROGRESSIVE HEALTH CARE HUMAN RESOURCES MANAGEMENT DEPARTMENT

A health care human resources management department should include professionals in several essential areas (see Figure 1.4). As mentioned earlier in this chapter, a favorite cliché in health care circles is "doing more with less—to the point of doing everything with nothing"—a bromide that can well apply to health care human resources management departments. It is not uncommon to see a complete human resources staff of fifteen members, including administrative and secretarial help, for a community health care organization of over two thousand employees. Although that ratio might represent a norm in health care, one would be hard-pressed to find a similar ratio in the for-profit business world. It is therefore essential that the human resources management department is well defined, well structured, and well staffed with professionals who see every day as an opportunity to increase their skill level, learn new strategies and approaches to their craft, and gain a competitive edge in the science of supporting efforts to attract, develop, and retain outstanding staff in each and every health care department.

Let's look at a general accountability overview of the key players on a health care human resources team, as represented in Figure 1.4:

Figure 1.4   Organizational Chart—Health Care Human Resources Management Department

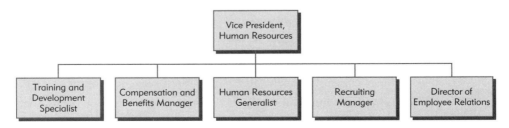

The *human resources generalist* should be capable of providing counsel effectively and efficiently in most human capital management situations. Examples of this would include insight into best recruiting sources for a new pharmacist, how to best resolve a manager-employee dispute, methods for conducting a quick but accurate wage comparison, and how to best explain a new benefits package to a befuddled food services employee. Although supported by specialists, the human resources generalist is often the individual who "directs traffic," is a "one-stop shop" on relatively uncomplicated issues, and is a "wise sage"—either individually or all at once, depending on the demand of the situation.

The *recruiting manager* has perhaps one of the most thankless tasks in health care human resources in the initial hiring process, but he or she can often garner one of the best intrinsic rewards available in health care human resources when excellent new employees prove their worth to the organization and provide an optimal return on investment over the long term of their employment. The frustration for this individual lies in the unbalanced supply and demand paradox that exists in nursing and other areas in which specialists are at a premium because of low supply (due to an assortment of academic and career development quandaries) but in high demand (due to increasing customer-patient expectations and needs). Recruiting managers, like all professionals in the health care human resources sector, act alternately as consultants who help lead line managers, or as leaders themselves in the process of recruiting, interviewing, and selection. A recruiting manager who is truly proactive will embrace a structured selection system (such as a targeted selection system) and also will work as an educator in the active and consistent use of an effective selection and hiring system.

The *compensation and benefits manager* has the vital responsibility of making certain that market-competitive salaries are counterbalanced across the organization with incoming revenue and other budgetary requisites.

The *training and development specialist* is the gatekeeper for the future development of the organization. Whether his or her title is manager of organizational development, human capital specialist, or director of education—or whether in reality the specialist assumes all of these responsibilities with perhaps only one of the titles—this individual holds the ongoing, continuous education and professional development of the entire health care organization as the mainstay of his or her professional responsibility. Providing training, for instance, can include offering management development; developing technical proficiency; or, less obvious but very important, facilitating certification of and academic education for employees using available tuition reimbursement funds and other resources.

The *director of employee relations* is responsible for workplace dynamics, which can include labor relations issues, management-employee dispute resolution, equal opportunity compliance matters, and other direct workplace management situations.

SUMMARY

Health care organizations occupy a truly unique place in society and business in the United States. Your local health care provider is a perceived public trust, yet probably does not receive direct public financial support. The organization itself could be a clinic, a major medical center, or an expanded suite of doctors' offices. It is likely that all three of these facilities are located nearby and could provide primary medical care for you. Accordingly, the mission, scope, and structure of a health care organization should be understood as completely as possible as the specific, singular charter of health care human resources management is assessed and developed through this text and in the balance of your professional and academic endeavors.

KEY TERMS

customer-patients	Spheres of Influence Model
nontraditional services	technical training

DISCUSSION QUESTIONS

1. This chapter included several examples of health care organizations, starting with examples from New Jersey. Cite three to five profiles of health care organizations within an hour's drive of your school or organization, and specify three to five points about each organization that make it unique.

2. This chapter discussed five dynamics that impel change in the health care environment and have an impact on the daily work lives of health care professionals at every level. What are some additional dynamics not covered in this chapter that you believe are significant?

3. The Spheres of Influence Model is a very useful graphic tool for organizational analysis. Draw spheres of influence charting the external-internal relationships between your local environment and an organization of your choice (for example, a school, team, community group, or current employer).

4. What are some additional causal relationships between the expectations and perceptions of health care customer-patients and health care professionals, in addition to the dynamics listed in this chapter?

5. Take a look at your local paper and some local television ads concerning health care, and list three to five factors in each that you believe would lead to negative or positive perceptions from customer-patients.

6. At least two hospitals or medical centers have closed in the past three years in your state or province. Research at least one and discern if some of the causes for the failure were in some way related to human resources issues (for example, poor leadership, wage problems, lack of staff, and so on).

2

Strategic Health Care Human Resources Management and Planning

LEARNING OBJECTIVES

- Describe the changing role of human resources management
- Define human resources planning and identify steps in the planning process
- Identify factors to be considered in forecasting the supply and demand for strategic human resources management (SHRM)
- Explain why SHRM is critical for health care organizations

STRATEGIC HUMAN RESOURCES MANAGEMENT (SHRM) is based on the belief that to be effective and able to adapt to changes quickly, organizations need realistic information on the capabilities and talents of their current staff—in essence, their human resources.

SHRM refers to the implementation of human resources activities, policies, and practices to make the necessary ongoing changes to support or improve the organization's operational and strategic objectives. Organization leaders need to understand how their workplace will be affected by impending changes and prepare for the changes accordingly. Such leaders should formulate objectives after reviewing relevant data on the quantity and potential of available human resources. Are human resources available for short- and long-term objectives? To be competitive, organizations must be able to anticipate, influence, and manage the forces that have an impact on their ability to remain effective. In the service sector, this means they must be able to manage their human resources capabilities. All too often agencies have relied on short-term service requirements to direct their human resources management (HRM) practices without giving much thought to the long-term implications.

By invoking SHRM, a health care organization is better able to match its human resources requirements with the demands of the external environment and the needs of the organization, ensuring that there is an appropriate staff and skill mix; it also serves to support the relationship between clinical outcomes and HR practices (Dubois & Singh, 2009; Khatri, Wells, McKune, & Brewer, 2006). Strategic planning, budgeting, and identifying human resources needs are linked in SHRM, the integrative framework that matches HRM activities with strategic organizational needs.

This chapter discusses SHRM, the changing role of HRM, and human resources planning, and illustrates the importance of all these concerns to organizational vitality and success.

THE CHANGING ROLE OF HUMAN RESOURCES MANAGEMENT

Health care organizations are facing some daunting challenges. For HRM departments to play a strategic role, they must focus on the long-term implications of HRM issues. For example, how will changing workforce demographics and workforce shortages affect the organization, and what strategies will be used to address them?

The downsizing and reorganization of public and nonprofit agencies, along with a strong focus on results, are forcing agencies to validate their business processes, reassess the role of the HR function, and evaluate the adequacy of the work performed by HR employees.

To be strategic partners, HRM departments must possess high levels of professional and business knowledge. They must establish links to enhance organizational performance and be able to demonstrate on a continuing basis how HRM activities contribute to the success and effectiveness of the organization.

A recent report by the Society for Human Resources Management (2010), titled *What Senior HR Leaders Need to Know: Perspectives from the United States, Canada, India, the Middle East and North Africa*, identified eighteen core senior HR leadership competencies (p. 4):

- *Business knowledge:* An understanding of the operations and processes of how business is conducted

- *Coaching/developing others:* Helping others to reach their potential

- *Credibility:* Being perceived by others as having the knowledge and experience to back up one's authority

- *Critical/analytical thinking:* Seeking information and using that information to inform decision and resolve problems

- *Cross-cultural intelligence:* Knowledge of and sensitivity to differences among cultures

- *Effective communication:* Being able to verbally or in writing convey messages in terms that make sense, and also to actively listen to others' interpersonal communication

- *Ethical behavior:* Perception of the moral appropriateness of individual and/or group conduct or behavior

- *Flexibility/adaptability:* The ability to adjust the approach as required by shifts within the organization and in the external business environment

- *Global intelligence/global mindset:* An overarching way of thinking about the nature of doing business that includes an understanding of and sensitivity to cultural differences among workers in other countries and legal issues inherent in operating a business multinationally

- *HR knowledge:* Understanding of tactical and strategic HR functions and processes
- *Integrity:* Honesty and doing the right thing
- *Leading change:* Charting the course for organization's stakeholders to navigate a shift in business processes, priorities, roles, and expectations
- *Organizational knowledge:* Understanding the business issues that are specific to the organization and having empathy for and an awareness of the impact of human capital issues on the organization as a system
- *Persuasiveness/influencing others:* The art of using interpersonal skills to convince others to share one's perspective or way of thinking
- *Results orientation/drive for performance:* The ability to link processes and practices to positive outcomes and to demonstrate the value that HR brings to the organization
- *Shaping organizational culture:* Creating values by which an organization operates
- *Strategic thinking:* Seeing the big picture, having a long-term line of sight and understanding the interconnectedness of decisions and activities within the various lines of the business
- *Technological savvy:* Knowledge of the unique solutions and challenges that new technology will bring to the organization and understanding of how talent management will be affected by a technologically enhanced business environment

Across all four geographical regions covered in the report, *effective communication* and *strategic thinking* were the two most highly rated competencies. In the Unites States the competencies HR professionals rated among their top five were (1) effective communication, (2) strategic thinking, (3) HR knowledge, (4) integrity, and (5) ethical behavior.

Unfortunately, many HRM departments have spent their time ensuring compliance with rules and regulations, so they lack the skills and competencies to act as strategic partners. For organizations to be successful in implementing SHRM, they need the collaborative effort of agency leaders and human resources professionals, who themselves need the knowledge and skills to undertake a more proactive role.

HUMAN RESOURCES OUTSOURCING

Another change in human resources management is the increasing use of human resources outsourcing (Coggburn, 2007; "*HRO Today,*" 2009). Many health care organizations often find it advantageous to outsource some or all of their HRM responsibilities. Many smaller organizations outsource such services as payroll and benefits functions, and in fact a variety of HRM activities can be outsourced. The journal *HRO Today* offers a resource guide with almost fifteen hundred providers in a number of service categories. HRM services that can be outsourced include these:

- **Benefits consulting services:** Benefits program design, cost containment, enrollment, actuarial analysis, and full-service administration. Other areas are health care strategy and plans, retirement plan design, life insurance, and long-term and disability plans.

- **Payroll software and services:** Payroll processing, withholding, and benefits accrual services.

- **Health benefits services:** Administration and management of health care plans that may include consumer-driven health care plans, health maintenance organization plans, preferred provider organization plans, point-of-service plans, health savings accounts, fee-for-service plans, and wellness programs.

- **Recruiting, staffing, and search services:** Provision of online recruitment technology, temporary staffing, and full-service recruitment process outsourcing.

- **Relocation services:** Helping employees move from one community to another. Relocation firms typically make their money through commissions from home sales and moves.

- **Screening and workplace security services:** Drug testing, background screening for applicants and existing employees, academic verification, review of resident work eligibility and employment history, and workplace security functions.

- **Human resources information systems and Web-based services:** Provision of HR services through human resources information systems and Web-based services.

- **Incentive services:** Developing employee recognition programs, measuring return on investment of such programs, providing technology support for incentive programs, and purchasing gift certificates and gift baskets for employees.

- **Information technology services:** Application development, architectural consulting, business intelligence, content management, data security and warehousing, enterprise resource planning, e-procurement, system integration, technology infrastructure, and Web hosting and development services.

- **Professional employer organizations (PEOs)** and **administrative services organizations (ASOs):** For example, where employees are paid under the PEO's federal employer identification number and placed on the PEO's benefits program and workers' compensation policy. ASOs offer many of the same services as a PEO but under a non-coemployment relationship.

- **Enterprise human resources outsourcing services:** Comprehensive HR functions, such as those pertaining to benefits consulting and administration, employee recognition and incentives, human resources information systems and human resources information technology, payroll, recruiting and staffing, relocation, screening, and training and development.

STRATEGIC HUMAN RESOURCES MANAGEMENT AND HUMAN RESOURCES PLANNING

Strategic planning is the process that enables a health care organization to guide its future activities and the use of its available resources. The process permits the external forces that affect the organization and the people in it to be identified. These forces may include workforce patterns, economic conditions, competition, regulation, social values, and technological developments. After the external factors are assessed, the internal strengths and weaknesses of the organization's incumbents must be identified. Factors to include in an internal assessment are current workforce skills, retirement patterns, demographic profiles, and employee capabilities.

The agency's vision, mission, and measurable goals and objectives drive the identification of future functional requirements, which in turn drive the analysis and elements of the workforce plan. The question to ask is, "What key functions need to be performed to move in the direction set out in the strategic plan?" This may include assessing many current functions, in addition to forecasting important future functions and activities. Such information can be used to forecast the organization's capabilities to confront its future opportunities and threats. The ultimate feasibility of strategic planning depends on the people who make it operational. Agency leaders need to understand how their workplace will be affected by impending changes and prepare accordingly.

Human resources planning, a critical component of strategic planning and SHRM, is the process of analyzing and identifying the need for and availability of human resources to meet the organization's objectives.

In an effort to prepare for the future, the U.S. Office of Personnel Management (2005) developed a five-step workforce planning model:

- *Step 1: Set the strategic direction.* This involves linking the workforce planning process with the agency's strategic plan, annual performance and business plan, and work activities required to carry out long- and short-term goals and objectives.

- *Step 2: Analyze the workforce, identify skills gaps, and conduct workforce analysis.* This involves determining what the current workforce resources are and how they will evolve through turnover; developing specifications for the kinds, numbers, and locations of workers and managers needed to accomplish the agency's strategic requirements; and determining what gaps exist between the current and projected workforce needs.

- *Step 3: Develop an action plan.* This involves the identification of strategies to close gaps, plans to implement the strategies, and measures for assessing strategic progress. These strategies could include recruiting, training and retraining, restructuring organizations, contracting out, succession planning, and upgrading technology.

- *Step 4: Implement the action plan.* This involves ensuring that human and fiscal resources are in place; roles are understood; and the necessary communication, marketing, and coordination are occurring to execute the plan and achieve the strategic objectives.

- *Step 5: Monitor, evaluate, and revise.* This involves monitoring progress against milestones, assessing for continuous improvement, and adjusting the plan to make course corrections and address new issues.

ANTICIPATING FUTURE NEEDS

Forecasting is used to assess past trends, evaluate the existing situation, and project future events. Forecasting and planning are complementary in that forecasts identify expectations, whereas plans establish concrete goals and objectives. An agency must consider how to allocate people to jobs over long periods and try to anticipate expansions or reductions in programs or other changes that may affect the organization. Based on these analyses, HR leaders can make plans for the recruitment and selection of new employees, the shifting of employees to different programs or units, or the retraining of incumbent employees.

A demand forecast anticipates the workforce that will be needed to accomplish future functional requirements and carry out the mission of the organization. Conducting a visionary staffing assessment to gauge future functional requirements can result in a forecast of the types of competencies, numbers, and locations of employees needed in the future. An important part of creating the demand forecast is examining not only what work the agency will do in the future but also how that work will be performed. Some things to consider include the following:

- How will jobs and workload change as a result of technological advancements and changing economic, social, and political conditions?

- What will the consequences or results of these changes be?

- What will the reporting relationships be?

- How will divisions, work units, and jobs be designed?

- How will work flow into each part of the organization?

Once these questions have been answered, the next step is to identify the competencies employees will need to carry out that work. The set of competencies provides management and staff with a common understanding of the skills and behaviors that are important to the agency. Competencies play a key role in decisions on recruiting, employee development, personal development, and performance management.

Forecasting HR requirements involves determining the number and types of employees needed by skill level. First, agencies need to audit the skills of incumbent employees and determine their capabilities and weaknesses. They must also audit positions. In most organizations, there are probably jobs that are vulnerable because technology or reengineering is ready to replace them. Job analyses can provide information on existing jobs. The basic requirements of a job should be defined and converted to job specifications that specify the minimum knowledge, skills, abilities, and other characteristics necessary for effective performance. The skill requirements of positions do change, however, so any changes that occur must be monitored and reflected in the job specifications.

It is not enough to monitor changes in positions; health care organizations must also keep abreast of the skills their employees possess. Human resources planning involves using data inventories to integrate the planning functions of SHRM. Data inventories are compilations of summary information, such as the characteristics of employees, the distribution of employees by position, and employees' performance and career objectives. Specific data that are typically catalogued are those related to age, education, career path, current work skills, work experience, aspirations, performance evaluations, years with the organization, and jobs for which one is qualified. Data inventories also track expected vacancies due to retirement, promotion, transfer, sick leave, relocation, or termination. Using a computerized **human resources information system (HRIS)** to compile these data makes information readily available for forecasting workforce needs.

Information technology enables organizations to maintain and retrieve information and records with greater accuracy and ease than older methods. An HRIS provides current and accurate data for decision making and broader applications, such as producing reports, forecasting HR needs, strategic planning, career and promotion planning, and evaluating HR policies and practices. Having accessible data enables HR planning and managerial decision making to be based to a greater degree on information rather than perceptions. Common applications of an HRIS include maintaining employee records; overseeing payroll and benefits activities; handling absence and vacation records; administering recruitment and training programs; communicating with employees; and tracking affirmative action data. Many agencies use intranets as part of their HRIS that allow employees to read current job openings and apply for positions online. They also provide information on employee benefits, training opportunities, and occupational safety and health.

Developing an HRIS can be expensive; it is therefore important that department managers and users, HRM professionals, and technology experts jointly develop it and plan for its implementation. Some factors to consider when developing an HRIS are the anticipated initial costs and annual maintenance costs, the ability to upgrade the system, the availability of relevant software packages for users, the compatibility of the HRIS with current information technology systems in place, the availability of technical support to maintain the system, the ability to customize the system for managing different information, the time required to implement the system, and the amount of training required for users to become proficient.

When forecasting the availability of human resources, agencies need to consider both the internal and external supply of qualified candidates. The internal supply of candidates is influenced by training and development and by transfer, promotion, and retirement policies. Assessing incumbent staff competencies is crucial. An assessment of employees' competency levels will provide information for determining the number of those available for and capable of fulfilling future functional requirements. It will also provide salient information as to what recruitment, training, and other strategies need to be deployed to address workforce gaps and surpluses.

With the assistance of human resources management representatives, unit managers should prepare a succession analysis that forecasts the supply of people for certain positions. Succession plans should be used to identify potential personnel changes, select backup candidates, and keep track of attrition. The external supply of candidates is also influenced by a variety of factors, including developments in technology, the actions of competing employers, geographical location, and government regulations.

SHRM attempts to match the available supply of labor with the forecast demand in light of the organization's strategic plan. A gap analysis involves comparing the workforce demand forecast with the workforce supply projection. The expected result is the identification of gaps and surpluses in staffing levels and competencies needed to carry out future functional requirements. A gap occurs when the projected supply is less than the forecast demand. It indicates a future shortage of needed employees. Such strategies as recruitment, training, and succession planning will need to be developed and implemented.

A surplus occurs when the projected supply is greater than the forecast demand. This indicates future excess in some categories of employees that may also require taking action. The surplus data may represent occupations or skill sets that will not be needed in the future or at least not to the same degree as other occupations or skill sets. Implementing retraining, transferring employees, or offering separation incentives may help address surplus situations.

If the necessary skills do not exist in the workforce, employees need to be trained in the new skills, or external recruitment must bring those skills to the organization. The employer must identify where employees with those skills are likely to be found and develop recruitment strategies accordingly. Organizations facing a worker shortage may be able to postpone the retirement of older workers. In an effort to retain their knowledge base or to better serve their clients, some organizations have developed creative ways to encourage retirement-eligible employees to remain on the job. They have improved training opportunities and technology to impart different skills, divided full-time positions into part-time work, and offered telecommuting as an option. Some organizations have phased in retirement plans that permit employees to reduce their hours or responsibilities so that they can ease into retirement. This provides an opportunity for experienced workers to mentor younger employees and transfer institutional knowledge. Organizations thus continue to gain benefits from soon-to-be-retiring workers' skills and expertise. Unless an organization has a mechanism in place to preserve worker knowledge, its loss can have a negative effect on the organization. Experienced workers often possess valuable knowledge and understand the cultural nuances of organizations.

An example of poor SHRM took place in 2007 in Atlanta, Georgia, at Grady Memorial Hospital, the state's largest public hospital. In an attempt to halt its declining revenue and increasing expenses, it offered early retirement to 562 employees: 422 employees took it, twice as many as anticipated.

One-third of the departing employees were nurses, nursing assistants, clerks, and other workers in patient care. Another 13 percent came from laboratories and radiology. "The impact of the buyout goes beyond the number of jobs involved," said Curtis Lewis, chief of Grady's medical staff. "In a cash-strapped hospital with aging equipment and a largely indigent patient population, people learn to make things work and maximize resources . . . . In addition, the senior staff developed long-term relationships. Those are the things you lose" (quoted in White, 2007, p. D11).

Strategies for halting the retirement of productive employees include offering part-time work with or without benefits (depending on the employee's need), training employees to develop new skills, transferring employees to different jobs with reduced pay and responsibilities, and addressing any age bias issues that may exist in the agency. Organizations that cannot halt the retirement of productive employees need to set up a system for transferring knowledge to younger employees.

EVALUATING THE EFFECTIVENESS OF STRATEGIC HUMAN RESOURCES MANAGEMENT

To evaluate the effectiveness of SHRM, SHRM audits and HR benchmarking and return on investment analysis can be used.

SHRM Audit

One method used to assess SHRM effectiveness is an HRM audit, an in-depth analysis that evaluates the current state of SHRM in an organization. The audit identifies areas of strengths and weaknesses and where improvements are needed. During the audit, current practices, policies, and procedures are reviewed. Many audits also include benchmarking against organizations of similar size or industry. A number of areas are typically included in an audit:

- Legal compliance (Equal Employment Opportunity Act, Occupational Safety and Health Act, Fair Labor Standards Act, Employment Retirement Income Security Act, Family and Medical Leave Act)

- Current job descriptions and specifications

- Valid recruiting and selection procedures

- Compensation and pay equity and benefits

- Employee relations

- Absenteeism and turnover control measures

- Training and development activities

- Performance management systems

- Policies and procedures and the employee handbook

- Terminations

- Health, safety, and security issues

HR Benchmarking and Return on Investment Analysis

Human resources management departments, like other units, are being asked to demonstrate their value to health care organizations. Human resources audits and HRIS are being used with greater frequency to obtain information on HR performance. Once information on performance has been gathered, it must be compared to a standard. One method of assessing HR effectiveness is comparing specific measures of performance against data on those measures in other organizations known for their best practices.

Employee costs in public and nonprofit organizations can be anywhere from 50 to 80 percent of expenses; therefore, measuring the return on investment (ROI) in human capital is necessary to show the impact and value of SHRM. According to Fitz-enz (2000, p. 3), "Management needs a system of metrics that describe and predict the cost and productivity curves of its workforce." Quantitative measures focus on cost, capacity, and time, whereas qualitative measures focus on more intangible values, such as human reactions. ROI calculations are used to show the value of expenditures for HR activities. Human resources activities and programs that have been subject to measurement include training programs, diversity programs, wellness and fitness initiatives, safety and health programs, skill-based and knowledge-based compensation programs, performance improvement programs, education programs, organizational development initiatives, change initiatives, career development programs, recruiting systems, and technology implementation (Phillips & Phillips, 2002).

Despite the belief that only for-profit organizations can evaluate ROI, public and nonprofit health care organizations can use such measures of performance as productivity, quality, time improvements, and cost savings through efficiency enhancements, as well as such qualitative measures as patient satisfaction, manner of performance, and responsiveness to clients.

PROBLEMS AND IMPLICATIONS OF STRATEGIC HUMAN RESOURCES MANAGEMENT

Research demonstrates the importance of SHRM. Why then is HRM often considered a secondary support function rather than a driver of an organization's future? A number of reasons may exist. There are also financial costs associated with SHRM. Some organizations may be reluctant to spend additional resources on employees. In some instances, leaders may want a greater integration of the HRM function with organizational strategy but often do not understand just what that means. Human resources management professionals may not have the flexibility to initiate new programs or suggest new organizational structures. This is especially true when organizational change issues challenge existing rules and regulations as well as embedded standard operating procedures.

The Government Accountability Office identified the following reasons why SHRM planning often fails (cited in Flynn, 2006, p. 6):

- Lack of ongoing support and interest from leadership.

- Succession planning is not seen as a priority.

- Funding is not sufficient.

- Recruitment and retention, particularly in critical management areas, is perceived to be sufficient to meet organizational needs.

- Resistance from middle managers who already feel overburdened with other "initiatives" not central to their job responsibilities.

- Employee suspicion toward unsure program goals, poor communication and organization is too small to sustain a full-scale program.

Another reason why SHRM is neglected is that often HRM professionals lack the capabilities and skills necessary to move HRM to a more proactive role. To be strategic partners, HRM departments must possess high levels of professional and business knowledge. They need to establish links to others in the organization who are working to improve performance and be able to demonstrate on a continuing basis how HRM activities contribute to the success and effectiveness of the organization. Unfortunately, many HRM departments have spent their time ensuring compliance with rules and regulations, so they lack the skills and competencies to act as strategic partners.

Organizational change also requires higher levels of coordination across functions and departments, and employees and management must be committed to continuous improvement. There must be greater interdepartmental cooperation. Trust and open communication across the organization will have to be developed. Organizations must encourage creativity and recognize such creativity through their reward systems. Change requires fairness, openness, and empowerment, but these may be contrary to an organization's existing culture and may require several incremental steps to achieve.

Some employees may be reluctant to change. Over the years, they may have acquired proficiency in the performance of their respective jobs. Changing their routines and standards of performance, requiring them to learn new skills, or obliging them to work with unfamiliar persons may be unsettling. Employees unwilling or unable to make the transition may choose to resign; some may even attempt to sabotage new initiatives.

Changes in policies and procedures take time to implement and are often not immediately apparent. To transform an organization requires chief executive and top administrative support, managerial accountability, fundamental changes in HRM practices, employee involvement, and shifts in agency culture.

SUMMARY

The future viability of an organization and its HR capabilities are interrelated and must be considered together. Strategic human resources management must be vertically integrated with strategic planning and horizontally integrated with other HR functions, such as training and development, compensation and benefits, recruitment and selection, labor relations, and evaluation of the HR planning process, to allow for adjustments to confront rapidly changing environmental conditions. Due to a projected budget shortfall of $229 million, Jackson Health System in Miami, Florida, is in the process of possibly closing two hospitals and laying off one-third of its employees (Dorschner, 2010; Skipp, 2010). Strategic human resources management guides staff in identifying and implementing the appropriate HR learning activities for resolving organizational problems or adapting to meet new opportunities.

Strategic human resources management determines the HR needs of the agency and ensures that qualified personnel are recruited and developed to meet organizational needs. Should there be a shift in demand for services, an agency must know whether there are potential employees with the requisite skills available to provide these services and whether the agency's finances can afford the costs associated with additional compensation and benefits. Forecasting an agency's HR supply reveals the characteristics of its internal supply of labor; it also helps to assess the productivity of incumbent employees, implement succession planning and salary planning, and identify areas in which external recruitment or training and development are necessary.

Training and development are essential to the effective use of an organization's human resources and an integral part of its planning. Training is used to remedy immediate needs, whereas development pertains to long-term objectives and the ability to cope with change. Training and development should be viewed as a continuous process. There will always be new employees, new positions, new problems, changes in technology, and changes in the external and internal environments that require a planned approach to training and development and their integration with other HRM functions. Training and development influence recruitment, selection, career planning, and the compatibility between agency goals and employee aspirations. Training and development programs must be integrated to complement the organization's mission and operations. An organization should use employees wisely with respect to its strategic needs.

An organization must anticipate and plan for turnover, including retirements. Human resources management departments must track the skills of incumbent employees and keep skill inventories. Health care organizations in particular need to develop talent from within if they wish to sustain a competitive advantage and business continuity (Collins & Collins, 2007).

Recruitment and training must be tied to the organization's mission. The availability and stability of financial support; the advancement of technological changes, new laws and regulations, and social and cultural changes; and the evolution of HR requirements must be considered when developing strategic plans.

At one time organizations hired employees to fit the characteristics of a particular job. Now it is important for an organization to select employees who fit the characteristics not only of the position but also of the organization. Human resources management professionals must serve as internal consultants, working with managers to assess HR needs. Together they must project the demand for services, develop new resources, and determine the appropriate reallocation of services. The SHRM process, once established, can be used to anticipate and prepare for major changes affecting the workplace.

Effective strategic human capital management approaches serve as the foundation of any serious HRM initiative. They must be at the center of efforts to transform the culture of an agency so that it becomes results oriented and externally focused. To facilitate these changes, HRM personnel and department managers must acquire new competencies to be able to deliver HRM services and shift toward a more consultative role for HR staff.

Health care organizations are driven by the knowledge and skills their employees possess. It is shortsighted for agency leaders to dismiss the importance of SHRM. Just as important, organizations must reinforce the importance of human capital and the contribution that knowledge management makes to the effective delivery of services. Human resources management departments must have the knowledge, skills, and authority to identify and facilitate changes.

KEY TERMS

administrative services organizations (ASOs)

benefits consulting services

enterprise human resources outsourcing services

health benefits services

human resources information system (HRIS)

human resources information systems and Web-based services

incentive services

information technology services

payroll software and services

professional employer organizations (PEOs)

recruiting, staffing, and search services

relocation services

screening and workplace security services

DISCUSSION QUESTIONS

1. Discuss strategic human resources management.

2. Define the five steps in human resources planning.

3. Discuss the process of implementing strategic human resources management.

4. What are some problems associated with strategic human resources management? How might these problems be overcome?

This chapter was adapted and updated from Pynes, 1997, 2003b, 2004a, 2004b, 2009a, 2009b.

3

Organizational Culture Standards for Health Care Human Resources

LEARNING OBJECTIVES

- Understand the elements of a progressive health care organization
- Be able to apply the Performance Matrix to a set of health care human resources concepts as a human resources consultant
- Recognize how the charter factors of pride, accountability, commitment, and trust set the foundation for the development of a health care organization
- Comprehend the role of a sound human resources management department in a progressive health care organization
- Be ready to identify the roles of a human resources professional in supporting line management and staff in a progressive health care organization

HUMAN RESOURCES PROFESSIONALS in health care are the stewards of the organization's culture, the all-important "how and why" of the organization's essential charter. This chapter explores standards and specific practical applications of health care organizational culture that inform organizational development and all human resources work across a health care organization. The discussion begins with the individual dynamics of health care organizational development, and then moves on to group dynamics.

PERFORMANCE MATRIX OF SUPERSTARS, STEADIES, AND NONPLAYERS

A central element of health care organizational development is the **Performance Matrix,** which is effectively a quality control and performance enhancement strategy for human capital. As indicated in Table 3.1, the essential composition of any organization is centered on three categories of performers—the superstars, or organizational drivers; the steadies, or organizational advocates; and, last and most pejoratively, the nonplayers, or organizational agitators. Rudimentary but accurate theories on positive and negative motivation have suggested that positive motivation works to drive superstars, whereas negative motivation works with nonplayers, and an artful combination of the two is needed to manage the steadies.

The Performance Matrix is often recognized as a tool for analysis that is resonant of the "80-20 rule" of 1960s management and leadership theory, which states that misguided managers spend 80 percent of their time on the 20 percent of their staff that comprises nonplayers. This theory has certain but limited application to health care—after all, a health care cadre featuring a core of 20 percent nonplayers would doom the entire organization to failure. However, the truth of this theorem as related to health care is that a manager determined to allocate a major amount of time toward "saving the nonplayer" is one who is likely to be unsuccessful in many important regards, as is discussed in further detail later in this book.

The top part of the Performance Matrix is composed of *superstars,* who usually are the "highest 20 percent" of any organization. The superstars thrive on change, as they see it as an opportunity to increase their skills while they make a larger contribution to the organization. These are usually the charismatic leaders of a group who have garnered the respect of their colleagues and peers by virtue of their consistently outstanding performance, a willingness to help those who need their expertise, and their leadership

Table 3.1   Performance Matrix

Category	Percentage of the Organization	HR Relevance
Superstars/Action Agents • Outstanding performance • Organizational exemplars	10–20 percent	• Top rating in performance evaluation • Models for selection • Should get maximum training and development
Steadies/Advocates • Largest opportunity for HR	60–70 percent	• Employee majority • Respond well to skill-based training • Organizational development base
Nonplayers/Agitators • Largest human capital risk • Worst return on investment in terms of management time and energy	10–15 percent	• Documentation to termination candidates • Performance improvement plans • Management consulting need

by example every day in the workplace. The superstars are individuals who understand not only the *what* of health care delivery but also the importance of the *how,* and who accordingly conduct themselves in an exemplary manner in dealing with patients and assisting colleagues, and in their approach to all of their assigned job components.

An additional term to describe these superstars, the best employees within a given health care organization, is *action agents.* They are the individuals who are first to try a new method, contribute positively to brainstorming sessions on improving customer-patient care, and invariably innovate solutions to existing problems that benefit both the organization and the customer-patient. Their daily actions are motivated by the desire to truly afford stellar health care to the customer-patient community, and they have an intrinsic desire to learn as much as possible, every day, about the health care business, their specific organization, and the technical and professional aspects of their particular specialty. They willingly act as mentors and educators to their peers, and are great facilitators of progressive discussion and positive action on a daily basis. Their job description is simply the fundamental overview of the job, consisting of the basic responsibilities of the work role; their daily actions and ongoing commitment to their professional responsibilities reflect a belief that their job is indeed a vocation, and that "going above and beyond" is a daily expectation.

To use an expression made famous by Richard Nixon, the *steadies* make up the "silent majority" of any health care organization. Their performance is usually consistent, and their behavior on the job is solid in most regards. Most steadies have one area of expertise in which they are outstanding, and they maintain a "meets expectations" level of performance on all of their assigned job duties. With the proper mentoring and development, a steady can become a superstar; in fact, one of the best contributions health care leaders can make to their organization is to develop an emergent steady into a bona fide superstar. Steadies will perform job responsibilities and assignments that are not under the established job description if asked by the supervisor specifically and given the reason why the extra work is needed. Conversely, if the steadies are not managed correctly and are not motivated through coaching and positive development, they can often slide down into the nonplayer sector.

Steadies can also be regarded as organizational advocates. According to the term's Latin root, an *advocate* is a "positive voice"; steadies are usually both positive voices and positive forces with an organization. In fact, they are often the backbone of a sound health care organization. Because they represent the largest group in the Performance Matrix, they also represent the greatest challenge to a health care leader. On occasion they can be swayed by the negative actions of the nonplayers. In other circumstances they can be motivated with nurturing, coaching, and mentoring by not only the health care leader but also superstars within their work group.

There are five ranges of steadies that a health care leader must consider artfully and manage ardently to attain the highest possible performance level given the steadies' individual potential. They include the following:

- *Hidden superstars,* who are steadies who could move into the superstar category with the right coaching and opportunities to flourish

- *Technical superstars,* who will continue to thrive in highly technical roles that have no supervisory or management requisites

- *"Steadies for life,"* who will always contribute a satisfactory work output sans flourish
- *Escalator-gravitaters,* who can heighten or slacken performance given a particular work role or job assignment
- *Borderline nonplayers,* who barely meet the assigned requisites of their job

Nonplayers represent the bottom part of the Performance Matrix and are easily its most problematic populace. Although they often seem to be the largest segment of an organization or work group, in reality they are a smaller segment that usually needs the greatest amount of corrective attention and management time. Nonplayers can exist at any level of the organization and can occupy any of the professional categories of health care, but they have in common the ability to negatively affect the customer-patient, impair the progress of their peers and coworkers, and eradicate the positive morale and progressive motivation of a work group—and in some cases, an entire health care organization.

Nonplayers can also be referred to as organizational *agitators.* They can create personal animosity among members of a work department—and in some extreme cases across the organization—with their penchant for gossiping and malicious verbal behavior. They can generate antipathy across the span of an organization as a result of their own personal apathy and ignorance of what is truly required in taking care of an ailing patient or handling a pressing situation. Perhaps most apparent, they generate acrimony toward management in general and toward their direct supervisor in particular by their lackluster work performance, constant questioning of work objectives, and inappropriate challenges to the authority of those charged with leading the organization.

One practical application for the three-level Performance Matrix in health care human resources can be found in the review of **performance evaluation systems.** For example, performance evaluation systems that use a five-level numerical system to rate performance often quickly degenerate into a de facto three-point system anyway. Performance evaluation systems that employ a ten-point system also usually degenerate into a three-tier allocation of ratings and rewards. The reason for this is that any given work assignment or job responsibility can only be assessed realistically in three ways—the individual meets the stated expectations of the job, the individual exceeds the expectations, or the individual does not meet the stated expectations. When individuals establish a pattern of work that involves consistently meeting expectations, which the majority of health care workers do most of the time, it is easy to naturally and justly classify these individuals as steadies.

Likewise, when individuals consistently exceed expectations, informed health care leaders know that they are fortunate to have superstars in their chain of command who are truly exemplary staff members. Conversely, when an individual consistently fails to meet standards and expectations, a nonplayer is making his or her deleterious impact evident to all, from peers to supervisors to customer-patients.

The Performance Matrix can also be applied as a foundational tool for selecting and interviewing job candidates. The Performance Matrix acts as a linchpin for learning about training and development, compensation, and other facets of health care human resources.

A unique inspiration for applying this concept comes from Casey Stengel, a baseball manager known as much for his wit as for his Hall of Fame skills. He is anecdotally said to have attributed his managerial success to understanding that in dealing with three types of people—those that love you, those that hate you, and those that aren't sure yet—the key is to keep those who are not sure away from those that hate you.

Employing strategies on how to fully develop your steadies—while heightening the contribution of your superstars and diminishing the pejorative impact of the nonplayers—stands as a major objective of the progressive health care organization.

PACT FORMULA

Pride, accountability, commitment, and trust (PACT) are the hallmarks of any successful health care organization, from the staff level to the overall corporate structure. The **PACT Formula** details the professional work strategies of health care workers at every level and in all technical roles (see Figure 3.1). As health care human resources professionals innovate their strategy, these factors should be an essential component of the overall organizational profile and should be incorporated into organizational culture analysis.

Figure 3.1   PACT Formula

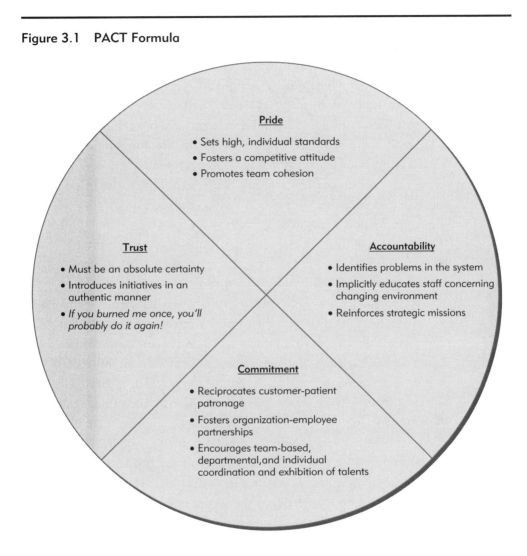

The PACT Formula, as per its acronym, has four categories of organizational culture, and each category has a set of couplets representing positive and negative management tendencies that can influence organizational culture. This system has been implemented as both a teaching tool and a foundation for human resources systems at many major medical centers, and it is a fundamental building block for establishing a leadership orientation that will facilitate the progressive human resources strategies contained in this text.

Pride

Pride is a characteristic relating to organizational development that pertains directly to the morale of the organization. Built on individual self-esteem, pride is evident in high-quality health care delivery and reflected in the dedication displayed by each and every staff member on a daily basis. Human resources professionals must ascertain if job candidates take pride in their work, are dedicated to their professional responsibilities, and have worked in organizations in which pride in performance and organizational achievement is a charter characteristic. This factor should also be evident in ongoing work performance and is integral to the success of work teams and of the organization as a whole.

Majority Versus Minority

As already discussed, all health care organizations consist of a majority of superstars and steadies. Unfortunately, many of the steadies tend to be quieter and more satisfied with their work role than are the nonplayers. As a result, their collective voice is usually lost in important work discourse and is muted whenever a major change or new work initiative is introduced. The positive majority of your staff will commit to your plan if they see actions and, over time, success; if you spend major time on the minor leaguers in your organization, you will surely get bush-league results.

One of the most important communication responsibilities of a health care leader, therefore, is to allow the voices of the steadies and superstars to squelch the whining tones of the nonplayers. The most important strategy for a health care leader in this regard is to make a conscious effort to ask all of the steadies and superstars for their opinions, perspectives, and suggestions—in group forums and on an individual basis—when undertaking a specific action.

Affecting Versus Annoying

All of us have personality characteristics that can be pleasant from one person's perspective yet less enchanting from another. As we have discussed, the nonplayers have a penchant for infusing their varied "personal issues" into every work situation possible. Because the spectrum of personality characteristics for nonplayers spans from whining to "acting out," it is quite likely that their personality quirks can be a source of great annoyance to both their supervisor and their colleagues, and can create destructive dissonance in employee relations.

Accordingly, it is important for the human resources professional to assist health care managers in dividing the nonplayer's personality characteristics into two categories: facets that are plain annoying from a personality perspective, and those more harmful behavioral characteristics that can greatly affect the perception of the customer-patient, influence negative performance throughout a given department, and inhibit the delivery of stellar health care. The proper documentation of the impact of negative behavior that impedes health care is essential for taking future corrective action.

Progress Versus Status Quo

Health care systems that are not progressive are doomed to quick failure, given the daunting confluence of financial issues, regulatory and political stress, and an array of other environmental factors. In the words of one health care leader, "Progress really is just reaching equilibrium with the current dynamic forces in the environment to maintain homeostasis, adaptation, and survival," according to Tal Ben Zvi, a thought leader in health care organizational dynamics. People working to maintain the status quo are really just nostalgic and looking into the past and avoiding looking into the present and future states.

Status quo advocates must receive a quick and effective education in the reality of today's health care forum as well as the guidance they need to help them become more adaptable. Otherwise, the best move would be for leadership to help them find a different business environment apart from health care in which they can pursue a paycheck in their own sedentary manner.

Wins Versus Losses

A primary malady for many health care organizations is the influence of the nonplayers, who seek to dominate most work discussions with laments about "what the organization does wrong"—that is, the organization's "losses." The steadies and superstars are, in a phrase, "too polite" to argue with the nonplayers, and they are more interested in quietly going about their everyday business of providing excellent health care to their community. Over time, however, the nonplayers' negative attitude can have a corrosive effect on organizational morale.

A remedy is to provide a time line of the positive accomplishments of this organization, which a CEO will be happy to present in a series of town hall meetings. The nonplayers invariably are silent during such presentations; in the words of one CEO, "You know, the nonplayers just hate it when things go right!"

Every health care leader should make a conscious effort to celebrate the wins at a level that supersedes the amount of time and energy spent in self-flagellation over the losses. Motivation and inspiration must be fed on a regular and consistent basis. Citing the wins and major accomplishments of a particular work group is vital to maintaining positive motivation that silences the nonplayers and, moreover, inspires the superstars and steadies. If health care leaders spend at least as much time on celebrating the wins as they do lamenting the losses, some nice, natural, positive motivation might be generated throughout the workplace.

The Department of Veterans Affairs (VA) medical centers use a time line system—whose implementation and innovation are led by educational experts in their human resources management departments—to engage all levels of leadership in creating **time lines** that cite wins the entire staff can appreciate and in which the superstars and steadies can take justifiable pride. This technique, as illustrated in Figure 3.2, has resonance in these facilities, which are always growing (as are many community-driven health care organizations in all categories across the nation) and have increased their patient population. An annual time line review of any facility's "biggest achievements" over the year can be presented fluidly on posters in the cafeteria, reviewed by individual managers in department meetings, and used as an educational tool with volunteers and other important—but sometimes missed—contributors.

Accountability

Accountability is an individual characteristic that is demonstrated by people who are responsible for their actions, responsive to new work challenges, and dedicated to new learning to increase their professional acumen. In health care settings, the job description is more of a general document than a pinpointed, pluperfect, step-by-step delineation of everyday responsibilities. Therefore, health care employees must be individually accountable for the daily responsibilities, making accountability a key characteristic in the selection process and, indeed, the entire chronology of employee development, as supported by health care human resources.

Customer Focus Versus Nonplayer Focus

The driving force of any of successful health care organization is the needs and demands, both established and emerging, of the community's customer-patients. The focus of leaders and all of their charges should therefore be on meeting the demands of the health care constituent as opposed to pandering to the needs of the nonplayer, whose perspective is skewed.

Accountability Versus Deniability

Accountable organizations and staff groups grow and thrive as they take care of their constituent community and regularly introduce new programs and services. Organizations and work groups that focus on deniability—the attitude of taking responsibility for nothing and blaming everything on others—at best become simply followers, and often become nonplayer havens. Hospitals that are committed to *genuine* process improvement and innovations that elevate the quality of patient care and community service are, by definition, organizations embracing accountability, not deniability.

Action Versus Discussion

The PACT factors of this chapter can be a good calibration tool for evaluating dynamics in your current work situation. As you conduct your analysis in this area, keep the phrase "all talk, no action" at the forefront of your thinking. Good leaders separate themselves from pretenders in this area by making certain that all communication opportunities have a dedicated focus based on specific agendas that end with plans of action—not just another scheduled meeting.

Consider great historical leaders who were successful because they knew how to get the best information available at the time and act on it efficaciously. Usually these leaders were expert at initiating action thanks to an early-career epiphany resulting from an error in judgment due to not taking action in a timely and focused manner. They learned a valuable lesson: a leader artfully balances input with decision making, and he or she understands that more discussion and deliberation are counterproductive to getting the job done. Action brings improvement, resolution, and results; talking,

Figure 3.2   Time Line Review of the Huntington VA Medical Center, West Virginia

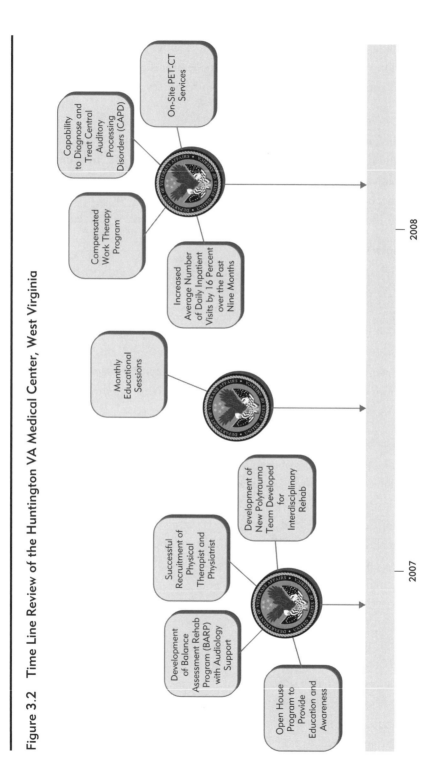

Capability to Diagnose and Treat Central Auditory Processing Disorders (CAPD)

On-Site PET-CT Services

Compensated Work Therapy Program

Increased Average Number of Daily Inpatient Visits by 16 Percent over the Past Nine Months

Monthly Educational Sessions

Successful Recruitment of Physical Therapist and Physiatrist

Development of New Polytrauma Team Developed for Interdisciplinary Rehab

Development of Balance Assessment Rehab Program (BARP) with Audiology Support

Open House Program to Provide Education and Awareness

2007

2008

discussing, and inordinately "processing" erode confidence and, in health care, can negatively influence life-and-death matters.

Practical Versus Conceptual

There are many phrases in the American business lexicon that have limited meaning in the health care setting, such as "in a perfect world," or "in theory." Unfortunately, health care does not operate in a perfect world, and theory has limited application when attempting to solve difficult dilemmas and resolving the daily challenges. The nonplayer often suggests conceptual solutions and theoretical conclusions that have limited value in the daily health care workplace.

Every group and individual health care work discussion should incorporate a focus on practical solutions. Emphasis should be placed on specific situations, particular environmental conditions, and an enumeration of the exact dynamics that the group or individual is confronting at a given time. The more specific the delineation of circumstances, the more likely it becomes that a specific, effective solution will be garnered for the benefit of the work group and the customer-patient community. Leaders must offer practical ideas and immediate solutions, not overblown theoretical concepts that have little promise for short-term implementation. The former notion leads to progressive action that benefits patients and employees alike; the latter notion represents both a waste of time and a quick route to lost credibility of and lost confidence in the leaders in the eyes of their reporting staff.

Closure Versus "Revisiting"

Without question, mistakes are made every day in the delivery of health care. A review of mistakes—and a discussion of new directions and new plans that will help avoid those mistakes in the future—is the best method to instill group pride and individual commitment to a given goal. This method brings a sense of closure to an unfortunate situation, and encourages a majority of the group to move ahead to new frontiers.

Conversely, the nonplayer revels in trying to bring work discourse back to unfortunate situations and past mistakes. This can quickly erode confidence and create apathy and distrust in the mind of the steady, who is committed to new action and to contributing to the greater good of the group. When confronted with a nonplayer who is intent on revisiting negative issues from the past, it is incumbent upon the leader to say something along these lines:

"Most of us would agree that we have learned from that mistake and moved on—I would encourage you to do the same." This exhibits the leader's commitment to closing negative issues, moving on to new challenges, and, perhaps most important, keeping the nonplayers' infectious negativity at bay.

"How" Versus "If"

No plan of action is totally foolproof. In fact, it is quite easy for a lazy person to take a cursory glance at a proposed course of action and make a general criticism of all the potential problems inherent in the plan. A detractor can easily cite the many ways in which a plan could "go wrong," and thus create apprehension in the conduct of the plan. Many individuals operating from a point of ignorance can use the word "if" exponentially ("If we do this, we will have a problem with . . . ").

A health care leader must elicit as many solutions as possible while emphasizing that the question at hand is not a matter of "if" but rather of "how" we will make this work. Coupled with a challenge to nonplayers to "top it or drop it"—that is, "Come up with a better plan, or we will undertake the proposed plan fully for the benefit of our customer-patients"—changing to a "how" mentality helps avoid unneeded apprehension and discord. Furthermore, the steadies and superstars are fully engaged in the conversation, and become true stakeholders as a positive plan is implemented. "How" encourages action and participation, whereas "if" breeds stagnation and consternation. "If" leads to all talk and no action, whereas "how" inspires a plan of work, and a motivation to propel that plan toward attaining its measures of success. "How" leads the action, whereas "if" sits and waits to criticize. Leadership demands detailed planning and astute execution using strong management expertise, not waiting for perfect scenarios that will never present themselves in the vexing world of health care. Being *innovative* rather than *inventive* in this respect means developing plans based on "how" to do it with resources available rather than saying, "If we only had (perfect amount of resources)."

Backstage Versus Onstage

In every health care organization, every day, there are situations that elicit emotional responses, such as laughing or anger. All health care staff members, at every level, must understand that a customer-patient is very circumspect and scrutinizes everything they say. Accordingly, there is no room for employees to "act out" in a deleterious manner in either the full view or the listening range of customer-patients.

It is therefore vital that human resources professionals support, and in many cases lead, consultative efforts to innovate and move forward into action policies that assist the organization by intelligently and appropriately embracing this tenet. Such policies can include providing management training that underscores the need to move emotional reactions and emotionally charged conversations away from patient traffic areas and into, for example, employee-only conference rooms or private offices. In addition, this practice should be featured in patient care education for all staff members.

Written Versus Verbal

Proactive documentation is the best method of ensuring accountability for everyone on your staff. When you have assigned a goal, consider sending an e-mail to each of the goal's main action agents. In this e-mail, specify the due date for the assignment, the amount of financial resources allocated, and a brief "vision" of what is expected as an end product. In addition, the e-mail should end with an encouraging offer for the recipient to contact you at any time that more explanation is needed and more guidance could be helpful.

By using this method, the nonplayer gets very specific, tangible direction, and a stated outcome is "on the record" as a basic reference and as solid documentation. For the superstars and steadies, the opportunity to shine is apparent, as they can now exceed stated expectations, and the documentation of their achievement can be integrated constructively into their performance evaluation. In all cases, clear accountability is assigned, monitored, measured, and assessed objectively. Moreover, clearly delineating the components of a goal removes the opportunity for nonplayers to evoke deniability of their responsibilities, as the pact factor of "written versus verbal" makes the assignment more vivid, more formal, and, in a very real sense, more serious.

Known Versus Unknown

Throughout the annals of psychology, fear of the unknown always seems to emerge as a major threat to an individual's comfort and basic lifestyle. For nonplayers, who enjoy fearmongering and drawing attention to themselves by creating discomfort, the presentation of "problems" and "issues" that are not completely defined—and that in some cases might not be real at all—becomes one of their favorite ploys.

The health care leader should therefore subscribe to a strategy that consists of a plan for all of the situations that are known to be part of the decision calculus and also contains some general preparation components that will help in confronting situations that are nebulous or unknown at the outset. Accordingly, for all dynamics that are known as a work group approaches a new situation, the leader should communicate a full and comprehensive plan. For the dynamics that are unknown at the outset, the leader should communicate an overarching tactic of preparedness for analyzing, confronting, and resolving any problem that arises.

Leaders Versus Leaners

Everyone who works in a health care facility must be a leader. As an example, consider a security guard or even a volunteer with a name badge who is asked numerous times in a given day to help "lead" a visitor to his or her loved one. Furthermore, because most health care staff members are experts in their particular field, they are in reality the true leaders within their area of expertise. As a result, there is no room within a health care facility for a chronic "leaner" who constantly needs direction and consultation to perform his or her job adequately. A leaner who cannot make decisions, cannot act quickly and effectively, and—perhaps most destructive—needs inordinate time and attention from coworkers and supervisors is unnecessarily draining resources that are already in short supply.

All staff members should be given strong, ongoing encouragement to act independently and take command appropriately in the interest of caring for the customer-patient; positive review and recognition of accomplishments should be consistent themes. For leaners, a strident review of their technical abilities as well as of their basic confidence should be enacted at the time of the selection interview if possible, and certainly at critical junctures in the performance evaluation cycle. For some leaners it is a matter of technical or job-related shortcomings—in these cases, additional training and point-specific mentoring could be the solution. In other cases, it is a matter of confidence or a byproduct of their orientation and adjustment to your organization, and perhaps your organization's management style. In any case, the problem of leaners must be addressed to ensure that your staff is operating at maximum efficiency and optimum effectiveness every day. Leadership involves imparting to subordinates the necessity of accomplishing the assigned tasks and enthusiastically accepting full responsibility for the results. Leaners will not take responsibility and often blame peers, the organization, their boss, and anything or anyone else conceivable for their shortcomings in regard to motivation and expertise.

Encouragement Versus Empowerment

During the "continuous quality improvement (CQI) craze" of the 1990s in health care, *empowerment* became a catchy buzzword. In a positive way, it encouraged leaders to empower all of their staff members with both the responsibility and the authority to make appropriate decisions and execute needed action. However, it was misappropriated by nonplayers who used it as a gambit to argue with their supervisors, with such phrases as "Well I'm the expert, I should be able to do this the way I want to, regardless of the needs of the organization and patient."

As a result, health care leaders need to use the word *encouragement* and focus on indeed encouraging their charges, while dropping the term *empowerment* completely from their management and leadership vocabulary. Thankfully this misappropriated term of *empowerment* has gone by the wayside, but its root of *power* should be replaced with the real force of employee encouragement. In this way, all health care professionals should have the courage to apply their skills, their devotion, and their abilities to the highest level, providing stellar health care in every situation, every day.

Note that leaders who encourage staff members but fail to provide the resources, authority, responsibility, and independence are falling short of their charter. Accordingly, solid leadership encourages staff, provides a realistic vision of objectives, and always asks, "What do you need from me to make this happen?" Risks are not taken unless rewards, recognition, and results are eminent. Encouragement also leads to a strong succession and promotion system, as the spirit of encouragement sparks long-term affiliation and growth in the organization.

Positions Versus Postures

Leaders who take a stand during times of adversity and change, rather than just maintaining a posture or "standing on ceremony," provide the commitment integral to PACT. All health care human resources professionals should incorporate the core organizational values depicted in Figure 3.3.

Figure 3.3   Defined Values of a Progressive Health Care Leader

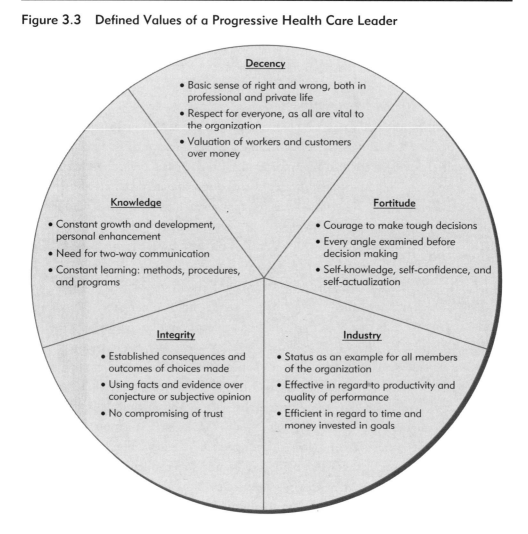

Commitment

Commitment is the characteristic that goes beyond the tenets of daily work contribution. The need to go the extra step, every day and in every way, is a job requisite for all health care professionals. Health care human resources must provide selection systems and performance evaluation counsel that help develop a workplace environment in which commitment is clearly evident in the work efforts of the overwhelming majority of managers and staff.

Majority Commitment Versus 100 Percent Consensus

Committed organizations understand that consensus, despite its importance, is not always possible, and that although people may sometimes "agree to disagree," the whole team moves on a set plan in the interest of the good of the organization and patient. Organizations seeking "100 percent consensus" will soon be unable to move because commitment to action never takes necessary form.

Need Versus Want

Health care professionals at every level should be focused on what they need to do as opposed to what they want to have in terms of resources or optimal job descriptions. It is important for leaders to always ask the critical question, "What do we want as opposed to what do we really need?" Leaders must parse demands and "must-haves" or "must-dos" essential to the mission from the "nice-to-haves" or "wish-we-coulds" that are often unrealistic and a waste of time. Gauging patient and community needs and considering the organizational strategy at hand can be good barometers in answering these questions.

Solution Formulation Versus Problem Reiteration

As discussed earlier, one of the favorite schemes of the nonplayer is to constantly draw attention to problems that exist within the work context. This technique, often referred to as derailment, is unfortunately facilitated unconsciously by new managers who believe that all employees should have an "equal voice" in work discussions. In their quest to be fair they are ironically unfair to the steadies and superstars who actually are very interested in improving the health care organization and the level of care that it provides.

An inherent responsibility of leaders is to conduct communication and planning sessions that move their charges to action-oriented solutions rather than squandering energy, time, and resources in facilitating nonplayer-led efforts to castigate the organization over old problems. Most exemplary health care organizations know any problem should be discussed in conjunction with a deeper conversation on how to solve the dilemma. When a problem is noticed, the opportunity for formulating a solution is always in the offing. All staffs consist of both problem generators and action-oriented problem solvers. An effective leader will garner a basic understanding of a problem and engage his or her staff comprehensively toward identifying a plan for problem resolution.

Accordingly, every health care leader throughout an organization should have a "house rule" that no one problem or challenge can be raised in departmental meetings or any other form of work communication without the person raising the problem at least suggesting a solution.

Specific Versus General

The nonplayer revels in generalities and specious statements. Presenting wide-sweeping perspectives that are often faulty in premise and context, the nonplayer seeks to create a Niagara of negativity that will impair the motivation of the steadies while creating an atmosphere of hopelessness across the workplace. Health care leaders seeking to be "politically correct" tend to keep work discussions very general, and as a result it takes more time than needed to specifically identify the problem and then try to innovate a particular solution.

Health care human resources professionals should try to encourage the use of directed questions, such as "Can you give me a specific example?" and the use of open-ended questions, such as "If I were a customer-patient, what three things that exist right now in our patient care delivery would I find most laudatory?" or "How about the three most deleterious aspects of patient care?" to get to the most pertinent, focused information possible, as quickly and effectively as possible.

Perspective Versus Perception

Perhaps the most overused and certainly misused word in health care management jargon is *perception,* which is consistently confused with the word *perspective.* Perspective in this case is loosely defined as a balanced view of a situation. Individuals who maintain perspective do not make mountains out of molehills, nor do they trivialize important situations. Perception alludes to the subjective view that an individual holds of a given situation. By definition, perceptions are important in understanding others' motivations and reactions. Perspective, however, is more important to maintain an objective, balanced view in holding work discussions and taking significant action.

Participants Versus Spectators

Fact—every health care organization in North America could use more staff immediately. Another fact—this is often used as an excuse among the nonplayers for their own individual nonperformance. Every employee of a health care organization is vitally needed in order for the organization to successfully attain its mission. All employees must participate in caregiving every day at an optimum level, while continuously improving their individual skills.

There is therefore no room at any health care organization for second-guessers. Many nonplayers enjoy simply watching the action, rather than making the action part of their daily work responsibilities. A leader should always seek to manage with careful consideration of each team member's abilities; provide boundless opportunities for educating developing steadies and superstars; and, as always, identify and diminish the impact of the non-players who are intent on undercutting work outcomes by being spectators rather than participants.

Outcomes Versus Opinions

Clear-cut results, particularly when supplemented by significant numbers and other quantitative indicators, are more essential to work discussions than the subjective, biased opinions of nonplayers. Health care leaders should try to incorporate resonant data in their planning and evaluate results based on clear criteria. The intrusion of nonplayers' subjective and often self-serving statements can cause a dangerous undertow in the organization, especially when these assertions are featured as "facts" by their promulgators.

Fact Versus Fiction

Leaders are always perceived as being "in the know" and must lead work discussions with outcomes that can be substantiated objectively; this infor-mation will then take natural precedence and priority over the supercilious opinions of the nonplayers. Nothing exposes a canard promoter more than being proven false by facts. The data that measure progress, validate success, and provide real-world standards to make comparisons to competitors and past achievements are the gold standard in implementing an "outcome-over-opinion" ambiance. Communicating with facts encourages the entire staff to operate in the real world of health care, not the doomed world existent in the warped perception of certain nonplayers—especially when these facts include significant metrics that objectively tell the real story.

Contribution Versus Criticism

A mistake that health care leaders often make almost unconsciously is to allow a monthly or weekly meeting to degenerate into a critiquing session led by the nonplayers. As experts on "everything that went wrong," nonplayers are very qualified to conduct this session, particularly when they are presented with an open forum. The health care leader should therefore prepare thoroughly before staff meetings and specifically use the time as an opportunity to provide encouragement and recognition for solid performance.

Taking a Stand Versus Having a Committee

As mentioned previously, several years ago health care endured a movement best described as the "CQI craze," when it seemed that every organization in the country underwent some sort of continuous quality improvement process. Unfortunately, this left a residual cultural problem of having a "decision-by-committee" approach to every pending organizational initiative.

When a health care work group of any size takes up a decision-by-committee style, the following ensues:

- Frustration sets in among the superstars, who want to take positive action.

- Time is spent unnecessarily.

- Steadies get discouraged and start to wonder if the nonplayers have a point about the organization's ineptitude.

- The credibility of leadership wanes, as people wonder who is *really* in charge.

- Good people waste energy and resent spending time researching and discussing an issue despite knowing that nothing good will come from the effort.

- Future organizational commitment from steadies and superstars becomes an unlikely commodity.

Telling Versus Selling

Many nonplayers enjoy using the phrase "I'm not sure I buy into that." The fallacy of the statement is that they are not being "sold" anything; as a matter of fact, they are being given work direction that they should follow as long as they are collecting a paycheck. They are not being presented with options relative to whether or not they are to accomplish the assigned task; instead they are being asked to use their discernment and expertise to determine the best course possible for accomplishing the task (not to debate its assignment).

Trust

Although there are no absolutisms in human behavior, trust is a workplace behavioral characteristic that embraces a number of absolutes. Whether it is between two employees or between a manager and a staff member—or among the members of the entire health care organization and its administrative and medical leadership—trust must be founded on clear communication, resolute action, progressive development, and outstanding service to the customer-patient community. The couplets in this section are designed to assist human resources professionals as well as line managers in understanding the functionality of trust in the health care work setting.

We Versus They

There is a ubiquitous "they" to whom nonplayers refer several times in a given day. On some occasions "they" are the customer patients; in other situations the "they" refers, usually negatively, to a hospital's administration. In all instances, the use of "they" is part of the blaming techniques of the nonplayer; "they" are responsible for everything that goes wrong within the health care facility, whereas the nonplayer has no accountability or responsibility.

Instilling the belief among staff that "we" are all "they" can be challenging, although ideally all organizations try to embrace a team-oriented "we" concept. Nonplayers always think that the "they" refers to the executive team; even some steadies subscribe to that thinking. Accordingly, both nominal leaders in the executive ranks and the charismatic leaders among the superstars and steadies have to exemplify a "we" team concept across the board so that their staff will commit to this notion.

Superstars and steadies are already committed to the mission, vision, and values of the organization, and always work toward elevating a team concept. Self-promoting and self-absorbed "I and they" nonplayers promote division when they refer to other team members in "they" terms; these individuals will usually also relegate the customer-patient to "they" or "the enemy" status. In the final analysis, as with many of the latter parts of these PACT couplings, the use of "they" is an exercise in nonaccountability. Great teams always function as a "we" and accept accountability, both positive and negative, for decisions and actions; these teams consistently apply a unified "we" or "team" approach, leading to the achievement of laudable goals and great outcomes.

Patient-Driven Versus Ego-Driven

The basic values of decency, fortitude, industry, integrity, and knowledge should be the driving factors not only for the health care leader but also for the entire staff. All too often decisions are made based on personal desire rather than on an examination of the defining ethics of effective health care action.

The prefix of *self-* is a good touchstone in understanding this particular leadership malady. Self-promoting nonplayers, at any level in a health care organization, maintain only a commitment to their own personal agenda and can quickly misdirect an entire organization. Self-aggrandizing non-players "wear out" all whom they come in contact with, from peers to patients. A self-absorbed leader who places a personal agenda above the mission of the organization unwittingly spawns a workplace environment in which apathy, deceit, and selfishness become the nefarious standards, supplemented by missed goals, fratricide, and high turnover of steadies and superstars who need a value-driven environment to strive and who have the skills and desire to seek another employer—which is exactly what the nonplayer should be doing instead.

Conversely, selfless leaders who epitomize the values presented in Figure 3.3—decency, fortitude, industry, integrity, and knowledge—are of great value to the organization, as their staff members do not have to won-der about their commitment or "personal agenda." Their plans and actions always reflect positively on the mission and values of the organization, and their leadership inspires a high quality in not only the *what* of organizational achievement but also the *how*.

Community Versus Family

The word *community* implies a common unity. The word *family,* used in a work setting, can imply that there are no limits to the "unconditional love" that a nonplayer can receive. In the community, people move in and move out on a regular basis. In a family, all behavior is acceptable, and unconditional love must be rendered—an unrealistic expectation considering that payment for effective action is the key to health care organizations' success.

Proactive Versus Reactive

When a health care leader neglects planning and preparation for his or her work group, the entire team is put in the disadvantageous position of always reacting to circumstances in a manner that brings to mind being constantly "behind the eight ball." The ability to see the entire "big picture" to devise thoughtful strategy relative to the existing work environment of health care gives the leader the opportunity to move the team forward and accomplish needed goals, rather than simply reacting erratically to the dictates of ever-changing situations.

Proactive leadership dictates action; reactive leadership only responds in a haphazard fashion. Proactive teams consider all possibilities and set an action plan; reactive teams are always caught short and are constantly surprised—and they have to continually put out fires that could have been avoided with some forethought. To truly establish trust across the span of a work group, action plans that consider patient needs and emerging dynamics must be in place and in a vernacular that is accessible to all members of the team.

Clarity Versus Complexity

The "KISS" theorem, which encourages a leader to "Keep it simple, stupid," should be part of the everyday approach of any health care leader. Although nonplayers enjoy making simple issues unnecessarily complicated, the greater good is better served when complex issues are simplified. For example, the exceptionally qualified neurosurgeon who can explain the dynamics of a complicated brain surgery to a supporting surgical staff in a way that a ten-year-old science student could grasp is as "people smart" as she is technically qualified. The ability to clarify vexing situations with logical communication is a management asset that cannot be overemphasized in the very complicated world of health care.

Running Toward Versus Running From

With good direction, focused planning, and timely communication from leadership, steadies and superstars at any level can see a direct relevance between their daily job accountabilities and their job's importance to the organization. Their commitment is enhanced as they see results that not only benefit the people they deal with directly but also help move the organization forward.

Assurance Versus Apprehension

There are difficult times in every organization, department, or group. People need to know that their work makes a difference. An effective leader will watch for apprehensive employees and guide them so that they do not lose focus. At the same time, a leader must not feel apprehensive about doing so, showing self-assurance and leading by example.

STRATEGIC REQUIREMENTS FOR A PROGRESSIVE HEALTH CARE HUMAN RESOURCES MANAGEMENT DEPARTMENT

The discussion now turns to specific characteristics and criteria that define health care human resources management departments and that are constructive cultural centerpieces of progressive health care organizations. The following criteria have been compiled for this text based on organizational scorecards from ten health care organizations that vary in size, medical mission, and location. It is interesting to note that each of the ten factors in this section was cited as "critically important" by all ten organizations without equivocation—the epitome of a "top ten list"—which helps make the case for incorporating all of these factors in your health care human resources strategy.

High Visibility

In health care organizations in which human resources is not considered a strong function, one of the major complaints is that the human resources office is either nondescript in general or "missing in action" when a crisis relative to human capital management occurs. The leadership practice of "management by walking around" is one that should be adopted by all members of the health care human resources staff, from administrative assistants to the vice president of human resources. When a situation requires a critical contribution from human resources, such as an employee relations crisis or a staffing shortage, it is imperative that the human resources management department be on the scene and in action immediately. In general, it is essential that the human resources management department be located not in the basement of the hospital but close to the main doors or central lobby for easy access for both employees and visitors. When there is a general perception that "you can never find human resources when you need them," the human resources function has rendered itself unimportant and irrelevant in the overall progress and development strategy of the health care organization.

Business Orientation

Human resources management departments are strategic business units in the purest sense. Pragmatic business decisions must be made in terms of staffing the human resources management department itself, and in terms of staffing and recruitment considerations for the entire organization. All members of the human resources management department must understand that health care organizations are not only community service organizations but also business entities that need to meet certain budgetary and fiscal requirements to be successful. Perhaps most important, all members of the human resources management department should believe—and demonstrate through their actions—that good people management is simply good business: inefficiencies, mistakes, and poor performance are among the most harmful threats to a health care organization, given that labor costs are approximately 65 percent of a typical health care organization's overall budget.

User-Friendliness

All members of a health care human resources management department, regardless of the organization's size or scope, must be available to all members of the organization at all times (typically known in the field as 100 percent coverage). Health care human resources management departments must have a strategy in which human resources services, counsel, and support are available as needed—which, given the reality of health care organizations, is all the time, seven days a week, twenty-four hours a day. Consider the fact that emergency rooms in a community hospital operate literally around the clock—because scores of skilled employees in addition to physicians and nurses are needed to work an emergency department, it is easy to understand the need for the human resources management department to be available, supportive, accessible, and adaptable in providing services effectively and efficiently. A human resources management department should never be "too busy" to talk to an employee needing assistance, nor should any follow-up action be allowed to fail due to lackluster time management.

Direct Communication

It is important that human resources professionals communicate clearly and in a manner that will enable the listener—often a troubled line manager or bewildered staff member—to understand strategies and resolution steps for whatever conundrum the human resources professional is addressing. The inability to communicate clearly and competently can make a puzzling situation even more problematic, while causing the requesting line manager or staff member's disenfranchisement and frustration in the process. The result of such a quandary can be a lack of trust between the health care professional and the human resources professional.

Responsiveness

Five "C Factors" of human resources interaction should be intrinsic to the communication style of all health care human resources professionals to maintain optimum responsiveness. First, human resources professionals should be *comprehensive* in their communication by providing a complete picture of possible solutions, critical data, and essential information. Second, all communication should be presented in a *cogent* manner, which means that applicable logic and facts are presented to help guide positive action while encouraging ownership and accountability. The third essential factor, and the most important in ensuring understanding, is *clarity*—brevity, thoughtfulness, and honesty are the ingredients vital to a clear message. Naturally, timing is everything in providing meaningful and useful assistance, so *clock management* is the fourth key element in maintaining trust and responding to requests for assistance. Finally, *compassion*—that is, the development of a "common passion," replete with sensitivity, tactfulness, and ardent listening—is a mainstay in demonstrating responsiveness in consultative situations.

Decisiveness

The organizational scorecards that helped provide the data for this section also gave respondents the opportunity to provide commentary and qualitative observations. A nurse leader, when discussing decisiveness, offered the comment that when a health care leader counters a challenge by saying, "We haven't made a decision yet on that issue," in reality the health care leader is

Figure 3.4   Decision-Making Criteria and Process

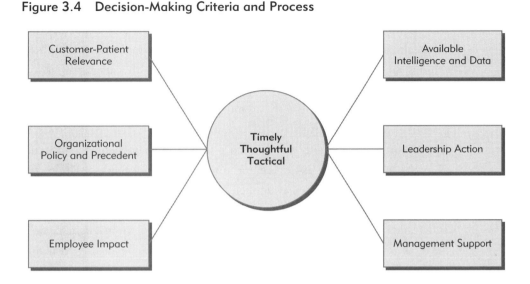

avoiding the challenge and has indeed made a decision—a decision not to do anything constructive or progressive, which will usually lead to dire outcomes. This nurse leader's view could lead to the development of a sound credo for health care human resources professionals—get your facts, ask the right questions, consider all options, make a decision, create a plan, and work your plan. As depicted in Figure 3.4, a sound decision-making process is needed to select the best possible option—with the knowledge that a pluperfect solution will never really exist for any situation—for the organization, the customer-patient, and the staff members affected by the decision. The science of decision making must naturally be augmented by the fortitude of appropriate leaders and the encouragement of all staff members to make the planned action a positive reality.

Knowledgeability

The health care human resources management department must have a wealth of knowledge in several critical areas. Naturally, a job requirement is strong emotional intelligence, or "people smarts." Communication ability, listening skills, perceptiveness, professional presence, and tactfulness are all subcategories of this important characteristic. Health care human resources professionals must know their craft, and even if they are not generalists they should have up-to-date knowledge and established expertise in the field of human resources. Organizational knowledge is also needed across the health care human resources management department. Knowing how "things are done around here" is vital, as each health care organization has its own culture and work personality, in addition to a set of practices and policies that are likely to be unique in their application with different personnel at varying levels of the organization. Management aptitude is also important in a health care human resources management department, as many management issues center on the time-honored discipline of management. Management is defined here as doing things right, whereas leadership is defined as doing the right things. Knowledge of management and leadership principles, along with general related knowledge in such fields as organizational ethics and labor law, should be readily available consultative resources in a health care human resources office. Moreover, all members of a health care human resources office should know how to get answers and specific information as needed in all of these critical areas to make them available to requesting line managers and other staff.

Action Orientation

Health care management tomes never fail to make a distinction between organizations that are proactive and those that are reactive. The distinction is often based on a health care organization's ability to anticipate emergent needs and growth opportunities as well as take quick and efficient action in the face of an unforeseen crisis. In a similar vein, health care human resources management departments should be able to put a premium on taking resolute action quickly and effectively, as opposed to simply pondering problems and "waiting for more data," or worse, "waiting to see what might happen next." Given the ever-escalating pace of the health care environment as well as the inordinate pressure to produce optimum results as a norm, a health care organization can ill afford to simply lay back and wait for the things that happen. Rather, the organization must constantly scan its environment for opportunities to improve performance in every conceivable manner and move accordingly. The human resources component must embrace that strategy fully—especially the critical areas of employee selection, talent retention, and organizational development—in order for the entire health care organization to be successful.

Strength

In the successful health care organizations, people make the difference. The health care organization is the exemplar of the "people business" among all businesses. A direct connection exists between a strong health care organization and a formidable human resources management department, as it is only logical that a premier organization is composed of outstanding people. Accordingly, a health care human resources management department in a progressive health care organization is a source of strength, and not merely a support department. By showing a sense of fortitude in helping line managers use the disciplinary process, for example, and by eliminating nonplayers from the organization and innovating development systems to maximize the encouragement of the steadies, the health care human resources management department becomes a central player. The ability to make tough calls during equitable labor relations negotiations that lead to win-win outcomes also is a testament to a strong health care human resources management department. A line manager responding to the organizational scorecard exercise made a defining statement for this "strength" attribute—"I know that the folks in my human resources management department back me up any time I'm trying to make the organization better, and provide me with the tools and expertise that I need to make a tough decision."

Pragmatism

A respondent in the scorecard exercise was much less complimentary to her human resources management department when she said, "I have gotten to a point where I do not trust my human resources colleagues, as they see themselves as social workers rather than businesspeople." This line manager believed that instead of being direct, thoughtful, and honest in dealing with unproductive and recalcitrant employees, the human resources generalists engaged in offering apologias and excuse making for the poor performance of nonplayers, usually centered on a set of spurious "personal issues" that supposedly are inhibiting the nonplayers' performance. This can, of course, encourage the nonplayers to continue to play the victim as opposed to actually doing their job, with a resultant negative impact on their assigned work group members, who must "pick up the slack." In another response, a line manager made this statement: "Our HR department seems more interested in promulgating policy than in resolving problems and helping me to do my job."

In both instances, a lack of pragmatic action and practical solution formulation belied the effectiveness and efficacy of the human resources management department and jeopardized organizational action. A sense of realism, balanced perspective, and integrity of purpose should be at the forefront of every health care human resources professional's work charter to provide pragmatic and practical services to the organization.

SUMMARY

Organizational culture is an essential component of any successful health care organization. Using standards for management and organizational development that reflect organizational pride, accountability, commitment, and trust is a critical leadership requisite. With guidance and education from human resources, organizational culture standards help inform the all-important "how we do business every day" foundation of a progressive health care organization.

The human resources team in an accountable care organization must be dedicated to making organizational culture standards a vibrant and viable part of every job and placing them at the forefront of every employee's job description. Specific and thoughtful innovation and application of the standards and strategies of this chapter help make this charter objective attainable.

KEY TERMS

PACT Formula	Performance Matrix
performance evaluation systems	time lines

DISCUSSION QUESTIONS

1. Considering a work team, school group, or any other entity of your choosing and membership, plot all of the members relative to performance using the Performance Matrix. What criteria did you consider when placing each in one of the three categories?

2. Select at least two of the PACT couplets that would apply to the entity you chose for the preceding question. What specific performance examples can you provide that would substantiate your selections?

3. Innovate at least three new PACT couplets that you think are essential for reviewing and enhancing an organization's culture.

4. Which human resources management role do you think is the most important to each of the following:

   • A major medical center

   • A local clinic of twenty to thirty employees

   • A multihospital health care organization

5. Construct a time line reviewing the work of an organization of your choice.

6. Decision making is a key to success in any health care organization. Considering health care human resources, cite five major decisions that have an impact on the entire organization and should be part of the organization's leadership charter (for example, human capital expenditures, types of training, layoffs). Supplement your answer with a specific three-to-five-point action plan that you would implement relative to an assumed decision.

4

Equal Employment Opportunity Laws and Health Care Human Resources Management

LEARNING OBJECTIVES

- Understand the federal laws related to equal employment opportunity and their implications for strategic human resources management

- Be able to explain the difference between equal employment opportunity and affirmative action

- Comprehend the religious exemption from Title VII protections provided to some health care organizations

- Know the difference between disparate treatment and disparate impact theories of employment discrimination

- Be able to understand and apply the constitutional protections provided to public health care employees

- Understand the concept of employment at will

UNDERSTANDING AND complying with federal equal employment opportunity laws and regulations is a requirement for all health
care administrators. Although this chapter will introduce you to important
federal laws, it is also important that health care administrators understand respective state and local laws that may govern equal employment
opportunity.

FEDERAL EQUAL EMPLOYMENT OPPORTUNITY LAWS

This section explains the federal laws governing equal employment opportunity. It is recommended, however, that you check with your state and
local governments' fair employment practice agencies for additional laws and
regulations that may have an impact on the equal employment opportunity
practices of your agency.

Civil Rights Acts of 1866 and 1871

The Civil Rights Act of 1866, based on the Thirteenth Amendment to
the U.S. Constitution, prohibits racial discrimination in the making and
enforcement of contracts, which includes hiring and promotion decisions.
Private employers, unions, and employment agencies fall under its coverage.

The Civil Rights Act of 1871 covers state and local governments.
Based on the Fourteenth Amendment, it prohibits the deprivation of equal
employment rights under state laws. It does not apply to private businesses
or federal agencies unless there is state involvement in the employment
practices in question.

Title VII of the Civil Rights Act of 1964

The Civil Rights Act of 1964, signed by President Lyndon B. Johnson,
covers all employers with fifteen or more employees except private clubs,
religious organizations, and places of employment connected to an Indian
reservation.

Title VII of the Civil Rights Act of 1964 deals specifically with discrimination in employment: it prohibits discrimination based on race, color,

religion, sex, or national origin. The passage of this law was not without controversy. Many politicians (mostly in the South) thought that a federal law forbidding discrimination would usurp states' rights. Congressman Howard Smith of Virginia tried to defeat the bill by including sex as one of the protected classifications. He hoped that the insertion of sex would render the bill foolish and lead to its defeat. The act passed with the inclusion of sex, and today litigation concerning sex discrimination is common.

The Civil Rights Act of 1964 created the U.S. **Equal Employment Opportunity Commission (EEOC)** to investigate complaints and try to resolve disputes through conciliation. The act was amended in 1972 by the Equal Employment Opportunity Act, which extended its coverage to state and local governments and to educational institutions. The EEOC was granted enforcement powers to bring action against organizations in the courts if necessary to force compliance with Title VII.

The EEOC requires that most organizations submit annual equal employment opportunity forms identifying the demographic breakdown of their employees. Data from these forms are used to identify possible patterns of discrimination in particular organizations or segments of the workforce. The EEOC may then take legal action against an organization on the basis of these data.

Title VII does not prohibit discrimination based on seniority systems, veterans' preference rights, national security considerations, or job qualifications based on test scores, background, or experience, even when the use of such practices may correlate with discrimination based on race, sex, color, religion, or national origin. Section 703(e)(1) of Title VII permits an employer to discriminate on the basis of religion, sex, or national origin in instances in which religion, sex, or national origin is a **bona fide occupational qualification (BFOQ)** reasonably necessary to the normal operation of that particular business or enterprise. For example, a BFOQ that excludes one group (for example, males or females) from an employment opportunity is permissible if the employer can argue that the essence of the business requires the exclusion—that is, when business would be significantly affected by not employing members of one group exclusively. One case that dealt with this issue was *United Automobile Workers v. Johnson Controls* (1991). Johnson Controls is a car battery manufacturer that excluded fertile women from jobs in which there was high exposure to lead. Fertile men were not automatically excluded and were given a choice as to whether they wanted to risk their reproductive health. The company argued that this policy fell within the BFOQ exception to Title VII. In its 1991 decision the U.S. Supreme Court disagreed. The court found that the policy was discriminatory because only women employees were affected by the policy:

> Respondent's fetal protection policy explicitly discriminates against women on the basis of their sex. The policy excludes women with childbearing capacity from lead-exposed jobs and so creates a facial classification based on gender.... Despite evidence in the record about the debilitating effect of lead exposure on the male reproductive system, Johnson Controls is concerned only with the harms that may befall the unborn offspring of its female employees.

The court stated that women as capable of doing their jobs as their male counterparts may not be forced to choose between having a child and having a job.

In general, the position of the courts in regard to BFOQs clearly favors judgments about the performance, abilities, or potential of specific individuals rather than discrimination by class or categories. The Supreme Court has said that the BFOQ exception to Title VII is a narrow one, limited to policies that are directly related to a worker's ability to do the job. The burden of proof is on the employer to justify any BFOQ claim.

For most public sector jobs, it is very difficult to substantiate the necessity of gender, race, religion, national origin, age, or disability as a BFOQ. Nevertheless, there are some instances in which a BFOQ case can be made. In *Dothard v. Rawlinson* (1977), the state of Alabama was permitted to exclude females from being guards in an all-male maximum-security prison in which 20 percent of the prisoners were sex offenders. In 1996 the U.S. Court of Appeals at Philadelphia ruled in *Healey v. Southwood Psychiatric Hospital* (1996) that gender can be considered a BFOQ for the purposes of staffing a psychiatric hospital unit that treats emotionally disturbed and sexually abused children. A female child care worker was assigned to work the night shift because the hospital needed a balance of men and women to provide therapeutic care to female and male patients who might want to talk with a staff member of their own sex. The court held that Title VII excuses discrimination that is justified as a BFOQ when it is reasonably necessary to the normal operation of business. The essence of the hospital's business requires consideration of gender in staffing decisions because if there are not members of both sexes on a shift, the hospital's ability to provide care to its patients is impeded.

The question of whether race, religion, national origin, color, or sex constitutes a BFOQ arises often in the nonprofit sector. Is gender a legitimate BFOQ for an executive director position at a rape and sexual abuse center? Can a qualified male perform the administrative and leadership tasks, or does the executive director need to be a female? Would race be a BFOQ for a leadership position in a community-based nonprofit that provides services to racial minorities? If a BFOQ is challenged, the burden is on the employer to justify any claim.

Laws That Address Religious Discrimination

Under Section 701(j) of Title VII, employers are obligated to accommodate their employees' or prospective employees' religious practices. Failure to make accommodation is unlawful unless an employer can demonstrate that it cannot reasonably accommodate the employee because of undue hardship in the conduct of its business. In *Trans World Airlines, Inc. v. Hardison* (1977), the Supreme Court ruled that the employer and union need not violate a seniority provision of a valid collective bargaining agreement, the employer has no obligation to impose undesirable shifts on nonreligious employees, and the employer has no obligation to call in substitute workers if such an accommodation would require more than de minimis cost.

Nonprofit organizations that provide secular services but are affiliated with and governed by religious institutions are exempt from the law under Section 702 of the Civil Rights Act of 1964, which states:

> This title shall not apply to an employer with respect to the employment of aliens outside any State, or to a religious corporation, association, educational institution, or society with respect to the employment of individuals of a particular religion to perform work connected with the carrying on by such corporation, association, educational institution, or society of its activities.

Educational institutions, such as universities, schools, or other places of learning, are also exempt from the law. Section 703(e)(2) of the Civil Rights Act of 1964 states:

> It shall not be an unlawful employment practice for a school, college, university, or other educational institution or institution of learning to hire and employ employees of a particular religion if such school, college, university, or other educational institution or institution of learning is, in whole or in substantial part, owned, supported, controlled, or managed by a particular religion or by a particular religious corporation, association, or society, or if the curriculum of such school, college, university, or other educational institution of learning is directed toward the propagation of a particular religion.

In *Corporation of the Bishop of the Church of Jesus Christ of Latter Day Saints v. Amos* (1987), the Supreme Court upheld the right of the Mormon Church to terminate a building engineer who had worked at its nonprofit gymnasium for sixteen years because he failed to maintain his qualification for church membership. The court claimed that the decision to terminate by the religious organization was based on religion and thus exempted from the Title VII prohibition against religious discrimination. The Section 703(e)(2) exemption is broad and is not limited to the religious activities of the institution.

Another change with an impact on how one manages religious diversity was the introduction of faith-based initiatives. President George W. Bush signed Executive Orders 13198 and 13199 in January 2001 and Executive Orders 13279 and 13280 in December 2002 requiring executive branch agencies to identify and remove internal bureaucratic barriers that have impeded greater participation in federal programs by faith-based organizations. The executive orders permit religious or faith-based organizations to receive federal funds for use in providing social services. Under the executive orders, these organizations have a right to use religious criteria in the selection, termination, and disciplining of employees. Providers of faith-based services are permitted to require applicants to be members of a particular denomination in hiring personnel, although they are still prohibited from discriminating on the basis of race, gender, disability, or national origin.

Pregnancy Discrimination Act of 1978

The Pregnancy Discrimination Act of 1978 prohibits employment practices that discriminate on the basis of pregnancy, childbirth, or related medical conditions. A woman is protected from being fired or refused a job or promotion because she is pregnant. She also cannot be forced to take a leave of absence as long as she is able to work.

Employers are obligated under the law to treat pregnancy like any other disability. For example, if other employees on disability leave are entitled to return to their job when they are able to work again, so should women who have been unable to work due to pregnancy.

The Pregnancy Discrimination Act requires that employers provide full benefits coverage for pregnancy. A woman unable to work for pregnancy-related reasons is entitled to disability benefits or sick leave on the same basis as other employees unable to work for other medical reasons.

States may pass their own laws requiring additional benefits for pregnant employees beyond the scope of the federal law. The Supreme Court upheld a California law that required employers to provide up to four months' unpaid pregnancy disability leave with guaranteed reinstatement, even though disabled males were not entitled to the same benefit (*California Federal Savings & Loan Association v. Guerra*, 1987).

Age Discrimination in Employment Act of 1967

The Age Discrimination in Employment Act (ADEA) was enacted by Congress in 1967 to prohibit discrimination in employment because of age in matters pertaining to selection, job retention, compensation, and other terms and conditions of employment. Congress intended to promote the employment of older persons based on their ability rather than age and to prohibit arbitrary age discrimination in employment. In 1974 the ADEA was amended to extend coverage to state and local government employees, as well as most federal employees.

The ADEA at that time protected workers between the ages of forty and sixty-five. Employers were granted four exemptions to the act: (1) where age is a BFOQ reasonably necessary to the normal operation of a particular business; (2) where differentiation is based on reasonable factors other than age; (3) to observe the terms of a bona fide seniority system or a bona fide insurance plan, with the qualification that no seniority system or benefits plan may require or permit the involuntary retirement of someone who is covered by the ADEA; and (4) where an employee is discharged or disciplined for good cause.

The ADEA was amended in 1978 by raising the upper limit to seventy years of age; that limit was removed in 1987, meaning that compulsory retirement for most jobs is now illegal. The ADEA applies to employers with twenty or more employees; unions of twenty-five or more members; employment agencies; and federal, state, and local governments.

On April 1, 1996, the Supreme Court ruled in *O'Connor v. Consolidated Coin Caters Corporation* (1996) that an individual claiming age discrimination must show a logical connection between his or her age and his or her discharge, but there is no requirement to show that the replacement was under forty years old. Justice Antonin Scalia wrote that "the fact that one person in the protected class lost out to another person in the protected class is thus irrelevant, so long as he has lost out because of age."

In 2000 the Supreme Court ruled in *Kimmel v. Florida Board of Regents* that the Eleventh Amendment to the U.S. Constitution bars state employees from suing a state employer in federal court for violation of the ADEA. This ruling does not apply to local government employees or employees working for nonprofit agencies.

The U.S. Supreme Court decision *Smith v. City of Jackson* (2005) held that evidence of an employment practice that is neutral on its face but has a disparate impact on older workers could be used in establishing a prima facie case of age discrimination. Defense against an ADEA claim involves showing that factors other than age were determining considerations.

On June 19, 2008, the U.S. Supreme Court ruled in *Meacham v. Knolls Atomic Power Laboratory* that the employer has the burden of proof in demonstrating that a layoff or other action that adversely affected older workers more than others was from "reasonable factors other than age."

Americans with Disabilities Act of 1990 and the ADA Amendments Act of 2008

In 1990 Congress passed the Americans with Disabilities Act (ADA). Title I of the ADA provides that qualified individuals with disabilities may not be discriminated against on the basis of disability in all aspects of the employment relationship, from the application stage through retirement.

The law took effect on July 26, 1992, for organizations of twenty-five or more employees and on July 26, 1994, for organizations with fifteen to twenty-four employees.

Employment practices covered by the ADA include job application procedures, hiring, firing, advancement, compensation, training, and other terms and conditions and privileges of employment. The ADA Amendments Act (ADAAA) of 2008 was signed by President George W. Bush on September 25, 2008, and became effective on January 1, 2009. It was the first major revision to the Americans with Disabilities Act. The new law overturned several court decisions and parts of EEOC regulations that limited the act's coverage. The Equal Employment Opportunity Commission issued final regulations and interpretive guidelines for the ADAAA on March 24, 2011. The ADAAA specifically states that all of its changes also apply to Section 501 of the Rehabilitation Act (federal employment); Section 503 of the Rehabilitation Act (federal contractors); and Section 504 of the Rehabilitation Act (recipients of federal financial assistance and services and programs of federal agencies). The Equal Employment Opportunity Commission has published a fact sheet on its final regulations for implementing the ADAAA, as well as questions and answers on the final rules for implementing the ADA Amendments Act of 2008 (www1.eeoc.gov).

The new legislation redefines "disability" so that more individuals receive protection under the law. The ADA recognized the following categories of disabilities:

- *Having a physical or mental impairment that substantially limits one or more major life activities.* Examples of physical or mental impairments that might be considered disabilities are speech impediments, learning disabilities, AIDS, mental retardation, chronic mental illness, and epilepsy. Under the ADAAA, the list of major life activities for courts to consider has been expanded to include caring for oneself; performing manual tasks; seeing or hearing; eating, sleeping, walking, and standing; lifting and bending; speaking and breathing; learning, reading, concentrating, and thinking; and working. Major life activities could also include functions of the immune system; normal cell growth; and digestive bowel, bladder, neurological, brain, respiratory, circulatory, endocrine, and reproductive functions.

- *Having a record of such an impairment.* This could include people who have recovered from a heart attack, cancer, back injuries, or mental illness.

- *Being regarded as having an impairment.* This would include individuals who are perceived as having a disability, such as individuals suspected of having HIV.

Under the ADAAA, the phrase "substantially limits" is to be viewed broadly; and an impairment that is episodic or in remission must be considered a disability as long as that impairment in its active state would be substantially limiting.

The ADAAA clarifies that the determination of whether an individual has a disability is to be made without taking into account the ameliorative effects of any mitigating measures, such as medication, medical supplies, equipment, or appliances. It prohibits courts from considering such mitigating measures as medication, prosthetics, and assistive technology in determining whether an individual is disabled. Prescription eyeglasses and contact lenses are excluded, and may be considered when assessing whether an individual is substantially limited in a major life activity.

To be considered qualified under the ADA, an individual must be able to perform the "essential functions of the position," meaning that the individual must satisfy the prerequisites for the position and be able to perform the essential functions of the job with or without reasonable accommodation.

Employers must provide the disabled individual with "reasonable accommodation" that does not place an undue hardship on the organization. "Undue hardship" is defined as an adjustment related to an employer's operation, financial resources, and facilities that requires significant difficulty or expense. Undue hardship and reasonable accommodation are to be determined on a case-by-case basis, taking into account such matters as the size of the employer, the number of employees responsible for a particular job or specific tasks, and the employer's ability to afford the accommodation.

Accommodations may include interventions, such as reassignment; part-time work; and flexible schedules, as well as modifications in equipment and the work environment, such as acquiring a special telephone headset or larger computer screen or moving a training workshop to a location accessible to wheelchairs.

In 2001 the U.S. Supreme Court, using similar reasoning to that in *Kimmel* (2000), ruled that the Eleventh Amendment to the U.S. Constitution bars state employees from suing their state employer for alleged violations of the ADA (*Board of Trustees of the University of Alabama v. Garrett*, 2001). This case, like the *Kimmel* decision, limits state employer liability and also limits congressional authority to implement antidiscrimination regulations in state government.

Immigration Reform and Control Act of 1986

Under the Immigration Reform and Control Act (IRCA), it is illegal for employers to discriminate with respect to hiring, firing, or recruitment or referral for a fee based on an individual's citizenship or immigration status, unless required to do so by law, regulation, or government contract. It also prohibits employers from preferring to hire temporary visa holders or undocumented workers over qualified U.S. citizens or other protected individuals, such as refugees or individuals granted asylum.

The IRCA requires employers to verify the identity and employment eligibility of all employees by completing the Employment Verification (I-9) Form and reviewing documents showing the employee's identity and employment authorization. Because of potential claims of illegal discrimination, employment eligibility verification should be conducted after an offer to hire has been made. The U.S. Equal Employment Opportunity Commission recommends that applicants be informed of the requirements in the preemployment setting by adding the following statement on the employment application: "In compliance with federal law, all persons hired will be required to verify identity and eligibility to work in the United States and to complete the required employment verification document form upon hire" (www.eeoc.gov/laws/practices/inquiries_citizenship.cfm).

Civil Rights Act of 1991

The Civil Rights Act (CRA) of 1991 was passed by Congress on November 7, 1991, and signed into law by President George H. W. Bush on November 21, 1991. The CRA provides additional remedies to protect against and deter unlawful discrimination and harassment in employment and to restore the strength of federal antidiscrimination laws that many felt had been weakened by several Supreme Court decisions.

The CRA amends five civil rights statutes: Title VII of the Civil Rights Act of 1964, the Americans with Disabilities Act of 1990, the Age Discrimination Act of 1967, the Civil Rights Act of 1866, and the Civil Rights Attorney's Fee Awards Act of 1976. In addition, three new laws were created: Section 1981A of Title 42 of the U.S. Code, the Glass Ceiling Act of 1991, and the Government Employee Rights Act of 1991. Compensatory and punitive damages were made available to the victims of discrimination committed by private employers. Public employees are now entitled to only compensatory damages. There is a cap on damages permitted under the law that is determined by the number of workers employed by an organization.

The CRA extended the application of Title VII and the ADA to U.S. citizens working abroad for U.S.-based employers. It extended the application of Title VII, the ADA, and the ADEA to previously unprotected Senate employees, allowing them to redress employment discrimination claims through internal procedures and a limited right of appeal in federal court.

Family and Medical Leave Act of 1993

The Family and Medical Leave Act (FMLA) was signed by President Bill Clinton shortly after his inauguration in January 1993 and took effect on August 5 of that year. The FMLA applies to all public agencies, including state, local, and federal employers; educational institutions; business entities engaged in commerce or in an industry affecting commerce; and private sector employers who employ fifty or more employees in twenty or more workweeks in the current or preceding calendar year, including joint employers and successors of covered employers.

Family and medical leave is available as the result of the birth or adoption of a child or the placement of a child in foster care; to care for a spouse, child, or parent with a serious health condition; or to accommodate the disabling illness of the employee. To be eligible for the leave, an employee must have worked for at least twelve months and for at least 1,250 hours during the year preceding the start of the leave.

The law requires employers to maintain coverage under any group health plan under the condition that coverage would have been provided if no leave were taken. When the leave ends, employees are entitled to return to the same job they held before going on leave or to an equivalent position. An equivalent position is defined as a position having the same pay, benefits, and working conditions and involving the same or substantially similar duties and responsibilities. Employees must be restored to the same or a geographically proximate worksite.

Not all employees are eligible for leave under the FMLA. An employee who qualifies as a key employee may be denied restoration to employment. A key employee is salaried and is among the highest-paid 10 percent of the employees at the worksite. An employee must be notified by the employer of his or her status as a key employee if there is any possibility that the employer may deny reinstatement. Employees are required to give thirty days' advance notice of the need to take family and medical leave when it is foreseeable for the birth of a child or the placement of a child for adoption or in foster care, or for planned medical treatment. When it is not possible to provide such notice, an employee must give notice within one or two business days of when he or she learns of the need for leave.

Employers can require a medical certification from a health care provider to support leave requests.

The FMLA does not supersede any state or local law that provides greater family or medical leave rights. Employers covered by both federal and state laws must comply with both. In *Nevada Department of Human Resources v. Hibbs* (2003), the Supreme Court upheld the right of state employees to sue their employer (the state government) in federal court for alleged violations of the FMLA.

On January 28, 2008, President George W. Bush signed into law the National Defense Authorization Act (NDAA) of 2008, which expands the FMLA for military families. An employee may take up to twelve weeks of unpaid FMLA leave for any qualifying exigency related to a spouse, son, daughter, or parent's active duty or notification of an impending call or order to active duty in the U.S. armed forces in support of a contingency operation. Also, an employee who is the spouse, son, daughter, parent, or next of kin of a covered servicemember is entitled to twenty-six workweeks of leave during a twelve-month period to care for the servicemember. The leave is available during a single twelve-month period. Other changes relate to how employees notify employers about FMLA leave and how employers certify the leave.

The Family and Medical Leave Act National Defense Authorization Act for FY 2010 Amendments were signed into law on October 28, 2009, by

President Barack Obama. These amendments expand the military family leave provisions added to the FMLA in 2008. The 2010 NDAA amendments to the FMLA provide that an eligible employee may take FMLA leave for any qualifying exigency arising out of the fact that the employee's spouse, son, daughter, or parent is on (or has been notified of an impending call to) "covered active duty" in the armed forces. The 2010 NDAA also expands the military caregiver leave provisions of the FMLA. Military caregiver leave entitles an eligible employee who is the spouse, son, daughter, parent, or next of kin of a "covered servicemember" to take up to twenty-six workweeks of FMLA leave in a single twelve-month period to care for a covered servicemember with a "serious injury or illness."

Under the 2010 NDAA amendments, the definition of "covered servicemember" is expanded to include a veteran "who is undergoing medical treatment, recuperation, or therapy for a serious injury or illness" if the veteran was a member of the armed forces "at any time during the period of 5 years preceding the date on which the veteran undergoes that medical treatment, recuperation, or therapy" (www.dol.gov/whd/fmla/2010ndaa.htm). In addition, the 2010 NDAA amends the FMLA's definition of a "serious injury or illness."

On June 22, 2010, the U.S. Department of Labor issued an "Administrator's Interpretation Letter" expanding the protections of the FMLA to require employers who are subject to the FMLA to provide gay and lesbian employees unpaid time off to care for a newborn or nonadoptive, nonbiological child with a serious health condition. Additional information concerning the FMLA is available at www.dol.gov/whd/fmla.

PROVING EMPLOYMENT DISCRIMINATION

Cases of alleged discrimination in violation of federal or state statutes can be made under one of two theories: disparate treatment and disparate impact.

Disparate Treatment

Disparate treatment occurs when an employer treats an employee of a protected class differently from a nonprotected-class employee in a similar situation. For example, deliberately using different criteria for selection depending on the candidate's sex or race would constitute disparate treatment, as when an employer asks female applicants but not male applicants questions about their marital status or child care arrangements, or when an employer requires African American applicants to take preemployment tests that other applicants applying for the same position are not required to take.

The following test, set forth in *McDonnell Douglas v. Green* (1973), permits plaintiffs to establish that an employer treats one or more members of a protected group differently from members of another group:

1. The applicant or employee is a member of a class protected by the statute alleged to be violated (sex, race, religion, color, national origin).

2. The applicant or employee applied for the vacancy and is qualified to perform the job.

3. Although qualified, the applicant or employee was rejected.

4. After rejection, the vacancy remained, and the employer continued to seek applications from persons of equal qualification.

The Supreme Court established that in disparate treatment cases, the burden is on the plaintiff to prove that the employer intended to discriminate because of race, sex, color, religion, or national origin. In *St. Mary's Honor Center v. Hicks* (1993), the court ruled that in addition to showing that all of the employer's legal reasons providing a job-related justification are false, an employee must prove that the employer was motivated by bias and show direct evidence of discrimination.

Disparate Impact

Disparate impact occurs when an employer's policy or practice, neutral on its face and in its application, has a negative effect on the employment opportunities of protected-class individuals. "Neutral" means that the employer requires all applicants or employees to take the same examination or possess the same qualifications for the positions. Unlike the examples provided under disparate treatment, in which the employer deliberately treated males and females or black and white applicants and employees differently, with disparate impact all applicants and employees are treated the same, but protected-class members are not hired or promoted. Such impact is illegal if the employment practice is not job related or is unrelated to the employment opportunity in question. For example, if an agency hired fifty whites and no Hispanics from one hundred white and one hundred Hispanic applicants, disparate impact has occurred. Whether the employer had good intentions or did not mean to discriminate is irrelevant to the courts in this type of lawsuit. After the plaintiff shows evidence of disparate impact, the employer must carry the burden of producing evidence of business necessity or job relatedness for the employment practice. Finally, the burden shifts back to the plaintiff, who must show that an alternative procedure is available that is equal to or better than the employer's practice and has a less discriminatory effect.

The Uniform Guidelines on Employee Selection Procedures were jointly adopted in 1978 by the EEOC, the U.S. Civil Service Commission, the Department of Labor, and the Department of Justice. Although they are not administrative regulations, they are granted deference by the courts. Their purpose is to provide a framework for determining the proper use of tests and other selection procedures. They are applicable to all employers: federal, state, local, nonprofit, and private.

The Uniform Guidelines and many courts have adopted the four-fifths rule as a yardstick for determining disparate impact: a selection rate, determined by the number of applicants selected divided by the number who applied, for a protected group should not be less than four-fifths, or 80 percent, of the rate for the group with the highest selection rate.

Disparate impact theory has been used in many cases involving neutral employment practices, such as tests, entrance requirements, and physical requirements. In 1988 the Supreme Court extended the use of the disparate impact theory in cases involving subjective employment practices, such as interviews, performance appraisals, and job recommendations (*Watson v. Fort Worth Bank and Trust*, 1988). Statistical data based on the four-fifths rule can be used in a disparate impact case to establish prima facie evidence of discrimination when decisions are based on subjective employment practices.

AFFIRMATIVE ACTION: EXECUTIVE ORDERS AND OTHER FEDERAL LAWS

This section explains **affirmative action** and the requirements imposed on employers through Executive Orders 11246 and 11375, the Rehabilitation Act of 1973, and the Vietnam Veterans Readjustment Act of 1974.

Affirmative action is the set of public policies and initiatives designed to help eliminate past and present discrimination based on race, religion, color, sex, national origin, disability, or military status.

Executive Orders 11246 and 11375

In 1965 President Johnson signed **Executive Order 11246,** which prohibited discrimination in federal employment or by federal contractors on the basis of race, creed, color, or national origin. In 1967 it was amended by **Executive Order 11375** to change the word *creed* to *religion* and to add sex discrimination to the other prohibited items. The executive order applies to all federal agencies, contractors, and subcontractors, including all the facilities of the agency holding the contract. Contractors and subcontractors with more than $50,000 in government business and fifty or more employees not only are prohibited from discriminating but also must take affirmative action to ensure that applicants and employees are not treated differently as a function of their sex, religion, race, color, or national origin. The order authorizes the cancellation of federal contracts for failure to meet the order's guidelines. It requires a contractor to post notices of equal employment opportunity and to document its compliance to the Department of Labor.

Executive Order 11246 is enforced by the Department of Labor through the Office of Federal Contract Compliance Programs (OFCCP), a branch of the Department of Labor's Employment Standards Administration. It promulgates guidelines and conducts audits of federal contractors to ensure compliance with the executive orders. The OFCCP is charged with processing complaints as well as compliance review. It can visit an employer's worksite in response to a complaint and can review the employer's affirmative action plans for compliance with the law. Minority availability is measured by the portion of qualified applicants (actual or potential) who are minorities. The OFCCP defines "underutilization" as having fewer minorities or women in a particular job group than would reasonably be expected by their availability. When a job group is identified as underutilized, the contractor must set goals to correct the underutilization. The goals for each underutilized group, together with the utilization analysis, become part of the written affirmative action plan. A federal contractor must monitor information about the status of employees when creating and using an affirmative action plan. The employer must demonstrate that its employment practices comply with Executive Order 11246 and the OFCCP's guidelines by documenting employment decisions on hiring, termination, promotion, demotion, and transfer.

If noncompliance is found, the OFCCP generally first tries to reach a conciliation agreement with the employer. Special hiring or recruitment programs, seniority credit, or back pay may be some of the provisions included in the agreement. If an agreement cannot be reached, the employer is scheduled for a hearing with a judge. If an agreement is still not reached during this time, an employer may lose its government contract or have its payments withheld. It may also lose the right to bid on future government contracts or be debarred from all subsequent contract work.

Whereas equal employment opportunity is a legal duty, affirmative action can be voluntary or involuntary. Although Executive Order 11246 applies only to organizations receiving federal funds, many public and nonprofit organizations have decided to implement voluntary affirmative action programs to redress previous discriminatory employment practices or make their workforce more representative. Involuntary affirmative action is permitted under the Civil Rights Act of 1964, Section 706(g), which states that if a court finds that an employer has intentionally engaged in an unlawful employment practice, it may order appropriate affirmative action. Affirmative action is not mandatory unless the employer has adopted the plan as a remedy for past discrimination or must comply with an executive order affirmative action as a condition of doing business with the government. Employers who are not the recipients of government contracts may be forced to develop affirmative action plans if an investigation by a state or federal compliance agency finds that an employer's personnel practices discriminate against protected-class members.

There are three types of involuntarily affirmative action plans, presented here in order from least restrictive to most restrictive:

- *Conciliation agreement.* After an investigation by a compliance agency, the employer may acknowledge that there is merit to the allegation of discriminatory employment practices and agree to change its practices to comply with the recommendations of the compliance agency.

- *Consent decree.* A consent decree is an agreement between an employer and a compliance agency negotiated with the approval of a court and is subject to court enforcement.

- *Court order.* Court orders result if a compliance agency must take an employer to court because neither a conciliation agreement nor a consent decree can be agreed on. If the court finds the employer guilty of discrimination, the judge may impose court-ordered remedies. These can include hiring or promotion quotas, changes in personnel practices, and financial compensation for the victims of discrimination.

Rehabilitation Act of 1973

The Rehabilitation Act of 1973 prohibits discrimination on the basis of physical or mental disability. A disabled person is defined as one who has an impairment that affects a major life activity, has a history of such an impairment, or is considered as having one. Major life activities refer to such functions as seeing, speaking, walking, and caring for oneself. Disabled individuals also include those with mental disabilities and may include those with illnesses making them unfit for employment, such as contagious diseases or other conditions (tuberculosis, heart disease, cancer, diabetes, drug dependency, or alcoholism, for example). The Supreme Court ruled in *Arline v. School Board of Nassau County* (1987) that individuals with contagious diseases who are able to perform their jobs are protected by the Rehabilitation Act of 1973. It stated that the assessment of risks cannot be based on "society's accumulated myths and fears about disability and disease." Most states have similar laws protecting disabled workers from discrimination.

Section 501 of the Rehabilitation Act requires the federal government, as an employer, to develop and implement affirmative action plans on behalf of disabled employees. Congress enacted this provision with the expectation that the federal government would serve as a model for other employers.

Section 503 requires all federal contractors or subcontractors receiving funds over $2,500 to take affirmative action for the employment of qualified disabled persons. Enforcement is carried out by the Department of Labor's Employment Standards Administration. Under the Rehabilitation Act, as under the ADA of 1990, a disabled person is considered qualified for a job if an individual analysis determines that he or she can, with reasonable accommodation, perform the essential functions of the job. Employers must make such an accommodation unless it can be shown that the accommodation would pose an undue hardship on the firm.

Section 504 prohibits federally funded programs and government agencies from excluding from employment an "otherwise qualified handicapped individual . . . solely by reason of handicap." The enforcement of Section 504 rests with each federal agency providing financial assistance. The U.S. Attorney General is responsible for coordinating the enforcement efforts of the agencies.

In 1993 the U.S. Court of Appeals for the First Circuit ruled that an individual who suffered from morbid obesity was denied a job in violation of Section 504 of the Rehabilitation Act of 1973 (*Cook v. State of Rhode Island, Department of Mental Health, Retardation, and Hospitals*, 1993).

Vietnam Era Veterans' Readjustment Act of 1974

The Vietnam Era Veterans' Readjustment Act of 1974, as amended, applies to employers with government contracts of $25,000 or more. Contractors are required to take affirmative action to employ and advance disabled veterans and qualified veterans of the Vietnam era. Enforcement of the act is done by compliance to the Veterans' Employment Service of the Department of Labor.

Uniformed Services Employment and Reemployment Rights Act of 1994

On October 13, 1994, President Clinton signed the Uniformed Services Employment and Reemployment Rights Act (USERRA). USERRA became effective December 12, 1994. Employees have a right to be reemployed in their civilian job if they leave their employer to be in the uniformed services, assuming certain requirements have been met (www.dol.gov/vets/programs/fact/userra_vets03.htm).

Table 4.1 summarizes the statutory laws discussed throughout this chapter.

CONSTITUTIONAL RIGHTS

Public employees have a broad array of constitutional protections that differentiate public employment from employment in the nonprofit and for-profit sectors. Public sector employees' rights and privileges to work are

Table 4.1   Federal Statutes Related to Equal Employment Opportunity

Statute	Provisions
Civil Rights Act of 1866	Prohibits intentional discrimination based on race and ethnicity.
Civil Rights Act of 1871	Allows individuals to sue state actors in state or federal courts for civil rights violations. This act prohibits public sector employment discrimination based on race, color, religion, sex, or national origin.
Civil Rights Act of 1964, Title VII	Prohibits employers from discrimination against employees in hiring, promotion, and termination decisions based on race, color, religion, sex, or national origin.
Age Discrimination in Employment Act of 1967, as amended	Protects workers forty and over in hiring, promotion, and termination decisions.
Rehabilitation Act of 1973	Makes it unlawful to discriminate against an otherwise qualified individual with a disability because of that disability.
Vietnam Era Veterans' Readjustment Act of 1974, as amended	Requires employers with government contracts of $25,000 or more to take affirmative action to employ and advance disabled veterans and qualified veterans of the Vietnam era.
Pregnancy Discrimination Act of 1978	Prohibits discrimination on the basis of pregnancy, childbirth, or related medical conditions.
Immigration Reform and Control Act of 1986	Makes it illegal for employers to discriminate with respect to hiring, firing, or recruitment or referral for a fee based on an individual's citizenship or immigration status, unless required to do so by law, regulation, or government contract.
Americans with Disabilities Act of 1990, and the **ADA Amendments Act of 2008**	Prohibits employment discrimination against qualified individuals with disabilities.

(Continued)

Table 4.1   *(Continued)*

Statute	Provisions
Civil Rights Act of 1991	Provides the right to trial by jury and emotional distress damages for discrimination claims.
Family and Medical Leave Act of 1993, and the **National Defense Authorization Act of 2008**	Requires employers of fifty or more employees and all public agencies to provide up to twelve weeks of unpaid leave to eligible employees for the birth and care of a child, adoption and placement of a child, or serious illness of the employee or an immediate family member. The National Defense Authorization Act of 2008 expands the Family and Medical Leave Act for military families.
Uniformed Services Employment and Reemployment Rights Act of 1994	Protects the employment rights of National Guard and Reserve members called to active duty.

to some extent protected by a broad umbrella of laws that either prohibit a government activity or create an individual right. Many of the constitutional protections afforded to public sector employees were originally enacted to protect free citizens from arbitrary government action in the areas of privacy, expression, association, contracts, and property. Because public sector employees work for the government, the protections are extended to them by operation of the employment relationship. Many of the rights under the U.S. Constitution are limitations on Congress and the states to exercise certain actions against citizens and employees. However, these constitutional limitations are not self-executing and therefore must be enforced through the Civil Rights Act of 1871, which was enacted by Congress as part of reconstruction legislation after the Civil War. In the public sector employment arena, it is important to note that Section 42 USC 1983 is the enforcement vehicle of the other constitutional rights and allows damages only against persons who act "under the color of law," that is, the government, where the government actor subjects any person to a deprivation of any rights, privileges, or immunities secured by the U.S. Constitution or the laws of the United States. Therefore, where a public sector employer acting "under the color of law" is within the employment relationship or otherwise deprives employees of certain constitutional rights, a cause of action against the employer or other employees may be available to protect the rights afforded. However, the employer may be held liable only when it has a policy, practice, or custom that deprives the employee of the right.

Today it is unlikely that employers have written policies that on their face would be a violation of the Constitution. However, many employment actions arise through incorrect policy implementation or in violation of the Constitution through supervisory personnel who deprive employees of their constitutional rights, giving rise to individual or, in some cases, employer liability. The legal concept of *respondeat superior* ("let the master answer") is generally not available under constitutional claims to hold the employer liable for nonsanctioned official actions of its employees (that is, actions that fall within employees' job responsibilities).

Expressive Rights

The First Amendment to the U.S. Constitution protects public employees against unwarranted employer interference with their freedom of speech, expression, association, and religion. It also protects the right of public employees to join a labor union or advocate the joining of associations, their right to speak out on matters of public concern, their right of access to a public employer's property, and their freedom from religious discrimination.

Prior to 2006 the prevailing legal theory under the First Amendment was that the interests of public employees in regard to free speech were balanced against the interests of the state, as an employer, in promoting the efficiency of the public services it performs through its employees. If a disciplined employee did engage in speech protected by the First Amendment through the balancing of interests, the disciplining could still be upheld if the employer could show that the employee would have been disciplined for other, legitimate reasons (*Connick v. Myers*, 1983; *McPherson v. Rankin*, 1987; *Mount Healthy City School District Board of Education v. Doyle*, 1977; *Pickering v. Board of Education*, 1968).

In 2006 the U.S. Supreme Court, in *Garcetti v. Ceballos,* pronounced a ruling that many feel has reduced the First Amendment protections afforded to public sector employees in speech cases (Hudson, 2008). The *Garcetti* decision created an additional hurdle for public employees by requiring them to show they were speaking as citizens on a matter of public concern and not simply doing their job when they expressed themselves. According to the court, public sector employees who speak as a result of the required duties of their job do so as employees rather than as citizens and will not be afforded First Amendment protections from subsequent disciplinary action by their employer as a direct result of the speech (Garry, 2007).

Ceballos was a deputy district attorney in the Los Angeles County District Office who was demoted after filing a deposition memorandum outlining alleged false statements by the police contained in an affidavit used to obtain a search warrant and informing defense counsel of those false statements. After being demoted Ceballos filed a suit alleging that his demotion was a result of his speech protected by the First Amendment. The U.S. Supreme Court held that the First Amendment did not apply because the deputy district attorney spoke as an employee and not as a citizen when he wrote his memorandum (Garry, 2007). The issue presented was not whether the speech was a matter of public concern, but whether it was made by a government employee in implementing his official duties. Ceballos spoke as a public employee and not as a citizen, so the court held that his supervisors had every right to criticize his performance and take disciplinary action.

Freedom of Association

Public employees are generally free to join organizations as long as their membership does not create a conflict of interest with their job or appear to invite impropriety. Public employees also have broad protections against being forced to join organizations. With limited exceptions, such as in executive policymaking positions, decisions to hire, terminate, train, transfer, promote, or discipline employees for partisan political reasons are not permissible. The Supreme Court reasoned that the contributions that patronage makes to the government's interests in loyalty, accountability, and party competition are outweighed by its infringement on public employees' freedom of association and belief (*Branti v. Finkel,* 1980; *Rutan v. Republic Party of Illinois,* 1990). Moreover, public employees cannot be required to join labor unions as dues-paying members, but may be included as bargaining unit members for the purposes of voting and contract application. Generally, dues-paying members are assessed fees to contribute to their fair share of contract negotiations, contract administration, and other privileges afforded under the contract, but bargaining unit members may not be.

Limits on Political Participation

Public employees can be restricted from participating in partisan political activities. The 1939 Political Activities Act, more commonly referred to as the Hatch Act, prohibits federal employees covered by it from taking an active part in political campaigns. The act prohibits federal employees from engaging in political activity while on duty, wearing campaign buttons in the office, and putting campaign bumper stickers on government vehicles. It also bans soliciting and accepting or receiving political contributions, and it prohibits employees from using their official position to influence or interfere with an election. In addition, the Office of Special Counsel (OSC), an independent agency that investigates and prosecutes allegations of improper political activities by government employees, has rendered opinions that limit persons from running for a partisan office where the individual is directly or indirectly responsible for funds arising from federal grants. In those cases, the individual may need to resign from public employment to run for a local office. Violators can be prosecuted under federal law and even lose their jobs.

An interesting issue has arisen as a result of the Internet. Today political messages, campaign solicitations, and cartoons come to an individual's e-mail inbox. The OSC notes that receiving an e-mail may not be under an individual's control; however, public employees should not forward an e-mail that urges a vote for a specific candidate or seeks to raise campaign money. Blogging about politics from work is not permissible, and blogging from home may also get a federal employee in trouble (Barr, 2008).

The political activities of most state and local government employees are also restricted by state or local governments' "little Hatch Acts." What is permitted and what is proscribed vary by state. Many of the state laws are less restrictive than the federal Hatch Act and permit state and local employees to engage in more political activity then federal counterparts are allowed. It is important for public employees to review current federal and state laws, along with local ordinances, resolutions, and regulations, to determine permitted political activity.

Privacy Rights

The Fourth Amendment to the U.S. Constitution bars unreasonable searches and seizures and essentially provides zones of privacy. However, not every intrusion on a privacy interest is a search, and employers can and do limit the zones of privacy in the workplace.

Public employees do not lose their Fourth Amendment rights against unreasonable searches or seizures because they work for the government instead of a private employer (*National Treasury Employees Union v. Von Raab,* 1989). Where employees have a "reasonable expectation of privacy" under employment circumstances, the Fourth Amendment provides protection, unless a search warrant is issued by a detached magistrate based on probable cause.

Due Process Rights

This area of the law is in constant development as societal values and ideologies ebb and flow. There are two concepts of recognized due process: procedural and substantive. Procedural due process is a concept adopting fundamental fairness as the rule of law to effect decisions that affect individual rights. Due process in this context is not necessarily a tangible right; rather, it relates to the preprocesses afforded to individuals before tangible rights are affected by government. Procedural due process essentially requires the government to provide reasonable notice and an opportunity to be heard within a fair forum under just conditions before a person's rights are negatively affected. Fairness is an objective standard and naturally depends on a multitude of considerations. Procedural due process is a check on arbitrary, capricious, or discriminatory decisions by government officials in individual cases. When invoked in the public employment context, it protects public employees from arbitrary discharge. If nothing else, procedural due process creates the opportunity for individuals to protect their rights and interests through the discovery of arbitrary or capricious government action. In order to comport with procedural due process, a public sector employer must give the affected employee notice, a meaningful opportunity for the employee to respond to charges and to present evidence, and access to an impartial decision maker.

Not all substantive due process rights are codified in the Constitution. The Fifth and Fourteenth Amendments' substantive due process provisions allow the courts to recognize tangible interests dependent on the concept of liberty. The Fifth Amendment applies to federal government action, and the Fourteenth Amendment applies to actions of the respective states. In limited circumstances, these amendments provide substantive due process rights to protect individuals against the deprivation of life, liberty, or property without the procedural due process of law. The concepts of life, liberty, and property are ever evolving, and therefore substantive due process rights are recognized on a case-by-case basis. In addition, at minimum, these amendments to the Constitution require a rational basis supporting government action. In the context of equal protection of rights not affecting a protected class of individuals, the government is not required to treat everyone the same, but it must treat similarly situated groups in a like manner unless it can establish a legitimate reason that is rationally related to the employment decision. Where a protected class of individuals is at issue—for example, members of a particular gender or race—the judicial scrutiny increases and therefore affords that class greater protection .

ADDITIONAL PROTECTIONS FOR EMPLOYEES

Constitutional employment rights are only provided to public employees. However, health care employees working for private for-profit or non-profit organizations may be protected by whistle-blower protection laws or employment- at-will statutes.

Whistle-Blower Protection

A whistle-blower is an employee, former employee, or contractor of an agency who reports agency misconduct. Generally the misconduct is a violation of a law, rule, or regulation or is a direct threat to the public interest, such as fraud, health and safety violations, or corruption. Whistle-blower laws and policies are designed to protect from retaliation employees who report wrongdoing, illegal conduct, internal fraud, and discrimination (Harshbarger & Crafts, 2007). The federal government and many state and local governments have some sort of statutory or common-law whistle-blower or antiretaliation laws. Many nonprofits have developed their own internal whistle-blower policies, as well. Harshbarger and Crafts note that internal whistle-blower policies can be used to identify problems in the workplace. With whistle-blower protections in place, intervention and prevention methods can strengthen and support a workplace culture of integrity, openness, transparency, and two-way communication. Even without internal policies, nonprofits have been advised to adhere to the whistle-blowing provisions of the Public Accounting Reform and Investor Protection Act of 2002, more commonly known as the Sarbanes-Oxley Act. The act was passed as a reaction to the Enron, Tyco, Adelphia, and WorldCom corporate scandals that cost investors billions of dollars and led to diminished confidence in the securities markets.

Public and nonprofit employers need to be aware of the Whistleblower Protection Act of 1989 and the state and local laws in jurisdictions in which they are located, and they must comply with any internal policies in regard to whistle-blowers. Public, nonprofit, and for-profit employees are typically covered by whistle-blower or antiretaliation laws. State and local governments have recognized with legislation—like the federal whistle-blower laws—a public policy exception to the doctrine of employment at will.

Employment at Will

The doctrine of employment at will provides that an employer may discharge an employee for any reason not prohibited by law, or for no reason. However, there are some exceptions:

- **Public policy exception**. Under the public policy exception, an employer may not fire an employee if it would violate the state's public policy or a state or federal statute.

- **Implied contract exception**. Under the implied contract exception, an employer may not fire an employee when an implied contract is formed between an employer and employee, even though no express, written instrument concerning the employment relationship exists.

    Proving the terms of an implied contract is often difficult, and the burden of proof is on the employee who has been fired. Implied employment contracts are most often found when an employer's personnel policy or handbook indicates that an employee will not be fired except for good cause or specifies a process for firing. If the employer fires the employee in violation of an implied employment contract, the employer may be found liable for breach of contract.

- **Good faith and fair dealing exception.** The exception for good faith and fair dealing represents the most significant departure from the traditional employment-at-will doctrine. Rather than narrowly prohibiting terminations based on public policy or an implied contract, this exception inserts a covenant of good faith and fair dealing into every employment relationship. It has been interpreted by some courts to mean either that an employer's personnel decisions are subject to a "just cause" standard or that terminations made in bad faith or motivated by malice are prohibited.

Employers may not fire employees for refusing to commit illegal acts, and if the employment handbook or agency policy outlines procedures that are necessary before an employee can be terminated, those procedures must be followed. If the employer fires an employee without following established procedures, the employee may have a claim for wrongful termination. Employers in all sectors must be aware of exceptions to the employment-at-will doctrine. These concepts are developed under the rubric of procedural and substantive due process as discussed earlier. In addition, the courts have found that public employees have a liberty interest (quasi–property rights) in their reputation as it relates to public employment. The liberty interest does not necessarily protect the job, but it allows the employee to invoke a liberty-interest hearing after termination. The hearing allows the employee to have the last word within the public personnel file.

SUMMARY

Equal employment opportunity laws have continued to evolve. They create legal responsibilities for employers and affect all aspects of the employment relationship. Recruitment, selection, training, compensation and benefits, promotion, and termination must all be conducted in a nondiscriminatory manner.

Whereas equal employment opportunity is a policy of nondiscrimination, affirmative action requires employers to analyze their workforce and develop plans of action to recruit, select, train, and promote members of protected classes and develop plans of action to correct areas in which past discrimination may have occurred. Affirmative action in the United States is jointly determined by the Constitution, legislative acts, executive orders, and court decisions. The Office of Federal Contract Compliance Programs is responsible for developing and enforcing most affirmative action plans, although the Equal Employment Opportunity Commission enforces affirmative action plans in the federal sector.

The federal government uses affirmative action to promote a more diverse workforce. Recipients of federal funds are required to develop affirmative action plans that encourage the recruitment, selection, training, and promotion of qualified disabled individuals; Vietnam War veterans; and individuals who may have been discriminated against because of their race, sex, color, or national origin. Affirmative action plans can be involuntary or voluntary. Involuntary action plans have increasingly come under intense scrutiny, and affirmative action itself is being challenged.

The focus on equal employment opportunity and affirmative action programs has increased the importance of strategic human resources management (SHRM) and planning. Compliance with equal employment opportunity laws and affirmative action regulations is essential to human resources planning and the effective utilization of all employees. One day affirmative action programs may be eliminated, and many of the paperwork requirements for compliance audits will no longer be necessary. However, organizations will still need to develop and implement progressive human resources management strategies if they wish to successfully manage a diverse workforce.

Employers must be aware of the legal environment under which SHRM is implemented. Employers must be aware of not only the laws governing equal employment opportunity but also other laws protecting employee rights. Public employers must be careful not to violate the constitutional rights of their employees. All health care employers must also be aware of legislation protecting whistle-blowers as well as employment-at-will exceptions.

KEY TERMS

ADA Amendments Act of 2008

affirmative action

Age Discrimination in Employment Act of 1967, as amended

Americans with Disabilities Act of 1990

bona fide occupational qualification (BFOQ)

Civil Rights Act of 1866

Civil Rights Act of 1871

Civil Rights Act of 1964, Title VII

Civil Rights Act of 1991

disparate impact

disparate treatment

Equal Employment Opportunity Commission (EEOC)

Executive Order 11246

Executive Order 11375

Family and Medical Leave Act of 1993

good faith and fair dealing exception

Immigration Reform and Control Act of 1986

implied contract exception

National Defense Authorization Act of 2008

Pregnancy Discrimination Act of 1978

public policy exception

Rehabilitation Act of 1973

Uniformed Services Employment and Reemployment Rights Act of 1994

Vietnam Era Veterans' Readjustment Act of 1974, as amended

DISCUSSION QUESTIONS

1. What types of discrimination in employment are protected against through federal law?

2. Define disparate treatment and disparate impact. How do they differ from each other?

3. What is the purpose of affirmative action? What office enforces Executive Order 11246?

4. Define whistle-blower protection and employment at will.

This chapter was adapted and updated from Pynes, 1997, 2004a, 2009a.

5

Managing the Unique Health Care Workforce

LEARNING OBJECTIVES

- Understand the unique dynamics of the health care workforce
- Calibrate human resources programs according to the specific needs of the health care workforce
- Specify particular dynamics, both external and internal, that have an impact on the health care workforce
- Categorize customer-patient cultural factors relative to the composition and daily actions of the health care workforce
- Apply the general concepts of psychographics to health care human resources management

THE HEALTH CARE workforce is unique in several ways. Figure 5.1 can be used as a working guide in understanding the nuances of the health care workforce.

To begin with, the health care workforce is singular among all industry groups in regard to the number of women a health care organization employs. The majority of the jobs in a health care organization have traditionally been staffed by females, starting with nursing and direct patient care. For

Figure 5.1 Unique Facets of the Health Care Workforce

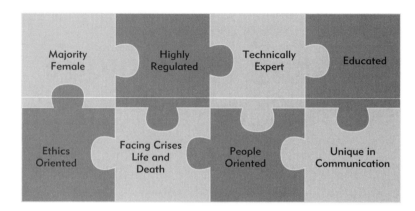

example, the **Visiting Nurse Association (VNA) Health Group** of New Jersey employs nearly 1,700 people, of whom 90 percent are female and 70 percent are involved in direct patient care. In addition, in many modern health care organizations the ancillary and related patient care service areas, such as physical therapy, pharmacy, and social work, have been staffed primarily by females.

The past twenty years have witnessed significant strides in the promotion of women in the executive ranks and leadership cadres of health care organizations. The proverbial "glass ceiling" has not prevented the ascendancy of women in health care leadership as it has in the service industries, manufacturing, and the political realm. For example, the president of the VNA Health Group is a female who had a stellar career in both nursing and leadership prior to becoming the CEO of the second-largest home health care organization in the United States. Furthermore, the executive director of the PG Chambers School, the largest and oldest dedicated special education and special health services school in the state of New Jersey, is also female and leads a professional staff that is 98.8 percent female. There have also been tremendous increases in the number of women in medicine, and several leading schools in that realm now indicate that in the premed and medical school enrollment areas their student base has almost equal numbers of males and females.

Given this dynamic, it is essential that health care personnel understand that such qualities as sensitivity, listening, patience, and selflessness—as well as the ability to extend the all-important human touch, or "tender loving care" (TLC), for patients, staff members, and coworkers—are requisites across the health care workforce. Although one can make a very subjective case that these traits are largely female, there's no question that as the vanguard elements of any effective health care provider they are essential to success in health care human resources analysis, planning, and development.

A second dynamic that is indigenous to the health care workplace, as indicated in Figure 5.1, is the highly regulated nature of the health care workplace and workforce. One can make a cogent argument that no other industry group or professional category is as regulated as health care. A prominent source of regulation and stricture in the health care workplace is **The Joint Commission (TJC),** which provides over six thousand hospitals and affiliated health care organizations with professional accreditation. This organization is both rigorous and vigorous in looking at standards and practices across the delivery of health care, and it has exacting tenets for health care delivery services in general and the health care workforce specifically. From a wider perspective, health care organizations regularly host inspections by organizations that regulate funding and reimbursement for patient care, such as Medicare, Medicaid, state reimbursement governance organizations, and often local authorities. In all cases the entire health care organization must constantly be prepared for inspections and on a daily basis must conduct all aspects of its business both effectively and efficiently relative to a wide array of regulations and strictures.

From a human resources perspective, individuals who work well with rules and regulations; maintain sharp attention to detail; and are not easily flustered by meeting detailed standards—and who are able to function under an administrative supervision style that can be easily misconstrued as "nitpicking" as efforts escalate to meet inspection standards—will probably succeed in the demanding, highly regulated health care business arena.

In many organizations, managers and supervisors are only tasked with the important but basic focuses of supervising their staff, maintaining a budget, widely using operational resources, and setting their department's work plans. As indicated in Figure 5.1, however, all health care personnel, and especially supervisors and managers, must also know a specific technical discipline based on their own expertise. For example, managers in respiratory services must have a strong command of the science of respiratory therapy, likely patient reactions to therapy, the procedure for delivering effective respiratory therapy, and a host of other areas of knowledge that not only will help guide their staff but also, when needed, can act as an expert in addressing specific, technical patient care issues. Health care supervisors must also make sure that their education is current; that they are aware of new breakthroughs in their particular technical area; and that they increase their acumen accordingly to act as educators to their staff, reporting executives, and others. In this respect the health care supervisor acts as the organizational expert in his or her specific field and in many cases as a lead internal consultant in a particular segment of medicine or health care services. In a similar vein, this individual is also a community expert in American health care. For example, at the time of this writing massive new federal legislation on health care has been enacted. On a daily basis health care managers and executives at all levels are being asked by community members, "What is in this health care bill?" "Will my taxes go to go up because of health care?" "Can I still use your hospital?" and a wide assortment of other queries—concerning all of which the average health care manager probably has only general knowledge to provide as a useful answer.

Health care human resources professionals must therefore ensure—for example, in an interview—that applicants for health care supervision and management positions are technically expert, an assessment that should be accomplished in consultation with line managers who are professionals in the subject area. In addition, it is imperative to ascertain in an interview the methods by which a health care manager keeps up-to-date on significant issues in health care in general, and on his or her specific area of expertise and supervision in particular.

For dire lack of a better expression, outstanding health care professionals at every level can be called "learning junkies." Education is a vital job requisite in each and every health care area. For example, one might think at first glance that housekeeping supervisors or environmental services managers do not need to maintain current and relevant knowledge in their particular area; after all, it just involves keeping the place clean, right? Nothing could be further from the truth—the movement to make health care workplaces environmentally and ecologically sound (made up of what are known as "green initiatives") mandates that environmental services managers and housekeeping supervisors be eminently aware of emergent regulations in this important area, in addition to fulfilling their more traditional, time-honored responsibilities. More obviously, individuals in areas of the health care organization that are centered on clinical and medical services require continuous educational development, including both formal off-site education as well as in-service education, as detailed in Chapter Twelve. Formal education that yields degrees, certificates, and continuing education units are also important facets of health care organizational education that are seldom mirrored in intensity or frequency in other industries.

Accordingly, a health care human resources cadre must first ensure that all the job applicants value education and are current on new trends and likely future initiatives in their particular professional area. An applicant's desire to learn on a formal basis, as well as his or her inclination to place a significant practical value on learning something new every day, should also be at the forefront of any interviewing process in a progressive health care organization. On a related note, the health care professional's ability to act as an educator in his or her particular area of expertise, as well as the overall impact dynamic of his or her particular technical area in regard to the overall delivery of health care, are also important features of a new job candidate or promotional candidate.

At the risk of being vainglorious, health care organizations often pride themselves on representing the epitome of ethical action. With the exception of schools, it is difficult to identify other professional organizations, especially in the for-profit arena, that have such a high regard for ethical action in every phase of their product delivery. Naturally, this is a hallmark of American health care, given all of the dynamics of public perception and constituency commitment discussed in Chapter One, and it is important to remember how increasingly aware customer-patients are of health care in every regard and how interested they are in how the organization operates from an ethical perspective. Most aggressive health care organizations not only embrace the values of decency, fortitude, industry, integrity, and knowledge, as detailed in Chapter Three, but also publish a values statement as an integral part of their mission statement.

In addition, many health care organizations have a credo that explains the set of beliefs that are their driving forces. Beyond the values and mission statements of a typical health care organization, the credo statement is a vivid declaration of the exemplars of work behavior that underscores the importance of an ethical orientation in a progressive health care organization at the employee level. Many health care organizations endeavor to practically incorporate their credo statement in daily action, strategic plans, and ongoing initiatives.

Discerning the ethical orientation of job candidates, therefore, becomes vital in the selection process at any progressive health care organization. Furthermore, there should be some ethical criteria established, validated, and communicated as part of the organization's performance evaluation program. This should be an important rating dimension in yearly evaluations, because ethical alignment is as important as the attainment of performance goals and other more quantitative aspects of employee performance.

In most health care organizations, life-or-death situations are part of the daily work flow; with the exception of certain law enforcement agencies, this is truly a unique aspect of health care organizations. Although this is an obvious dimension in direct patient care areas, such as emergency rooms, operating rooms, hospices, and oncology centers, almost all segments of the health care organization work with the dynamics of life and death in one fashion or another. As a result, the pace at which tasks must be accomplished is extraordinarily fast, and can increase proportionally given the dire circumstances of a particular work situation. The pressure on all health care employees to perform their job effectively is also abnormally high in comparison to other professions, given the very nature of life-or-death circumstances.

Health care human resources professionals must determine if a new job applicant who does not have experience in health care will be able to contend on a daily basis with this extraordinary dynamic. If an individual has worked in a health care organization previously, the hiring determination should still be based on open-ended questions about the candidate's ability to read, react to, and respond effectively in a given critical situation. It is important at this juncture to understand that the inability, either suspected or proven, of a candidate to cope successfully with the life-or-death nature of a health care workplace is a disqualifier for employment, and that inaction by an individual who cannot thrive in this unique environment is unacceptable. An inability to cope with this dimension can result in the unwarranted death of or harm to a patient, and, less important, in the organization's fiscal and legal peril.

Health care organizations are people oriented. Consistent people contact occurs from the minute a health care employee arrives at his or her workstation on any given day. Communication can be incoming, as indicated in the Spheres of Influence Model introduced in Chapter One, from a variety of sources ranging from patients to coworkers. Perhaps the prevailing factor in customer-patients' perception of quality health care is the TLC a professional provides during the delivery of health care. Customer-patients' evaluation of their experience, whether positive or negative, is in fact based largely on their interpersonal interactions with health care professionals. In contrast, certainly a consumer at a car dealership expects the exact opposite, when the expectation is centered on getting as good a deal as possible while enduring questionable sales ethics and other nefarious behavior. In a health care setting, the customer-patient will seldom remember the name of the procedure, but in all cases will remember the name of the individuals who were primary in their health care experience.

Clearly, someone who exhibits antisocial tendencies in any regard should not be employed in a health care organization. Less obviously, someone who enjoys talking more than listening and, furthermore, is ineffective in reading, assimilating, and applying significant information, should not be employed in a health care organization. These attributes must surely be evaluated and appraised in both the initial job interview and in performance evaluations conducted regularly by the line manager in concert with the human resources professional.

Relative to communication, health care organizations employ a vernacular that is unique to their industry, as do most types of organizations. However, health care organizations use more acronyms than most organizations to describe everything from the way that a patient might pay his or her bill (PHO, COBRA, HMO, and so on) to the type of equipment that was used in that patient's care (MRI, CHAPS, and so on). Acronyms also extend to certain governing bodies, such as TJC, as well as other governance structures and regulatory laws that are part of the everyday of a health care organization. Another communication nuance is the amount of emotionalism that is intrinsic to a health care environment, which is most apparent in emergencies and in situations that customer-patients perceive to be emergencies or crises (which is how most customer-patients perceive every need).

Accordingly, certain "C Factors" of communication, some mentioned in a different application in Chapter Three, must be present in all communication across the health care organization, and especially in the identification of suitable job candidates, successful promotional candidates, and individuals who should receive outstanding performance evaluations from a human resources perspective:

- *Clarity,* which ensures that the message is delivered quickly and clearly

- *Comprehensiveness,* which provides the complete picture and all essential information effectively

- *Closure,* which frames a significant message as a clear call for action leading to an effective conclusion

- *Compassion,* which demonstrates an appropriate sensitivity and humanity

- *Coordination,* which leads to efficient cooperation in the provision of health care

These five factors not only clearly indicate the unique nature of the health care workplace but also provide significant requisites for human resources action that supports the sacred mission of health care in any setting.

CULTURAL FACTORS RELEVANT TO HEALTH CARE HUMAN RESOURCES

Extrinsic to the progressive health care organization are a series of cultural factors that have an impact on health care human resources on a daily basis. Given the size of most health care organizations, it is logical that culture would play a major role in the formation, conduct, and evaluation of a health care organization, and many subcultures exist within health care organizations that influence their daily actions. Furthermore, the diversity of cultures in a progressive health care organization's service community also makes true the axiom that "cultural awareness is simply good business." From a health care human resources perspective, culture does not just relate to ethnocentric differences or mere demographics, but in fact extends to behavioral dimensions, community belief systems, region-based affiliations, and other factors that are apparent in Figure 5.2. As seen in that diagram and as delineated in this section, a fundamental understanding of culture as it relates to health care human resources is essential to organizational development, organizational growth, and the span of human resources action.

Figure 5.2   Cultural Composition Foundations

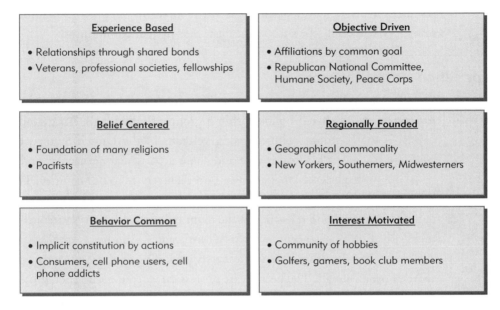

Experience Based

- Relationships through shared bonds
- Veterans, professional societies, fellowships

Objective Driven

- Affiliations by common goal
- Republican National Committee, Humane Society, Peace Corps

Belief Centered

- Foundation of many religions
- Pacifists

Regionally Founded

- Geographical commonality
- New Yorkers, Southerners, Midwesterners

Behavior Common

- Implicit constitution by actions
- Consumers, cell phone users, cell phone addicts

Interest Motivated

- Community of hobbies
- Golfers, gamers, book club members

There are many profound examples of how culture can have an impact on a health care organization in a general sense. For example, the borough of Queens in New York City is quantitatively the most diverse county in the United States based on ethnic origin. In this relatively small area, 168 languages are spoken on a daily basis by an assortment of recently arrived Americans and, in many cases, second-generation Americans who also work in the county, pay taxes at an exorbitant rate, and thus demand premier health care. Accordingly, the plurality of cultures in Queens should be reflected in the stellar health care organizations across the borough, several of which have been in business for over seventy-five years based on a strong medical reputation as well as a true commitment to the community. Understanding the cultural nuances celebrated by specific groups of the service community in Queens that have been there for generations, such as Greek Americans in Astoria, as well as new cultural groups, such as Korean Americans in Flushing, is key to success in progressive health care organizations in regard to both customer-patient relations and community development and marketing as well as internal development, based on the recruitment, retention, and development of employees who either share a similar cultural background with many of the customer-patients or have a firm understanding of and ability to relate to their community's unique culture. In all cases, the human resources management department is at the forefront of efforts to maintain resonance with and relevance to the customer-patient community.

Experience-Based Cultures

Our discussion begins with experience-based cultures, which are based on relationships and shared bonds within a group of individuals. An example of this is the common culture among veterans in the United States who have specific needs for health care and share a particular vernacular and a set of unique experiences that are based on their service to our country. The **Department of Veterans Affairs (VA) Health Care System** strives to maintain both currency and relevance in the manner in which it serves veterans in the nearly 120 medical centers across all fifty states. Another example of an experience-based culture is that of a society providing education to a specific cadre of professionals. The health care profession is replete with such professional societies. For example, the American Nephrology Nurses' Association, which at first glance seems to be a small, highly specialized organization but in reality has nearly four thousand members, provides meaningful education to nurses and patient care professionals in the areas of renal and kidney medicine and is a stellar example of an experience-based culture.

In regard to the first example of an experience-based culture, it is important from a human resources perspective that new employees understand veterans, their unique needs, and their expectations clearly in order to best serve them. What is more, every culture has a subculture—for example, Vietnam-era veterans have different needs than do veterans of World War II. In the former case, medical attention and outpatient services are major demands; in the latter case, services for the aging, which include the Domiciliary Program (which is the VA's particular parlance for a long-term care unit), are a major need. In fact, the National Association of State Veterans Homes is an example of an experience-based culture that serves an experience-based culture in the same manner as the national VA system, as it includes the state veterans homes funded by state taxes in all of the fifty states. It is interesting to note that all of these state veterans homes are separate and distinct from the national VA system, and that each takes pride in creating an organizational and institutional tone that reflects the environmental and regional tone specific to its state, which in turn makes the customer-patient as comfortable and "at home" as possible.

Objective-Driven Cultures

Objective-driven cultures are founded on affiliations dedicated to the achievement of a common goal. For example, members of the Peace Corps, advocates of animal humane societies, and members of many political groups could easily be considered part of an objective-driven culture. The relevance to health care from a general perspective can be easily seen: for example, a group devoted to fundraising for cancer care is an objective-driven culture with a distinct link to health care. An objective-driven culture that would not fit in certain health care organizations might be a group that believes in pro-life legislation or a group that believes in pro-choice tenets. In either case, depending on the services provided by the local health care organization and the belief systems of the local community, this objective-driven culture could have a profound effect—either constructive or harmful—on its local health care organization.

In regard to human resources, identifying membership in objective-driven cultures can be a tricky business (as is often also the case with belief-centered cultures, discussed in the next paragraph). Given equal opportunity employment law, a health care human resources professional cannot ask specifically about personal convictions or about avocations that are not directly related to the workplace. However, the bona fide occupational qualification statute in equal opportunity legislation could come into play in certain cases. For example, if a job applicant discloses that she is a cancer survivor, belongs to a fundraising organization dedicated to cancer research, and has a distinct interest in working in the oncology pavilion, a concordant and synergistic tie can be made to an open position in the oncology pavilion. Conversely, if a job applicant freely discloses that he is pro-choice, belongs to several groups that are adamantly pro-choice, and would have a problem with the ethical orientation of a Catholic hospital, it would be wise for the human resources professional to consult the staff attorney on the need to interview other candidates who might be equally (if not more) qualified for the position based on skills—candidates who might not have a strong personal belief that could preclude complete commitment to the organization's goals and values.

Belief-Centered Cultures

This leads to the topic of belief-centered cultures, which include religious organizations. These also include many health care organizations that have a specific religious affiliation, which is common, particularly in urban settings across the United States and Canada. In such an organization, such as the Franciscan Health System or Bon Secours Health System, the mission of a religious order can be a prominent organizational dynamic and a major marketing and business advantage. As stated by an administrator of a Catholic hospital in Oklahoma, "Folks around here look at Catholic health care the way that they look at Chinese food—in both cases you get a little more, something better than average, and you expect top quality!" This admittedly subjective viewpoint is actually substantiated by customer-patient evaluations of many religiously affiliated health care organizations, which are commonly rated higher in customer-patient satisfaction than their secular counterparts.

It is essential from a human resources perspective to take special care in interviewing new job candidates relative to their religious affiliation and other aspects of personal belief. As noted earlier, labor law has many statutes, primarily in the category of equal opportunity, that help govern proper interviewing technique in these areas. Again, however, free and full disclosure by job candidates can be helpful in determining both their alignment with organizational values and their suitability in regard to the more qualitative aspects of a given job position.

Regionally founded cultures are perhaps the easiest to understand, as they are purely quantitative in nature and scope. Regionally founded cultures also have the clearest relevance to a specific health care organization. For example, Baptist Hospital in Louisville, Kentucky, is a perfect match to its community, as Southern Baptists make up the predominate religious culture in the area. Also, the majority of the employees at the facility are Kentuckians— and, more specifically, Louisville denizens—as are the majority of the organization's customer-patient base. The Long Island Jewish Hospital, which has been in business for nearly seventy-five years on the Queens–Long Island border, is a large regional health care organization that, like Baptist Hospital, has a laudable reputation and continues to be the most easily identifiable community hospital in one of the most competitive regions in the nation.

Regionally Founded Cultures

Understanding the relevance to human resources of the regionally founded cultures in health care is easy enough. In the selection process, it is paramount to remember that in most community health care organizations nearly 92 percent of the workforce also lives within the organization's service area. Less obvious is that any strategic education plan for employees should involve the leading educational institutions in the local area, which signifies to all interested applicants that the organization is serious about providing top-notch education as a reward to the employees and in return for their well-earned tuition reimbursement benefits. Furthermore, the prominence of the health care organization, supported by its human resources management department, in local career days, health fairs, mall health exhibitions, and other community-driven educational events in the region becomes integral to the development and the continuance of the health care organization as a true community health care provider, despite any dissonance that might be occurring in the local media, national news, and other sources of attacks on the American health care system.

Behavior-Common Cultures

The next culture category of which the human resources professional needs to be aware is behavior-common cultures, which comprise individuals implicitly grouped by their actions or behavior. Clear examples at present include cell phone addicts and, more specifically, individuals who seem to be unable to live without constantly stroking the keyboard of their Blackberry device (is it any wonder that they are considered "crackberry" addicts?!?). It is vital for a health care organization to understand from a business perspective that individuals in behavior-common cultures receive information in a certain manner and through specific avenues of communication that could be the primary mode for conveying the services, pertinent news, and strategic future plans of the health care organization. For example, Internet banner ads are likely to be more successful, especially in urban and exurban areas, than signage at the local commuter rail station, as commuters are more likely to be working on their Blackberry device than looking at a static poster, no matter how appealing the images or how clever the advertising argot.

There is a wonderful opportunity for human resources professionals to use behavior-common cultural dynamics in their daily work. A primary example of this pertains to organizational communication. For example, at Newark Beth Israel Medical Center, the human resources management department has innovated The Beth Blog, which is available to all employees and provides information ranging from new parking opportunities to news about medical services to updates and improvements to employee benefits, including on-site education provided by Stevens Institute of Technology. Another, perhaps more typical example is the use of text messages during times of inclement weather, which are sent to employees at a health care facility using a list of employee cell phone numbers. In a progressive health care organization there are boundless opportunities to focus on behavior-common cultures in the interest of providing stellar human resources services.

Interest-Motivated Cultures

The sixth and final category is interest-motivated cultures, which can include golfers, surfers, book club aficionados, and, prominent among teenagers and college students, competitive gamers. In each case, a specific malady or set of medical concerns can be directly related to the activities of the culture, especially when considering dynamics in the customer-patient community. For example, competitive gamers or others who excessively use personal computers can experience carpal tunnel syndrome. Certain terms in the medical lexicon, such as *tennis elbow,* have a clear connection to an interest-motivated culture. The increase in instances of many skin diseases—including the escalation of melanoma over the past thirty years as a result of excessive sun tanning and exposure to the sun, especially in areas of the country that only enjoy three to four months of great weather—is yet another specific example of how certain interest-motivated cultures endure particular maladies.

On a lighter note, understanding interest-motivated cultures can be a wonderful benefit to a health care human resources professional charged with arranging the medical center's bowling night or finding sponsorship for the medical center's coed softball team. In regard to work roles, understanding the avocations and particular interests of individual members of the workforce can provide direct benefits in regard to the placement of volunteers. For example, if a new volunteer enjoys photography, there is a natural opportunity for her to help contribute to an e-media advertising campaign using her talent and interest.

PRACTICAL APPLICATION: A TALE OF TWO JERSEY CULTURES

Using **psychographics,** loosely defined here as charting dynamics and nuances of culture within a business context, is a most effective practical application for the material in this chapter. As depicted in Tables 5.1 and 5.2, this section employs psychographics to compare two cultures that coexist peacefully and progressively in the Garden State of New Jersey.

We'll begin by taking a look at how to construct a strategic cultural assessment, which is a handy tool that you can use in charting cultural dynamics as they affect your particular health care human resources responsibilities. As shown in the titles of the first columns in Tables 5.1 and 5.2, you start by determining a general label that best depicts your subject culture in common parlance that will be recognizable to and respected by any target audience, as in the profiles of both the Hoboken Gen X crew and the New Jersey retirees. These examples, which were developed by a focus group of health care managers, also include the following components:

- *Values,* which can quickly be detected as common within a culture, or as an answer to the question "What does this particular culture value?"

- *Worldview,* which delves into the political and popular perceptions commonly held by the particular culture

- *TV/media/social networking,* which addresses the communication input and preoccupations of the particular culture

- *Heroes/anti-heroes,* which helps typify the belief system of the particular culture from an array of perspectives

- *Avocations/pastimes,* which can provide clues into both the type of maladies the culture endures as well as "hot-button issues" that might provide insight into the proclivities of customer-patients and employees alike

- *Communication,* which helps delineate the syntax, jargon, and other keys to communication that can enhance one's understanding of the culture's group norms

After setting up columns and then filling in each column with pertinent information based on the input of at least three to five individuals from

Table 5.1 Cultural Dynamics of the Hoboken Gen X Crew

Hoboken Gen X	Values (Verb/ Noun)	Worldview (Politics/ People Perceptions)	TV/Media/Social Networking	Heroes (+)/ Anti-Heroes (−)	Avocations/ Pastimes	Communication
• a.k.a. "Yuppies"	• Condo ownership	• Global	• Facebook	• Jon Stewart (+)	• Bars in Manhattan	• "Awesome"
Quantitative:	• Interdependent via texting	• Independent	• *The Bachelor*	• Lady Gaga (+)	• Bars in Hoboken	• "Hook up"
• About thirty-four years old	• Friendship	• Interconnection	• *American Idol*	• Usher (+)	• Hooking up	• Any texting jargon
• Pay off student loans	• Networking	• Eco/green	• *Lost*	• Bon Jovi (+)	• Gaming	• "I'm just saying"
• Limited savings	• "Cashless" society—credit cards and e-commerce	• Urban	• *Twilight*	• Eli Manning (+)	• Sports (for example, lacrosse)	• "Dude"
• Credit cards		• Multicultural	• No newspapers	• Bernard Madoff (−)	• Movies	• "Really??"
Qualitative:		• Experimental foodie (sushi)	• iTunes		• Travel	• "You know"
• Not "interpersonal"			• Kindle		• Hot cars with gadgets	• "Friend" (verb)
• Job stability			• iPhone/iPad			• "Sick"
• Immediacy			• Books on tape			• "Cool"
			• *Sex in the City*			• "Googled"
						• "Shoddy"
						• "Like"

Table 5.2 Cultural Dynamics of New Jersey Retirees

New Jersey Retirees	Values (Verb/Noun)	Worldview (Politics/People Perceptions)	TV/Media/Social Networking	Heroes (+)/Anti-Heroes (−)	Avocations/Pastimes	Communication
• a.k.a. "Real Jerseyans"	• Patriotism	• State/local	• *The Price Is Right*	• Jon Wayne (+)	• Bingo!	• "Swell"
Quantitative:	• Golf courses	• Medicare Good old days	• "You know who called me?!?"	• Lady Gaga (−)	• Golf	• "Keep it clean"
• Over sixty-two years old	• Financial security	• Taxes are too high	• Local newspaper	• Ronald Reagan (+)	• Bowling	• Anything said with good manners
• Pensions/Social Security/reverse mortgages	• Pride in New Jersey and local towns	• Polarized politics	• Radio talk show	• Jimmy Carter (−)	• Sailing	• "Darn"
Qualitative:		• Disillusioned with New Jersey politicians	• Romance novels	• Colin Powell (+)	• Gardening	• "Shoot"
• Largely blue-collar			• Relating to the TV anchor	• Mickey Mantle (+)	• "Early Bird Special"	• "Shore" (to refer to the beach)
• Downsizing			• *The Weather Channel*	• Arnold Palmer (+)	• Bridge	• "The Bridge"
• Must have been born here			• *60 Minutes*	• Past New Jersey Governors (−)	• Volunteering	• "The City"
			• Reruns of old shows	• New York Giants (+)	• Church	
			• *CSI*	• Meryl Streep (+)	• Spectator sports	
			• *Dancing with the Stars*	• Barbara Streisand (+)	• Child care	
				• Frank Sinatra (+)		
				• Frankie Valli (+)		

the human resources management department, line management, or other groups that truly understand the customer-patient and employee community, you can mine the gathered data to develop insight into potential strategy. For example, you can identify the following elements for strategic use:

- Employee needs

- Employee wants

- Volunteer needs

- Possible service areas (For example, it is apparent that substance abuse and alcohol treatment are a concern for the Hoboken Gen X crew; therefore, in crass business terms, treatments make up a good product line for Hoboken University Medical Center.)

- Media icons, which could be used in employee communication as well as advertising

Psychographic analysis, when applied logically, can be a useful starting point for strategic planning in health care human resources: "It ain't who you know, it's what you know about 'em!"

SUMMARY

Because the human resources management department acts as the guardian of the most important asset of any health care organization—its people—it is imperative that health care human resources professionals consider the intrinsic and extrinsic dynamics of culture in all of their activities, programs, and daily accountabilities. A focus on the specific needs of the employee as an individual must be complemented with a continued understanding of the group cultural dynamics both internal and external to the organization in order to position the progressive health care organization to provide the best health care in every situation.

KEY TERMS

Department of Veterans Affairs (VA) Health Care System

The Joint Commission (TJC)

psychographics

Visiting Nurse Association (VNA) Health Group

DISCUSSION QUESTIONS

1. Based on your own observations and perspective, what unique facets of the health care workforce might be missing from Figure 5.1?

2. Credo statements attest to the common beliefs of the members of a health care organization (for example, "Our diverse strengths and perspectives provide a powerful, positive ability to provide care to our diverse community"). Craft a credo statement that would reflect the common beliefs of an organizational culture of which you are a member.

3. Why is it "good business" for a health care organization to have an organizational culture that reflects its customer-patient community?

4. Cite six cultures from your frame of reference that could match each of the cultural composition foundations charted in Figure 5.2 and discussed in this chapter.

5. Consider your own experience; of how many of the six cultures mentioned in this chapter are you a member?

6. Construct a psychographic cultural analysis, similar to those in Tables 5.1 and 5.2, of a customer-patient community group from your frame of reference.

7. Considering psychographics, chart a group that reflects a subculture that relates to your life at work, at home, or at play.

6

The Importance of Volunteers in Health Care Organizations

LEARNING OBJECTIVES

- Understand the critical importance of volunteers in a health care organization
- Determine how to best use volunteers as integral and productive components of your health care organization's human resources management department
- Incorporate management methods for the selection and specific placement of volunteers within a progressive health care organization
- Strategically plan work activities for volunteers that augment the continuous efforts of health care organizational development
- Implement and maintain communication systems for health care volunteers

THE IMPORTANCE OF volunteers in people-intensive health care organizations cannot be underestimated. There are many work roles that qualified volunteers can fill competently to help the progressive health care organization in meeting its mission and operational objectives. In the customer-patient's ever-important subjective perception, anyone with the name badge is probably an employee of the health care organization. Therefore, the expertise, discernment, and thoughtfulness that go into the selection and placement of an employee should be equally applied to the selection of volunteers and their placement within a health care organization by health care human resources professionals and participating line managers.

This chapter reviews the importance of volunteers in a health care organization, with particular emphasis on their selection and strategic placement, and the communication and organizational development responsibilities of human resources professionals that are intrinsic to maximizing volunteer performance.

SELECTION AND PLACEMENT STRATEGY CONSIDERATIONS FOR VOLUNTEERS

Specific selection criteria should be used throughout the interviewing process for volunteers who work in a progressive health care organization. Three major background categories—experience, acumen, and skill sets—should be evaluated to ensure maximum return on investment from selected volunteers (see Figure 6.1).

Experience

Professional experience should be the first priority in the volunteer selection calculus, and the human resources professionals conducting volunteer interviews (with line managers participating in the process) should seek to ascertain a volunteer's work-life experience in the health care business arena, basic business, and leadership. Health care experience of any kind can be a strong asset for volunteers, as they will have an established frame of reference and foundation for working in the unique health care environment: coping with emergency situations, meeting high customer-patient expectations, communicating precisely and effectively, and other requisites of the health care workplace will be familiar to these volunteer candidates. Not all health care organizations are exactly the same, however. Accordingly, health care human resources professionals should be certain in an interview situation that the applicant does not come into a voluntary work role with

Figure 6.1   Identifying Background Strengths of Health Care Volunteers

Experience	Health Care	Business	Leadership
Acumen	New Learning	Teaching/Training	Child Care
Skill Sets	Customer Service	Technology	Communication

a potentially detrimental subjective opinion or contrary outlook on health care organizations based on previous experience. Such a bias or firm negative perspective can prove counterproductive because the volunteer—even with good intentions—will see his or her new work role through a prism that is inaccurate or discordant in the new volunteer position.

The health care human resources professional should ask open-ended questions that accurately evaluate the type of health care experience volunteer candidates possess and make a determination on where their particular base of experience might best serve the organization. For example, if a volunteer candidate has had experience in direct patient care and possesses a good attitude, evident people skills, a solid managerial aptitude, and a strong team orientation, he might be a suitable candidate for a physician's office, at the front desk of a clinic, or in another high-traffic patient area, such as a gift shop or radiology center in a major medical center. If a candidate is a retired nurse and has all of the aforementioned personal characteristics that are required for any employee at the health care organization, she can be invaluable both in direct customer-patient contact as well as in particular sectors of patient education—provided she keeps her knowledge base current by attending the organization's in-service educational forums.

In all cases, individuals who have previous health care experience should be evaluated to ensure that their frame of reference about the health care industry is still pertinent, as everyone knows that trends in health care are constantly changing, and a state of daily fluctuation exists due to improved technology, patient care enhancements, and other new variables. Any volunteer candidates, including those who are retirees from a health care career, who are insistent on not needing to increase their current education relative to health care or a particular aspect of patient care are often more of a detriment than an asset as volunteers.

Individuals who possess a strong background in business, particularly in such areas as service support, accounting, technology systems, and even human resources, can be stellar volunteers provided they are properly evaluated in the interview and placed intelligently within the organization. Indeed, progressive health care organizations are businesses that have complicated business systems, and although they might be nonprofit in nature, there is still revenue that must be processed and operational systems that must work effectively and efficiently in order for the organization to thrive. Individuals with a sterling business background can thus be of invaluable assistance, with proper guidance and leadership, in improving performance in these key areas. In this regard, it is important to note that not all volunteers are retirees. For example, someone who has a terrific business background but is now a stay-at-home mom can dedicate some valuable hours to a local clinic to help it in its business practices. From another angle, there are many hospitals on the East Coast that have volunteer positions for students of various culinary institutes who complete voluntary training practicums. This can benefit not only student volunteers in regard to their practical education but also all who get to enjoy extraordinary cuisine that is the antithesis of the pejorative stereotype of "hospital food"!

Finally, hospital volunteer candidates who possess leadership experience can become essential contributors to a progressive health care organization. Although it would be ideal for volunteer candidates to have leadership experience in the realm of health care or nonprofit organizations, any sound range of leadership experience can be a distinct addition to the volunteer corps of a progressive health care organization. For instance, if an individual has had leadership experience as a Girl Scout coordinator, which would reflect

confluent skills in communication, leadership, administration, and organization in a nonprofit setting, she can be a terrific volunteer contributor in children's health awareness, community outreach, and numerous other areas. In a similar vein, individuals who have spent considerable time serving in the armed forces not only have acquired very useful leadership experience but also are likely to have developed—both formally and informally—leadership skills that would be relevant to the fast pace and high pressure of a progressive health care organization. A savvy human resources professional should ask for examples of leadership success and practical application of leadership skills, interviewing all volunteer candidates who appear to have leadership experience with an intent to place them in areas in which they must "lead the action" relative to customer-patient services, as well as in areas in which they will supervise, organize, and manage other volunteers.

Acumen

The second area for consideration in assessing volunteer potential is the category of acumen, which here translates to expertise and aptitudes that are areas of strength for the volunteer candidate. As discussed in the previous paragraphs, it is vital for any volunteer at a progressive health care organization to be able to understand, assimilate, and apply new learning. Volunteer candidates, regardless of age or years of experience in health care work roles, must learn new practices, procedures, and their new health care organization's particular "way of doing things." Every health care organization has its own mission, values, and vision, and in almost all cases has a specific standard operating practice (SOP) and particular methods for treating patients and conducting its daily business. Every volunteer must be able to understand the organization's SOP and be able to apply it fluidly in his or her new volunteer work role. In addition, the new volunteer must be able to learn the critical job requirements of—and the daily communication responsibilities intrinsic to—the volunteer role. An individual who values new learning, and in fact wants to be a volunteer within the health care organization because she values intellectual engagement, is indeed an ideal candidate for becoming a health care organizational volunteer. Conversely, individuals who believe they "know it all already" are destined to be stuck indeterminately with only what they know now. Furthermore, they will not be long-term assets as health care organizational volunteers and will probably become sources of negative motivation and reduced volunteer corps morale.

The ability to teach and train others is certainly a skill, but it is often based on a natural proclivity for making information user-friendly and on an intrinsic desire to help educate others. Accordingly, candidates who have acumen in teaching and training can be strong candidates for volunteer placement within a progressive health care organization, as they can fill a variety of work roles in which significant information must be imparted to customer-patients as well as employees and internal volunteers. Individuals who apply for health care organizational volunteer roles who have a background in teaching, even at the elementary school level (or perhaps especially at the elementary school level, given the number of children present every day on most health care campuses) can be exceptional candidates to work in any area in which health awareness and education are needed. Likewise, any applicants for volunteer positions within a progressive health care organization who have had experience and have truly enjoyed their work as corporate trainers, organizational educators, or one-on-one mentors can also be invaluable to a health care organization that needs individuals to help in the preventive wellness program. In addition, they can be placed effectively in positions in which general individual communication is needed but that do not require medical or health care expertise, in such areas as community drives to supply a blood bank or annual flu inoculation events. Someone who has both the acumen and proclivity for communication or education can be invaluable in quickly and effectively educating community members on how to complete certain forms to donate blood or receive a flu shot.

With appropriate training, these volunteers can experience professional growth within the health care organization, because the organization's provision of medical and health care knowledge can enhance their basic skills in communication and education. These volunteers can then perhaps move into more challenging volunteer roles suited to their interests and the organization's need, and in the process gain more knowledge of health care. This type of development, which can be led by educators within the health care human resources management department, can both increase volunteers' motivation and provide a wonderful, long-term, and free resource for the progressive health care organization.

Anyone who has spent any time with new parents knows that a common question is, "Where can I buy a complete instruction manual on raising children?" As we all know, this particular tome is yet to be written, but parenting and child care skills are clearly among the most important resources in our society. In health care, the overwhelming majority of organizations have child care centers that can be excellent placement locations for qualifying volunteer candidates. Starting with the initiative in the 1980s pioneered by The Hospital for Special Care in New Britain, Connecticut, many health care organizations have used **intergenerational day care** as a featured benefit for new employees. An intergenerational day care facility is usually staffed by volunteers who forge constructive relationships with not only the children but also their parents, who work at the health care organization. Furthermore, many health care organizations have significant pediatric services; in some cases, such as at the Children's Hospital of Philadelphia, the entire organization is dedicated to the wellness of children and the cure of pediatric-specific maladies. It is easy to see, therefore, that child care experience can be an excellent qualification for a volunteer candidate at a progressive health care organization.

Skill Sets

Skill sets, which are the third category of selection criteria for health care volunteers, might be the easiest and most objective to understand and apply as a health care human resources professional. For example, an individual who has experience in customer service can work in any part of the health care organization with great effectiveness, because skills in dealing with people—particularly in tough situations in which understandable emotionalism is the order of the day—can be useful in almost any outpatient area and in any patient areas that have a front desk operation. Customer service skills are also invaluable in any business office, even in a clinic, in which customer-patients must have a clear understanding of billing procedures as well as of their rights and responsibilities as health care consumers. Customer service skills can also be used relative to fundraising, which is the lifeblood of many nonprofit health care organizations. Individuals who are not afraid of picking up the phone to ask for donations, for example, can become some of the most esteemed members of a health care organization that relies greatly on community support to keep its doors open.

In addition, every health care organization worth its salt has an information line or similar major communication mechanism to provide general information, ranging from responses to patient inquiries to answers to questions about the types of services that the organization provides for the community. Again, individuals who have customer service skills and can maintain a patient and professional demeanor in answering all inquiries can become critical links in the health care organization's daily operations, as their skill sets can make both volunteers' and employees' work lives more productive. When a volunteer can handle a call gracefully, gratefully, and effectively—and thus alleviate the time pressures of direct care providers so they can actually handle medical issues, everyone in the health care organization benefits.

Technology is certainly part of the fabric of every health care organization, from small clinics and doctors' offices to health care systems that employ thousands of people in multicampus settings, such as The Florida Hospitals or the Mayo Clinics. Communication, patient information, medical records, and employee data are just a few of the many areas in which technology has become a major change dynamic over the past ten years. Accordingly, any volunteer candidate who has expertise in technology, including data entry capabilities, software skills, and knowledge of certain programs, such as Excel, can be placed by a progressive human resources professional not just in one department of a hospital but perhaps in a specific volunteer team consisting of several other individuals who have similar skills in particular technical areas. Consider this example: a stay-at-home mom who once worked in a corporate information technology department, a retired military dependent who was the first on her base to learn how to use Excel spreadsheets, and a retired school superintendent who is an expert at PowerPoint can collaborate wonderfully to manage most of the data and communication responsibilities at a small clinic in the form of a special projects team—all at absolutely no cost to the organization's all-important bottom line.

Communication is the linchpin of health care organizational success. External communication with the customer-patient community that can help enhance the image of a health care organization, and internal communication, when effective, timely, and efficient, can be defining factors in organizational excellence. Volunteer candidates who demonstrate strong communication skills within an interview, as well as those who have excellent written communication skills, can be placed in any area of a progressive health care organization in a similar manner to those who have viable skills in technology and customer service. In fact, as project management becomes a major focal point in health care organizational management, the volunteer with strong communication skills can be assigned to assist any department that needs help in compiling reports and presentations. The department would benefit greatly from volunteer expertise in this area, and would definitely welcome this assistance.

MAXIMIZING HEALTH CARE VOLUNTEER PERFORMANCE

The strategic placement of volunteers in a major medical center by health care human resources professionals can enhance the organization's performance quickly and constructively. This section explores placement opportunities for volunteers in a typical medical center setting in the areas of organizational support, patient care, business operations, and community relations. Although the focus example of this section is a medical center, it will be easy for you to understand how these placement opportunities can exist in any progressive health care organization regardless of size, from a doctor's office of a dozen employees to major health care organization consisting of a medical center, physician complex, teaching component, and wellness facility, as any health care organization possesses many of the components delineated here.

Organizational Support

In the area of organizational support, the lobby is perhaps the most important physical space in any health care organization, as it is the area in which the customer-patient begins to form a perception, which in turn will become a firmly set belief relative to the organization's effectiveness and efficiency. It is therefore vitally important that the lobby area is staffed with individuals who are courteous, caring, competent, and knowledgeable about the basic operations of the health care facility. Volunteers placed in this area should be able to embody these characteristics successfully, and should receive training in critical dimensions of this important work. Furthermore, volunteers should not be excluded from any customer-patient services seminars; in fact, they should be among the prime participants in an in-service educational event at the health care facility that addresses how to deal with difficult customers, how to handle objections, and how to get an assist when needed from a health care professional or supervisor. Many health care organizations, such as the Mercy Hospital System in Oklahoma, make sure that all volunteers working in direct patient care areas have certain guidelines on the flipside of their name badge that help them remember key facets of their work role, namely:

- Noise annoys; please do not engage in loud conversations or unnecessary chats in view or earshot of our patients and guests.

- Answer any and all patient inquiries promptly, professionally, and personally; if you do not know the answer to a question, simply tell the patient, "I will get an answer for you immediately," and contact the supervisor or any other individual who you know will be able to give you a prompt and accurate answer.

- It is nice to be important, but is more important to be nice; the Mercy Way is to be courteous, caring, and compassionate in every situation, and that is a daily objective for all of us who have the privilege to work here.

This simple triad of customer service principles should be encouraged in every health care organization, as these tenets are integral to customer-patient satisfaction starting in the lobby area.

Volunteers can also be very useful at special events sponsored by the health care organization. These can include such community events as health awareness fairs, mobile health presentations, and other occasions in which extra manpower is needed. In many cases volunteers may have an intrinsic advantage in their work role because they are usually residents of the medical center's service community and thus are likely to have personal ties and relationships with many of the attendees. They also probably know enough about the community to handle unforeseen circumstances that may arise unexpectedly at the event. Fundraising events, such as summer carnivals, bake sales, and fund drives for particular diseases, such as multiple sclerosis or autism, are also natural venues for volunteer assistance.

Outpatient clinics represent another opportunity to engage qualified volunteers in organizational support. Outpatient clinics typically handle a lot of traffic from the front desk to the conclusion of the caregiving cycle, and thus tend to require a lot of manpower. Work responsibilities in an outpatient clinic may be daily in nature, or in many cases may include specific projects and responsibilities that only need to be accomplished once a week. For example, certain bookkeeping and record maintenance tasks can be conducted competently at an outpatient clinic with only five to ten hours of work a week. Accordingly, an innovative employ of volunteers at an outpatient clinic would involve scheduling a once-a-week contribution for volunteers who do not want a daily role. From the perspective of the outpatient clinic manager, he or she would have supervisory responsibilities concerning each of these volunteers only once a week as opposed to every day, as would be the case for someone working in the lobby or other area that must be staffed on a daily basis.

Facility tours are part of the everyday action at any health care facility. Tours can be arranged for community groups, school groups, Scout field trips, church groups, and, in facilities that provide long-term care, potential residents and family members. If volunteers possess good people skills and abilities in the realm of guest relations—or are skilled in educating or communicating with others—they could be ideal candidates for conducting facility tours.

Patient Care

As depicted in Table 6.1, patient care areas also offer opportunities to put volunteers to good use. Outpatient front desk operations, as indicated previously, can provide natural placement options for volunteers on a daily basis. General service areas, such as radiology and other diagnostic units, also need individuals to staff the front desk and handle patient flow. Recordkeeping, patient transport, and internal mail delivery can also be some of a volunteer's responsibilities.

Physicians' offices in many cases are strategic business units (SBUs) and often welcome as much help as possible. The administrative leadership of a progressive health care organization can increase goodwill among physician members by extending the range of volunteer services to their individual facilities. Given that most credentialed physicians have offices within the service area of a major medical center, finding a volunteer to participate fully at a physicians' office under the aegis of the major medical center is not a daunting proposition. In addition, positions at physicians' offices in

Table 6.1   Progressive Placement of Medical Center Volunteers

Organizational Support	Patient Care	Business Operations	Community Relations
Lobby	Outpatient front	Finance	Gift shop
Special events	desk	Information technology	Fundraising initiatives
Outpatient clinic	General services	Project management	Youth liaison programs
Facility tours	Physicians' office	Food services (for	Blood drives
	Intergenerational	example, in a coffee	Community outreach
	day care	shop)	events
		General health care	

doctors' park facilities, which are often run by the medical center and are near—if not part of—the main medical center campus, can also offer easily accessible, maximum-benefit opportunities for placing volunteers.

Intergenerational day care, as indicated in Table 6.1, also represents a natural opportunity for volunteers. As stated earlier, assisting in direct child care responsibilities can be part of a volunteer's contribution to the medical center. For example, a guest reader or play group leader for children at a day care center, therapy group, or special education or medical assistance class can be a very rewarding and significant volunteer role. In many organizations, enlightened human resources professionals specializing in education have arranged training opportunities for volunteers to learn how to work with children with special needs who attend day care at the medical center, such as children with autism or children who have learning disabilities or are hearing impaired.

Business Operations

Business operations could also take advantage of volunteers' expertise in such areas as finance, information technology, and other traditional aspects of business expertise. Project management has become a major staple of health care organizations, and again affords a wonderful chance for individuals of varied backgrounds to participate as important volunteers in a medical center. Volunteers in food services can extend beyond the culinary students already mentioned to include individuals who can work on the food line, handle a cash register, or sign people up for varied activities as they enjoy the medical center's cuisine. General health care operations, such as eye exams and dental exams for children participating in the local Head Start program, also have seasonal and special staffing needs that can otherwise be a strain on medical center administrators. Again, volunteers can truly ride to the rescue and assist in some very meaningful endeavors that can immediately enhance the health of their fellow community members.

Community Relations

Community relations activities, such as fundraising events, are great opportunities not only to involve ongoing, current volunteers at the medical center but also to enlist new volunteers and to engage individuals who might be "one-time" volunteers, depending on the nature of the activity. For example, if a medical center sponsors a walk for breast cancer, many current volunteers who are cancer survivors will naturally want to be engaged in the activity; furthermore, they might bring along fellow breast cancer survivors (as they are all part of a specific experienced-based culture) who might become volunteers for a day or, optimally, join their friends as regular volunteers at the medical center.

Youth liaison programs are a major part of any progressive health care organization, especially in community-driven medical centers. These programs can take the form of sports injury centers, field trips from local schools, career days both at the medical center as well as in school settings, and other programs that link the community's youth population to the medical center. In this regard, it is important to remember that volunteers do not necessarily have to be retirees, but can be youth volunteers ranging from the traditional candy striper nurse aspirant to premed college volunteers who want to see how a real medical center operates. Again, the medical center has an opportunity to engage a set of new volunteers in a very attractive and appropriate manner. Likewise, blood drives and other community outreach events, particularly when organized in collaboration with other community nonprofit organizations, such as volunteer fire departments, can be natural opportunities for volunteer recruitment across the medical center.

AGENDA TOPICS FOR VOLUNTEER SUMMITS

As discussed throughout this chapter, purposeful communication is central to the development and maintenance of volunteer corps cohesion and strong group performance. Organizations that assist medical centers in volunteer group development, such as the Iroquois Healthcare Alliance in upstate New York, suggest that quarterly meetings for the volunteer corps in any sizable progressive health care organization present critical components that help maintain good communication, increase positive morale, and garner useful feedback. Such meetings are offered to the volunteer corps to enhance an enlightened and unique perspective on the progress of both the health care organization and its service community. The following list acts as a strategic guide for developing and delivering efficacious volunteer summits on a quarterly basis.

- *Time line updates,* to include progress made on significant organizational goals, as well as new initiatives within the organization.

- *National and regional trends,* including an exploration of significant impact factors that have particular pertinence to the health care organization in a general sense, and perhaps particular relevance to the volunteer corps and a majority of the volunteer work roles.

- *Annual reports,* which have become standard publications in most progressive health care organizations. In an effort to make volunteers feel as though they are indeed as important as "regular employees," some organizations have actually hand-delivered newly published annual reports to volunteers at the first quarterly summit of the year, or at the final quarterly summit of the year in conjunction with a nice holiday party in which all the volunteers receive a special guest visit from the hospital CEO as well as a freshly minted copy of the annual report.

- *Award presentations,* which can take place at the initial meeting of volunteers in the first quarter of the calendar year or, perhaps more traditionally, during the fourth-quarter volunteer summit in conjunction with a holiday party. As opposed to merely presenting a "Volunteer of the Year" award, which could be too exclusive and a bit trite, it might be useful to enhance the award titles using such words as "Spirit of . . . " For example, recipients of outstanding volunteer service awards at Hoboken University Medical Center who work in conjunction with Stevens Institute of Technology's nonprofit health care consortium receive an award called "The Spirit of Castle Point"; everyone in the neighborhood knows "Castle Point" was George Washington's designation for the riverside section of Hoboken (although many only know that part of the city as the childhood home of Francis Albert Sinatra).

- *The strategic plan,* the unveiling of which not only contributes to the summit's status as a special event but also immediately empowers the volunteers as ambassadors of the new strategic initiatives to their service community, as they are now "in the know" before anyone else.

- *New services,* such as those of a new ambulatory care area or a new clinic. Introducing new services at a volunteer summit can enhance their word-of-mouth campaign launch potential; it can also enhance volunteers' pride in the organization and their accountability to act as ambassadors; reengage their commitment to their growing organization; and clearly demonstrate leadership's trust in the volunteers to act as advocates of, and active members in, the organization's forward progress.

- *Policies and procedures,* the discussion of which is often considered a necessary evil, but which can be quickly and easily introduced and implemented as "last items" on the agenda at volunteer quarterly summits.

- *New health care initiatives,* discussed from a global perspective and then related specifically to the service community.

- *Community imperatives,* such as the need for particular services and major change dynamics within the customer-patient sphere of influence. The discussion of such imperatives can elicit meaningful and very useful feedback, suggestions, and communication. Volunteers often have knowledge of prevailing sentiments among customer-patients because many often live within the service community.

TEN ESSENTIAL RULES FOR VOLUNTEER PLACEMENT

 1. Do not hire volunteers who you suspect are "know-it-alls," as they probably have no interest in learning and growing within a health care organization, which by definition must grow and provide learning experiences daily to prosper and survive.

2. Make certain that the volunteers know the mission, vision, and values of the organization, so that they understand how their work behavior must reflect positively and progressively a set of meaningful principles in all their activities.

3. Communicate frequently and informally with all volunteers, so that the volunteers not only stay motivated but also are provided on a daily basis with meaningful feedback.

4. Ensure that a mentor is selected, either from the corps of volunteers or from the professional staff, to help in the orientation and ongoing training of each volunteer. This ensures that good learning becomes the rule of the day and that volunteers each have a designated superstar to help them as they contribute to the organization.

5. Be firm and resolute in addressing volunteer malfeasance, such as gossiping, rumormongering, and other inappropriate behavior that could reflect poorly on the health care organization. A volunteer can have a negative impact on an organization as quickly and deleteriously as can a full-time employee.

6. Reward outstanding volunteer performance with appropriate awards and recognition at every opportunity; as is the case with performance evaluation, simply waiting until an annual review or quarterly summit to give positive feedback and encouragement wastes an opportunity to provide continuity and consistency to volunteer performance development and growth.

7. Have a set performance evaluation policy in place, developed with the director of volunteer services if one exists at your organization, that

can help in the performance improvement process for volunteers. Such a policy should document the clause that if an employee continues to demonstrate detrimental, inconsistent performance, removal from the organization is a possible course of action.

8. Try at every opportunity to match volunteer expertise and acumen with any emergent needs within your health care organization so that the pace and pressure of the organization are matched by thoughtful placement of skills and talent across the volunteer corps (as is ideally the case across employee staff ranks).

9. Be as creative as possible while maintaining effectiveness and efficiency in aligning volunteer capabilities and potential with needs and growth initiatives within the organization. Such an effort not only helps the growth and development of each volunteer but also increases the aptitude of the health care human resources professional.

10. Consistently embrace every opportunity to encourage and recognize the superstar and steady performance of each and every volunteer at your health care organization. In a very practical sense, doing good by your volunteers in every conceivable way will ultimately help your organization do some real good in providing stellar health care throughout your community.

SUMMARY

Volunteers are a natural wellspring of talent for any health care organization, specifically organizations that are community centered. With purposeful planning and thoughtful volunteer placement, health care organizations can maximize volunteers' contribution as an artful counter to the oft-heard lament of being "short staffed."

KEY TERMS

confluent skills   youth liaison programs

intergenerational day care

DISCUSSION QUESTIONS

1. What interviewing questions and overall strategy would you employ in selecting volunteers for a health care organization?

2. What five specific features would you incorporate in an orientation program for new health care organizational volunteers?

3. For a local organization in your community, what specific recruitment targets—groups or individuals—would you focus on for new volunteers?

4. What other areas and work roles in a health care organization, in addition to those cited in this chapter, would you earmark for volunteers?

5. What risks do you see associated with the use of volunteers in a health care organization? How would you minimize or eliminate the potential harm?

6. List at least five major benefits of smartly using volunteers in a health care organization.

Methods and Accountabilities of Health Care Human Resources

7

Critical Job Analysis and Design

LEARNING OBJECTIVES

- Understand the importance of job analysis to strategic human resources management (SHRM)
- Understand what a job analysis is
- Discuss the different SHRM purposes and uses for job analyses
- Discuss commonly used methods used to conduct job analyses
- Explain the different types of information about performing a job that are identified through job analysis techniques

THERE IS A need for a human resources management (HRM) department to assist its organization in improving organizational effectiveness. Strategic job analyses are integral to strategic human resources management (SHRM) planning. Such analyses recognize that most jobs will not remain stable but will change to meet future demands.

Job analyses provide the foundation for most HRM activities. Following is a brief introduction to each area of activity:

- **Recruitment and selection.** Job analysis identifies the knowledge, skills, abilities, and other characteristics (KSAOCs) required for each position. It identifies the minimum education, certification, or licensing requirements. It also identifies the essential tasks and responsibilities of the job. This information helps identify the skills of the people the agency needs to recruit and hire. A job analysis is critical when an organization uses preemployment examinations for selection and promotion. Tests must be job related; the knowledge, skills, abilities, personality variables, and constructs to be tested need to be identified through an up-to-date job analysis. An organization does not know what knowledge, skills, and abilities to test for unless it knows what competencies are required for successful performance.

- **Developing compensation systems.** Compensation is typically related to a job's requirements, such as education the employee must possess, the skills and experience needed to perform the job, and whether or not the employee is working in hazardous conditions. A job analysis provides a standardized procedure for systematically determining pay and other benefits across the organization. It provides all employees with a basis for gaining a common understanding of the values of each job, its relationship to other jobs, and the requirements necessary to perform it.

- **Human resources planning, career development, and training.** Job analysis information can help employers design training and career development programs by identifying the skills required for different jobs. Identifying the knowledge, skill, and responsibility requirements of each job makes it possible to train and develop employees for promotional opportunities. Available information helps all employees understand promotion and transfer requirements and recognize career opportunities.

- **Performance evaluation.** Performance standards should be derived from what employees actually do on the job. A job analysis identifies the tasks and responsibilities that employees perform in the course of their work. Areas of accountability can be identified and evaluation standards developed.

- **Risk management.** A job analysis can help identify job hazards, such as exposure to flammable materials or complicated machinery. Employers should use this information to develop training programs to alert employees to possible dangers, including health, safety, and security issues.

- **Job design.** Jobs are arranged around a set of work activities designed to enable the organization to carry out its mission. External and internal changes, however, often force an organization to rearrange or restructure work activities. The traditional tasks associated with a particular job change over time, and a job analysis is necessary to identify and accommodate these changes.

This chapter discusses the legal significance of job analysis, the types of information obtained through a job analysis, the factors to consider when designing a job analysis program. It concludes with a look at some of the job analysis techniques commonly used in health care organizations.

LEGAL SIGNIFICANCE OF JOB ANALYSIS

To demonstrate the validity and job relatedness of an employment test, the Uniform Guidelines on Employee Selection Procedures (1978) require that the test-validation strategies be based on a thorough and up-to-date job analysis. When used as the basis for such personnel decisions as promotions or pay increases, performance evaluations are also considered to be examinations and fall under the same rigorous scrutiny as employment tests. Furthermore, the Americans with Disabilities Act defines a qualified applicant as one who can perform the essential functions of the job. Essential functions are the primary job duties intrinsic to the position; they do not include marginal or peripheral tasks that are not critical to the performance of the primary job functions. It is important that employers analyze each position to identify these functions. The applicant must then satisfy the prerequisites for the position and be able to perform the essential functions of the job with or without reasonable accommodation.

The most common reasons for conducting a job analysis are so that a job description can be written, job specifications can be identified, and the job can be placed within a job family classification. A **job family** is a collection of jobs that require common skills, occupational qualifications, technology, licensing, and working conditions. A **job description** is a summary of the most important features of a job. It states the nature of the work and provides information about tasks, responsibilities, and context. Information typically found in a job description includes job title, job family, job summary, task statements, reporting relationships, and job context indicators.

The Americans with Disabilities Act does not require employers to develop written job descriptions. However, a written job description that is prepared before advertising a position or interviewing applicants for the job should be reviewed to make sure that it accurately reflects the actual functions of the job. The Equal Employment Opportunity Commission and the Civil Rights Division of the Department of Justice recommend that job descriptions focus on the results or outcomes of a job function, not solely on the way it is customarily performed. This is because a person with a disability may be able to accomplish a job function, with or without reasonable accommodation, in a manner that is different from the way an employee who does not have a disability may accomplish the same function.

Job specifications contain information about the KSAOCs of the position. Whereas each job description is specific to a particular job, job specifications may be more general. They contain the minimum qualifications that a person should possess to perform the job.

Job analysis is used as the basis for many HRM activities. However, different types of job analysis information, instruments, and procedures lend themselves to different purposes. The first steps in conducting a job analysis are to define the purpose behind the analysis and to determine what information is required.

JOB ANALYSIS INFORMATION

During a job analysis, information is most commonly collected on job activities, education requirements, types of equipment or tools used, working conditions, supervisory or management responsibilities, interpersonal or communication skills, agency contacts, external contacts, and the KSAOCs. *Knowledge* is the information required for the position. It can be factual, procedural, or conceptual and is related to the performance of tasks, such as a general knowledge of accounting principles or of fund accounting as used in nonprofit organizations. *Skills* are the observable competencies required to perform the particular tasks of the position, such as the ability to input data accurately at one hundred characters per minute or to diagnose and repair problems with personal computers. *Abilities* are the applicant's aptitudes for performing particular tasks—what the applicant is able to do and how well—such as the ability to prepare and make presentations or to read city maps. *Other characteristics* include attitudes, personality factors, or physical or mental traits needed to perform the job.

Job analysis information can be obtained through a variety of methods. The method of data collection depends on the nature of the positions being analyzed, the number of incumbents in and supervisors of the positions, the geographical dispersion of jobs, and the time available, as well as the types of information needed and the purpose of the analysis. The job analyst and the agency supervisors must work together to determine the most effective method for collecting information. The job analyst can be an employee from the HRM department; an employee working for a consulting firm hired to perform job analysis studies; or, in a small organization, a support staff employee, such as the administrative assistant to the city administrator or the executive director of a nonprofit agency. Following are the most common methods used for data collection:

- *Interview.* The analyst interviews the incumbent performing the job, the immediate supervisor, or another subject matter expert (SME), or a combination of all three, about the essential functions of the position.

- *Questionnaire.* Subject matter experts are asked to complete an open-ended questionnaire (see Figure 7.1). The job incumbent usually is asked to complete the questionnaire first, and then the supervisor is asked to review it to add anything that may have been neglected or to clarify statements made by the incumbent.

- *Structured checklist.* This is another form of questionnaire (see Figure 7.2). The SMEs are asked to respond to information presented on the checklist. They then check the responses most appropriate for their respective positions.

- *Observation.* The analyst observes the incumbent performing the job and records what he or she sees. This method works primarily for jobs in which activities or behaviors are readily observable. This method would not work well for intellectual or cognitive processes.

- *Diary or log.* Employees are asked to keep track of and record their daily activities and the time they spend on each.

Figure 7.1   Example Job Analysis Questionnaire

Name: Date completed:

Job title:

A. Please list the activities and tasks you perform daily, and specify the percentage of your total time spent in performing each task.

Essential Activities	*Tasks*	*Percentage of Time*

B. Indicate with a check mark the types of interactions you regularly have with individuals you come into contact with. Also indicate the primary means by which you contact these individuals.

Within Agency (Employees)

- ☐ Contact mainly within one department or office
- ☐ Regular contact with other departments or offices, furnishing and obtaining information
- ☐ Regular contact with other departments or offices, requiring tact and the development of utmost cooperation
- ☐ Regular contact with major executives on matters requiring explanations and discussions

Means of Contact

- ☐ Personal conversation   ☐ Telephone   ☐ Letter
- ☐ Other (specify):

Outside Agency (Nonemployees)

- ☐ Regular contact with persons outside the organization, involving effort that necessitates a great deal of tact and diplomacy
- ☐ Regular contact with others by presenting data that may influence important decisions
- ☐ Regular contact with persons of high rank, requiring tact and judgment to deal with and influence these people

Means of Contact

- ☐ Personal conversation   ☐ Telephone   ☐ Letter
- ☐ Other (specify):

C. What types of errors are possible on your job, and what would be the consequences of such errors in terms of additional expense to the organization, the time wasted in and cost of repeating or improving upon the work, or the loss of goodwill?

Figure 7.2 Example Structured Checklist

For each question, three responses are required:

A. Indicate the *frequency* with which this function is performed in this position.

B. Indicate how *important* this function is to the position.

C. Indicate whether *knowledge* of this function is essential for a newly hired employee in this position.

Frequency	Importance	Knowledge
0 = Never	0 = Not applicable	0 = Not required for job
1 = Rarely	1 = Not important	1 = Essential for newly hired employees
2 = Sometimes	2 = Somewhat important	2 = Not essential at time of hire (can be learned on the job)
3 = Often	3 = Important	
4 = Very often	4 = Very important	

Typing

	Frequency	Importance	Knowledge
1. Type letters from handwritten rough drafts.	☐	☐	☐
2. Type letters to students, faculty, staff members, applicants, or outside individuals or companies.	☐	☐	☐
3. Type inventory reports or budget reports.	☐	☐	☐
4. Type monthly status reports.	☐	☐	☐
5. Type general office forms (such as purchase requisitions, work orders, travel vouchers, or printing requisitions).	☐	☐	☐
6. Compose various letters and memos without written or verbal instructions.	☐	☐	☐
7. Proofread for spelling, grammar, and punctuation on all correspondence and reports.	☐	☐	☐
8. Type or edit manuscripts or drafts for supervisors.	☐	☐	☐
9. Prepare manuscripts for publication, including correction of errors and consultation on other editing matters.	☐	☐	☐
10. Lay out format and spacing for tables, charts, or other illustrations in preparation for typing.	☐	☐	☐

- *Critical incident technique.* Job experts generate a list of good and poor examples of performance that job incumbents exhibit. The purpose is to gather information about specific behaviors that have been observed, not to develop judgmental or trait-oriented descriptions of performance. These behaviors are then grouped into job dimensions. The final list of job dimensions and respective critical incidents provides information about a job and the behaviors associated with success or failure. A critical incident should possess four characteristics: it should be *specific,* focus on *observable* behaviors that have been exhibited on the job, describe the *context* in which each behavior occurred, and indicate the *consequences* of the behavior.

- *Combination of all methods.* Depending on the purpose of the job analysis and the targeted jobs, it may be necessary to use a combination of all of the methods introduced here. Not all jobs lend themselves to observation. Many public and nonprofit incumbents sit behind desks, use personal computers, and talk on the telephone. An analyst can observe those behaviors but will not understand the cognitive processes that accompany them or the requisite educational background and knowledge that may be specific to each position.

Many health care organizations have a variety of positions, ranging from very skilled to unskilled. For example, a hospital will have doctors, nurses, and physical therapists; experts in information technology and computer applications; budgeting and finance personnel; clerk-typist positions; and custodial and maintenance positions. The analyst will use different methods of data collection for different positions. For example, the custodial and maintenance positions may require limited reading and writing skills. To ask incumbents who may lack those skills to complete an open-ended written questionnaire may not provide the analyst with useful information. Instead, interviews and observation might be more appropriate data collection techniques. The finance personnel, however, might be asked to complete a questionnaire, followed by an interview to clarify any jargon or statements that the analyst does not understand. A follow-up interview also allows the incumbent to add information that she or he forgot to provide when completing the questionnaire.

In large organizations with many incumbents in the same position, or in state or federal organizations with geographically dispersed locations, the analyst may want to meet with a small number of incumbents and supervisors and ask them questions or have them fill out an unstructured questionnaire. The analyst could then develop a structured questionnaire based on the information provided, distribute it to all of the incumbents who hold that position, and then analyze the data for common work activities and responsibilities.

DESIGNING A JOB ANALYSIS PROGRAM

Why are you collecting job information? For what purpose will the data be used? The answers to these questions are important because different purposes require different information. For example, if the job analysis is to serve as the basis for determining compensation, the analyst would need to obtain information about education requirements and the level of experience and training needed. However, if the analysis is to serve as the basis for developing performance appraisal instruments, the job analyst will need to identify levels of task proficiency.

Another consideration is that employees may be sensitive to some of the purposes behind the job analysis. For example, employees are likely to be more concerned about a job analysis when it will be used to develop a compensation system than when the information will be used to develop training and orientation materials for new employees. Employees are thus likely to emphasize different information depending on the purpose of the job analysis.

The analyst should work with representatives of the organization to determine the most effective methods and procedures for collecting information. It is important for the analyst to understand how the organization operates and the best time to obtain information from incumbents and supervisors because not all jobs or tasks require the same intensity at the same time or for forty hours a week. Different tasks are likely to be performed on different days or at different times of the month or year. Also, some jobs have busy cycles during which the incumbents cannot be interrupted to visit with an analyst or take the time to complete an extensive questionnaire.

The following factors should be taken into consideration when deciding on the most effective way to collect information:

- *Location and number of incumbents*. Will a particular method or procedure enhance or restrict data collection because of a job's location? Many jobs are geographically dispersed throughout the city, state, or country. It might be too expensive and time-consuming for an analyst to visit and interview, for example, all of the clinical social workers across a state. Asking the incumbents to complete a questionnaire instead would be more feasible.

- *Working conditions and work environment.* Would work need to shut down during interviews because of a dangerous work environment? Would the incumbent or analyst be at risk if work were disrupted? Are there distractions in the work environment, such as noise, heat, hazardous materials, or risk management requirements, that would impair the data collection?

- *Knowledge, technological skills, and personal factors.* Do the knowledge, technological skills, or personal characteristics of the incumbents lend themselves to a particular method or procedure? Not all jobs or aspects of jobs are conducive to observation. A nurse's interactions with a patient can be observed. But what about the preparation? What would an analyst see? Can the thought processes or the knowledge required to prepare a lesson be observed? Other factors to consider are whether the job consists of routine or unpredictable tasks and whether the complexity of the job favors a particular method of collecting information. Will the SME prefer a particular method? Are there peer or organizational factors that influence whether or not a data collection procedure will be effective? For example, will a group interview inhibit employees from speaking up because they are intimidated by the presence of others? If supervisors and incumbents are asked to collaborate, will the supervisors dominate the conversation with the analyst?

After considering the factors just presented, the analyst needs to identify the jobs to be studied and choose the types of instruments he or she will use to obtain relevant data and information. Management should notify the incumbents and supervisors in advance that a job analysis will be undertaken and explain to them the purpose or purposes behind the endeavor. The quality of the data collected depends on assistance from SMEs.

JOB DESCRIPTIONS AND JOB SPECIFICATIONS

Often the information obtained from a job analysis is used to develop a job description and its job specifications. A job description identifies the tasks, duties, and responsibilities of a job. The job specifications list the KSAOCs individuals need to possess to perform a job successfully. Most job descriptions contain the following sections:

- *Identification of the job position.* This section provides the job title, reporting relationships, department, and location. It may also include the job code, pay grade, exempt or nonexempt status under the Fair Labor Standards Act, and Equal Employment Opportunity Commission classification.

- *General summary.* This is a brief statement of the general responsibilities and components that make the job different from others.

- *Essential functions and duties.* This identifies the major tasks, duties, and responsibilities performed.

- *Job specifications.* This provides the qualifications needed to perform the job successfully. Usually noted are the KSAOCs, the education and experience needed, physical requirements, and working conditions. Figure 7.3 provides an example of a job description.

Advances in information technology have changed many health care organizations. Positions are being redefined to mesh better with new missions and services. Organizations have become less hierarchical as many managerial responsibilities have been transferred to employees and work teams. Positions have become more flexible in an attempt to capitalize on improved information management capabilities as well as the changing characteristics of employees. Today many employees are expected to plan and organize their own work. One result of these changes is that employees are expected to perform a variety of complex tasks that go beyond formal job descriptions.

Traditional job analysis tends to focus on the KSAOCs required for performance of a position as it currently exists or as it has existed in the past. However, if agencies want to prepare for future changes, they must integrate into the job analysis strategic issues that may affect jobs in the future. To adopt a future-oriented approach to job analysis, agencies should convene a panel of SMEs to discuss the types of issues that are likely to challenge positions as well as the organization in the future.

Recommended SMEs include job incumbents, managers, supervisors, strategic planners, human resources staff members, and experts in a technical field related to the job to be analyzed. After potential future issues have been identified, tasks and KSAOCs need to be revised in anticipation of possible changes. Implementation of this **strategic job analysis** process can

Figure 7.3   Example Job Description

Job Title: State nursing home administrator

Job ID: 50001542

Full- or Part-Time: Full-time

Regular or Temporary: Regular

Salary Range: $61,648 to $80,000 annual salary

Position Information

This position involves managerial work planning, supervising, or coordinating activities in medicine and health services in hospitals, clinics, or public health care organizations, or in administrative health functions.

Examples of Work and Job Duties

- Administers fiscal operations, such as by planning budgets, authorizing expenditures, and coordinating financial reporting
- Coordinates or supervises activities of medical, nursing, technical, clerical, service, and maintenance personnel of the health care facility or mobile unit
- Develops or expands medical programs or health services for research, rehabilitation, and community health promotion
- Develops or recommends organizational policies and procedures and establishes evaluative or operational criteria for the facility or medical unit
- Implements and manages programs and services for the health care or medical facility
- Manages the establishment of work schedules and assignments for staff, according to workload, space, and equipment availability
- Manages the preparation of the status reporting of programs, services, and quality initiatives
- Recruits, hires, and evaluates the performance of medical and management staff and auxiliary personnel
- Reviews and analyzes facility activities and data to aid and improve service utilization
- Consults with medical, business, and community groups to discuss service problems, coordinate activities and plans, and promote health programs
- Designs instructional materials and develops in-service training programs for employees and community members

- Inspects facilities for emergency readiness and compliance with access, safety, and sanitation regulations, and recommends building or equipment modifications
- Provides technical assistance to other agencies concerning health services
- Manages all activities relating to the inspection and testing of agricultural products for fitness for human consumption

Required Education

A bachelor's degree in public administration, finance, or a related field, or its equivalent, is required. A master's degree in public administration, business administration, health care administration, or a closely related field is preferred.

Required Experience

The position requires eight years of management-related experience in health care facilities. Professional or managerial experience with public or nonprofit health care organizations is preferred.

An equivalent combination of related education and experience may be considered.

Other Requirements

There may be supplemental questions that must be answered and submitted with your application to complete this process. These questions will be e-mailed to you after the posting deadline.

Background Check

The state has determined that a criminal background check and qualifications check will be performed for this position.

Affirmative Action/Equal Opportunity Employment

This state is an affirmative action/equal opportunity employer.

assist HRM practitioners by helping them anticipate and forecast future organizational needs.

Changing responsibilities require employee flexibility. Employees are more involved in planning and controlling their own work. For organizations adapting to change, job descriptions are likely to be short-lived, so there needs to be a system of continuous work analysis. The shift to teamwork and self-managed groups requires greater emphasis on interactive activities.

Organizational citizenship behaviors and contextual performance have become more important as employees interact with a greater variety of people. Managing the emotional aspects of work, such as by displaying sensitivity toward culturally diverse individuals, is important. Emotional stability and other personality attributes have received little attention in conventional job analysis compared to cognitive and technical aspects of the job. However, interpersonal, team, and customer-oriented attributes can be decisive in many of today's work assignments and in such cases should be acknowledged.

An organization may want to not only review the way it analyzes work but also focus on the level of general characteristics important for success in the organization's culture and for dealing with change. For example, the emphasis could be on general categories of competencies important for success, such as adaptability, self-motivation, and trainability, in addition to job context and specific technical skills. The job description could incorporate a broader set of KSAOCs instead of specific tasks or behaviors.

COMPETENCY MODELING

Whereas typical a job analysis breaks a position down into KSAOCs, competency modeling is a method of collecting and organizing job information and worker attributes into broad competencies. **Competencies** are characteristics and qualities that a person needs to possess to perform a job successfully. A competency model incorporates a set of competencies that are necessary for effective performance, and it typically covers a broader range of jobs than traditional job analysis. Many organizations adopt a critical set of core competencies that are required of organization members across all jobs and all levels. Bartram (2005) has identified eight competencies for managerial positions (p. 1187):

- *Leading and deciding,* described as telling other people what to do and deciding what action to take

- *Supporting and cooperating,* described as working well with other people and being a team player

- *Interacting and presenting,* described as persuading others and possessing social confidence and presentation skills

- *Analyzing and interpreting,* described as effectively analyzing problems and being comfortable with data

- *Creating and conceptualizing,* described as dealing effectively with change and moving things forward according to the larger environment
- *Organizing and executing,* described as planning to meet objectives and ensuring customer satisfaction
- *Adapting and coping,* described as handling pressure and bouncing back after setbacks
- *Enterprising and performing,* described as focusing on results and understanding finances

Competencies have also been identified for positions in health care organizations (Accrediting Commission on Education for Health Services Administration, 1997; Affara, 2009; Pillay, 2008; West, 2002). The Accrediting Commission on Education for Health Services Administration (1997) has identified nine competency domains for health care managers:

- Structuring and positioning health organizations to achieve performance
- Financial management of health organizations under alternative financing mechanisms
- Demonstrating leadership, interpersonal, and communication skills in managing human resources and health professions in diverse organizational environments
- Managing information resources and collecting, analyzing, and using business and health information in decision making
- Application of statistical quantitative and economic analysis in decision making
- Legal and ethical analysis applied to business and clinical decision making
- Organizational and government health policy formulation and implementation
- Assessment and understanding of the status of populations and determinants of health and illness, and managing health risks and behaviors in diverse populations

- Developing, organizing, financing, and measuring the performance of health systems in diverse communities, drawing broadly on the social and behavioral sciences

The International Council of Nurses has identified competencies for the nurse specialist (Affara, 2009). They are grouped under three headings:

Professional, Ethical, and Legal Practice
- Accountability
- Ethical practice
- Legal practice

Care Provision and Management
- Health promotion
- Planning
- Evaluation
- Assessment
- Implementation
- Therapeutic communication and relationships
- Interprofessional health care
- Maintaining a safe environment
- Delegation and supervision

Professional, Personal, and Quality Development
- Enhancement of the profession
- Quality improvement
- Continuing education

JOB ANALYSIS TECHNIQUES

A variety of job analysis approaches have been developed over the years. These approaches gather information on job content and worker characteristics that are common to jobs across a wide spectrum. They might describe how the incumbent does the job, the behaviors that are required to perform the job, or the activities that are performed. Let's look at some of the common approaches analysts use.

Position Analysis Questionnaire

The Position Analysis Questionnaire (PAQ), developed by researchers at Purdue University, is a structured job analysis questionnaire consisting of 187 worker-oriented job activities and work situation variables divided into six categories:

- *Information input.* Where and how does the worker get the information that is used in performing the job?

- *Mental processes.* What reasoning, decision-making, planning, and information-processing activities are used in performing the job?

- *Work output.* What physical activities does the worker perform, and what tools or devices are used?

- *Relationships with other people.* What relationships are required in performing the job?

- *Job context.* In what physical and social contexts is the work performed?

- *Other job characteristics.* What activities, conditions, or characteristics other than those already described are relevant to the job?

The PAQ items are rated using different scales, including importance, amount of time required, extent of use, possibility of occurrence, applicability, and difficulty. It is scored by a computer, and a profile for the job is compared with standard profiles of known job families. The quantitative nature of the PAQ enables it to be used for evaluating job worth and for identifying applicable exams for screening applicants.

Department of Labor Procedure and Functional Job Analysis

The Department of Labor Procedure and Functional Job Analysis are comprehensive approaches that concentrate on the interactions among what an employee does with respect to data, people, and things (see Figure 7.1). In addition, the Functional Job Analysis considers the goals of the organization, what workers do to achieve those goals as part of their job, the level and orientation of what workers do, performance standards, and training content.

Comprehensive Occupation Data Analysis Program

The Comprehensive Occupation Data Analysis Program is a task inventory developed for U.S. Air Force specialties by the Air Training Command. Detailed task statements are written to describe their work. Each statement consists of an action, an object of the action, and essential modifiers. Incumbents are asked to indicate the relative amount of time they spend on each task. Responses are then clustered by computer analysis into occupational groupings so that jobs with similar tasks and the same relative time-spent values are listed together.

Job Element Method

The purpose of the job element method, developed by Ernest Primoff of the U.S. Office of Personnel Management, is to identify the behaviors and accompanying achievements that are significant for job success. A combination of behavior and achievements is referred to as an element. Elements may include job behaviors, intellectual behaviors, motor behaviors, and work habits.

A panel of SMEs identifies tasks significant to the job and then the KSAOCs necessary to perform the job. At this stage, the job tasks are turned into job elements. For example, the task "writes computer programs to perform statistical analyses, interprets the data, and writes reports" is transformed into the element "ability to write computer programs to perform statistical analyses, interpret data, and write reports."

The SMEs then rate the elements on four factors (Primoff, 1975, p. 3):

- *Barely acceptable.* What relative portion of even barely acceptable workers are good in the element?

- *Superior*. How important is the element in picking out the superior worker?

- *Trouble*. How much trouble is likely if the element is ignored when choosing among applicants?

- *Practical*. Is the element practical? To what extent can we fill our job openings if we demand it?

The ratings on these four factors are analyzed to identify the elements with the greatest potential for selecting superior applicants. The premise behind the job element method is that the same elements may traverse different tasks and different jobs. The federal government uses this method to establish selection standards and to validate selection examinations (Primoff & Eyde, 1988).

Occupational Information Network

The Occupational Information Network is a database compiled by the U.S. Department of Labor to provide basic occupational data. Its framework is organized around six sets of descriptors: worker requirements, experience requirements, worker characteristics, occupational requirements, occupation-specific requirements, and occupation characteristics. The information is available online (www.onetcenter.org/overview.html) and can be used to develop job descriptions, job specifications, and career opportunity information.

Contextual Performance Analysis

Contextual performance refers to aspects of performance unrelated to specific tasks. These include activities directed at enhancing the interpersonal and psychological environment that facilitate task completion. Borman and Motowidlo (1993) note that contextual activities are different from task activities or job performance. Whereas task activities contribute directly to the technical or core of an agency's or department's production of goods and services, contextual activities contribute to the social environment. Task activities may differ across jobs, and contextual activities are common to many if not all jobs. Task activities are also associated with skills or abilities, whereas contextual activities are associated with motivational or personality variables. Some examples of contextual behaviors are coming to work on time, working overtime on short notice when unexpected problems arise, helping others when needed, minimizing or solving conflicts within the work group, and training or mentoring newcomers (Guion & Highhouse, 2006).

Personality-Based Job Analysis

In an attempt to identify behaviors associated with contextual performance, researchers have developed personality-based job analysis instruments. Raymark, Schmit, and Guion (1997) developed an instrument based on twelve personality dimensions: general leadership, interest in negotiation, achievement striving, friendly disposition, sensitivity to others, collaborative work tendency, general trustworthiness, adherence to work ethic, attention to details, desire to generate ideas, tendency to think things through, and emotional stability. Other instruments used to identify personality measures are the Self-Descriptive Index (Guion, Highhouse, Reeve, & Zickar, 2005); the International Personality Item Pool (Goldberg, 1999); the NEO PI-R Job Profiler and NEO Job Personality Inventory (Costa, McCrae, & Kay, 1995; McCrae, 2002; McCrae & Costa, 2004); and the Position Classification Inventory (Gottfredson & Holland, 1994).

Team-Based Job Analysis

Because working in teams has become more important, job analysis questions and measures need to be developed to identify the job elements and competencies for successful collaboration and teamwork. The following issues are important in understanding what is required to successfully perform a job:

- *Task interdependence*. Within the team, jobs performed by team members are related to one another.

- *Goal interdependence*. Work goals come directly from the goals of the team.

- *Interdependent feedback and rewards*. Performance evaluations are strongly influenced by how well the team performs.

- *Communication and cooperation among groups*. Teams cooperate to get the work completed on time.

For a comprehensive compilation of different types of job analysis techniques and job analysis studies across a variety of occupations, refer to *The Job Analysis Handbook for Business, Industry, and Government* (Gael, 1988).

SUMMARY

Forecasting human resources needs is a critical component of SHRM. Organizations must assess past trends, evaluate their present situation, and project their human resources needs. Before they can make decisions on recruitment and selection or training and development objectives, organizations need to audit the skills and positions of their incumbent employees. This audit will provide information on the inventory of KSAOCs and positions available within the agency and will call attention to any KSAOCs or positions that may be missing. Jobs change, and the KSAOCs required to perform them also change. To remain competitive, agencies must keep abreast of changing skill and position requirements.

A job analysis not only is required for the planning and development of recruitment and selection strategies and for planning training and development programs but also provides the foundation for other HRM functions. A job analysis is essential for the development of compensation systems, for identifying job-related competencies that can be used to objectively evaluate employees' performance, for restructuring work activities, and for assessing risks in the workplace.

KEY TERMS

competencies

developing compensation systems

human resources planning, career
    development, and training

job description

job design

job family

performance evaluation

recruitment and selection

risk management

strategic job analysis

DISCUSSION QUESTIONS

1. Define job analysis.

2. Explain how job analyses affect the following areas: recruitment and selection; developing compensation systems; human resources planning, career development, and training; performance evaluation; risk management; and job design.

3. What types of information are usually collected during job analysis?

4. Discuss the most common methods of data collection for job analysis.

5. What types of information do job descriptions typically include?

6. What is competency modeling?

7. Describe two types of contextual performance analysis.

8

Recruitment, Interviewing, and Selection Strategies

LEARNING OBJECTIVES

- Understand the importance of recruitment and selection to strategic human resources management
- Recognize the opportunities for health care human resources maximization through effective recruitment and selection
- Understand how to proactively employ a targeted selection approach
- Be able to assist health care line managers in the selection process
- Discuss how technology is affecting the health care recruitment and selection process
- Understand how tests and techniques are used in selecting health care personnel

ONE OF THE most important concerns of health care human resources management is the selection of promising candidates for open positions who will contribute to the progressive improvement of performance across the organization. A high-performing new addition to a health care work team can provide inspiration and enhance team members' motivation as they benefit from the new addition's stellar performance. Conversely, the hiring of a lackluster new team member can create a recognizable performance gap because the deleterious work habits and absent motivation of this nonperformer will act as a contagion throughout the work group. Moreover, the effort required to motivate this individual—and ultimately to terminate his or her employment—will be extremely time-consuming, and this negative episode will become fodder for gossip among your already existent nonplayers.

Strategic planning for acquiring select new human capital for a progressive health care organization centers on truly proactive, progressive innovation throughout the hiring process, from job component analysis to interviewing, selection, and, finally, orientation of a new employee. Health care organizations that have not mastered these essential elements are constantly plagued by the trauma created by poor performers, whereas enlightened organizations that have successfully mastered the selection and orientation process diminish the likelihood that they will constantly have to terminate poor performers or address performance problems, instead allowing them to focus their management efforts on developing motivated, talented human resources.

The intent of this chapter is twofold: to directly provide counsel that will help health care human resources professionals hone their recruitment, interviewing, and selection strategies as well as to offer information that can help health care human resources professionals in providing targeted counsel and formal training to line managers in these important leadership capabilities.

PRESELECTION PROCESS

A common mistake among health care line managers in conducting their first interviews is to jump into the process without preparation. Frequently this happens because a new manager is immediately presented with a department that has several openings and a short time in which to fill them. Consequently, the new manager may review résumés without any forethought as to the type of individual needed or the long-range consequences of the selection decision. The next six subsections outline six recommended stages to incorporate into the preselection planning process:

1. Compiling a wish list

2. Compiling a list of expectations

3. Reviewing the job description

4. Reviewing recruitment tactics

5. Undertaking application and screening procedures

6. Reviewing résumés and setting an interviewing slate

Compiling a Wish List

The preselection process should begin with the compilation of a wish list through a true brainstorming process. This should start with a review of everything known about the open position, considering such criteria as the success-to-failure ratio of prior efforts to fill the position, line manager and human resources knowledge of the position, and any other significant input that can help determine critical needs for the position. In addition, gaining insight from individuals who have worked in that job position or have supervised a similar position about what makes for a successful performer in that particular job is a great first step in this process.

Outcomes from compiling this wish list should be both quantitative and qualitative, and should include the following:

- Job requirements (past, present, and future)

- Past success and failures associated with the position

- Potential expansion of the position

- Collective insights (from self, staff, and peers)

- Quantitative and technical requisites (things that can be measured by numbers, such as the typical jobholder's number of years in the field, total years' education, number of technical degrees and accreditation licenses, and number of years employed in the specific technical area)

- Qualitative factors (work personality, attitude, and ethic)

Qualitative outcomes incorporate factors that are not clearly measurable numerically but are nonetheless essential to the job; quantitative information indicates whether the individual *can* do the job, qualitative information indicates *how* he or she will do the job. For example, in filling the position of staff pharmacist, quantitative indicators would include a candidate's number of degrees, the number of years he or she has been a pharmacist, the number of licenses held in your organization's state (and number of years licensed overall), and the number of years working in the unique setting of a hospital pharmacy. Qualitative indicators would include attitude, such as the candidate's flexibility, persistence, and basic work ethic, and the people skills needed for interpersonal relations, such as communication skills, the ability to listen and perceive information, and the innate ability to create a positive presence and conduct daily interactions with customer-patients and fellow organization members with an appropriate, professional attitude.

A candidate's managerial aptitude would also be important, including the ability to use good judgment, be creative on demand, and plan daily activities. Furthermore, you would want to ensure that an applicant is a team player, is able to support other staff professionals, acts as a resource to other team members, and contributes to the group process. A values orientation, including strong loyalty to an organization, a sense of compassion for the customer-patient, and an intrinsic desire to respect the dignity of others, is also an essential qualitative criterion.

Compiling a List of Expectations

The next step in the preselection process is to establish a list of expectations consisting of the responsibilities that a prospective jobholder is expected to fulfill on a daily basis. A good strategy for this effort is to try to make this a "top ten" list of basic job elements that can subsequently provide the reporting line manager with a sound frame of reference in monitoring and measuring performance. The job description—if available and current (see Chapter Seven)—is a solid starting point, as is input that helps to craft a big-picture perspective on how the job position supports the entire organization.

As you analyze the particular job position, for example, try to use time proportions to determine its major activities. List all elements of the job that take up at least 10 percent of a "typical" day (given the unpredictable nature of the health care setting). In the case of the hospital pharmacist, for example, consider that a typical pharmacist spends at least 40 percent of the day actually filling prescriptions; "filling prescriptions" would be a paramount component of the expectations list. List all work activities that are undertaken daily and are essential parts of the basic job profile, and also consider which work contributions are most critical to overall departmental activity.

Use a wide variety of sources in compiling your analysis by garnering the input of others and, once you have established a draft of expectations, seeking the opinions of past holders of the job position. Outside review will provide you with a final checkpoint to ensure that your list is valid. Remember, use current top players as guides, as anyone currently in the position who consistently provides stellar performance and seems to do "all the right things" in the job position is a most useful model.

Reviewing the Job Description

The job description can be extremely helpful in the preselection planning process, as already mentioned. However, the current job description might not be accurate, might not reflect all the activities the job requires, and might have changed so much that it is only 50 percent (or less) accurate. As a result you might have a great constructive opportunity to review and restructure the job description's content and application by comparing your wish list and expectations to the prevailing job description to update it for accuracy. The new job description can act as the foundation for the employee's orientation and will be used throughout his or her work experience in each performance evaluation cycle.

Reviewing Recruitment Tactics

Recruitment is the process of attracting qualified candidates to apply for vacant positions within an organization. **Selection** is the final stage of the recruitment process, when decisions are made as to who will be selected for the vacant positions. Both recruitment and selection require effective planning to determine the human resources needs of the organization. The organization must determine its immediate objectives and future direction, and it must forecast its employment needs so these are aligned with the organization's strategies.

To fill positions, health care organizations have a wealth of choices relative to recruitment sources, as illustrated in Figure 8.1. They can recruit new employees, they can promote or transfer incumbent employees who possess the skills necessary for the vacant positions, or they can provide training or educational support to lower-level or paraprofessional employees in anticipation of future needs.

Recruitment is an ongoing process in most organizations; however, often it is not planned and is therefore less successful than it could be. For recruitment to be successful, planning is essential. Recruitment efforts must be consistent with the agency's mission. Employers must understand how to determine the job requirements, where to seek applicants, and how to screen them so that qualified and competent individuals are selected.

As already discussed, before recruitment for candidates begins, the human resources management (HRM) recruiter and the line manager should review the qualifications needed for the vacant position or positions. This review enables them to identify the knowledge, skills, abilities, and other characteristics (KSAOCs) they will be looking for in the applicants, and it will guide them in developing an accurate job bulletin or advertisement.

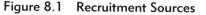

Figure 8.1   Recruitment Sources

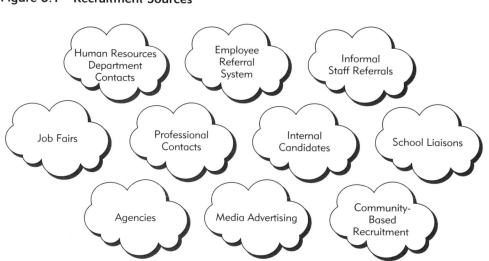

They should also identify different career patterns that can fit within the department or agency's framework. Many prospective employees have expectations, needs, and interests that are different from those of previous generations, which means agencies must offer a wider variety of employer-employee relationships and recruit differently than they have in the past (U.S. Office of Personnel Management, 2006).

Recruitment is certainly one of the most difficult endeavors for a progressive health care organization due to the unfortunate shortage of qualified personnel in virtually all health care positions. The past two decades, for example, saw immense shortages in both the United States and Canada in the ranks of nurses, pharmacists, physical therapists, and dietitians. This mandates creative and comprehensive work by health care human resources professionals to generate a good roster of candidates and as many recruitment sources as possible. There are ten recruitment resources, described briefly in the following subsections, that will resonate with your line managers.

Human Resources Management Department Contacts

The human resources management department should already have a network of contacts that can assist in recruiting, from placement agencies to local schools, and certainly a bank of résumés from individuals who have contacted the department for employment opportunities or who were past candidates for previously open positions at your health care organization.

Job Fairs

Job fairs can provide good opportunities for meeting contacts and identifying potential talent, and health care human resources staff members should endeavor to attend job fairs in specific high-demand technical areas. This will help build a data bank of talent in your technical specialty areas. Although certain job fair attendees are simply shopping around and are not interested in immediate employment, collecting résumés and obtaining information on potential candidates is a continuous process, and one that should be undertaken at every opportunity.

School Liaison Programs

Many health care professionals maintain contact with the school (or schools) they graduated from, whether a nursing school, four-year university, or other accredited academic institution. Establish a list of alma mater ties across your line manager cadre, and contact the placement offices at the schools accordingly to see what "up-and-coming talent" might be suitable for your organization. The placement and alumni staff at these schools certainly will know alumni in the field who might be suitable candidates for your open positions. In a similar vein, if you are seeking to fill an entry-level position or an unskilled job role, you might contact a guidance counselor at a local high school or vocational school and inquire about possible candidates.

Employee Referral System

Most organizations have an employee referral system that assists in recruitment. Basically, this is a system through which employees refer qualified individuals to the personnel office for openings in the organization that have been posted by the human resources management department in a central area and on the organization's Web site. If your organization does not have an employee referral system, or if you work in a small health care organization, implement a system in which a monetary reward (or extra day of vacation!) is extended to any employee who recommends a candidate for an open position who is successfully hired. Employee referral systems give individuals the opportunity to participate in their organization's selection process, to have a hand in selecting their fellow workers, and to earn recognition.

Professional Contacts

Many health care managers have regional and national professional contacts. If you have a need for a physical therapist (PT), for example, contact your organization's PTs who have worked at other health care organizations. You can enlist your PTs to contact these other institutions and check with their former colleagues as to the availability of potential candidates; you can then inquire into their knowledge of sharp people in the field who might be looking for a job.

Agencies

Many health care recruiters frown on placement and search agencies, largely because of a perception that agencies require the largest expenditure out of all recruitment sources for a marginal return on investment. However, agencies that have proven track records, make an effort to understand the unique needs and nuances of your particular health care organization, and have demonstrated a consistent ability to provide the desired quality of talent should certainly be considered in your recruitment effort. You should therefore spend as much time as possible with the primary recruiter in reviewing your wish list, expectations list, and revised job description. This will help to weed out unqualified candidates while saving time, money, and energy.

Media Advertising

Health care institutions run employment advertisements regularly. Media advertising can be somewhat expensive and unfortunately does not provide consistently good results. When taking this route, efforts should be made to ensure that the advertisement is run in such a way as to yield the best advantage possible. This involves ensuring good placement within the newspaper or magazine; having a catchy logo; and including a three-to-five-sentence depiction of the job, the salary range, and the name of a specific contact person in the human resources office. These elements will eliminate candidates who are simply job shopping or who are not seeking the salary range established for the position.

Informal Staff Referrals

Current staff members probably know of someone who might be qualified for the open position. However, unless they are asked, they may assume you are not interested in their recommendations. Furthermore, because they are busy and preoccupied with their own job responsibilities, human resources professionals must make a concerted effort to ask appropriate department staff members for recommendations. In many cases they can be the most knowledgeable about the position as well as possible successful applicants, so encouraging their participation can be a particularly efficacious strategy.

Internal Candidates

Health care organizations should first look at current staff to fill vacancies. For **internal recruitment** to work, progressive health care organizations need to be proactive and incorporate strategic planning into their human resources practices. Organizations must track the KSAOCs needed for the various jobs within the organization, and they should identify employees who possess the needed skills, whether administrative, managerial, or technological. Human resources management departments and department managers should work together and make workforce projections based on employees' current skill levels. They should review transfers, retirements, promotions, and termination patterns and do succession planning to identify individuals who might fill positions when incumbents leave. This requires keeping track of and updating the records of each employee's KSAOCs and the demands required of each position. A human resources information system can sort employee data by education, career interests, work histories, occupational fields, and other factors.

Many organizations favor internal recruitment because administrators have the opportunity to review and evaluate the KSAOCs of internal applicants prior to selection. Choosing internal candidates also enables agencies to recoup the investment they have made in recruiting, selecting, training, and developing their current employees. Promoting qualified incumbent employees rewards them for their performance and signals to other employees that the agency is committed to their development and advancement.

Before organizations limit recruitment efforts to internal recruitment, however, other factors should be considered. Some positions in health care organizations require specialized skills that may not be found within the agency or unit, and for such positions it may be necessary to recruit and hire from outside.

A qualified applicant for an open position may already be somewhere within your organization, perhaps in another department or at an affiliated facility. Some individuals might have applied directly for a new position, or might have indicated an interest in a new job on their performance evaluation. Internal promotion is a great morale builder when an outstanding employee is the beneficiary; ignoring or excluding a qualified internal candidate is a morale buster. To ensure the former, build a file of qualified internal candidates for certain job positions and use personal development plans so that when a position opens you have a file folder of immediate possibilities.

Community-Based Recruitment

Smaller health care providers, particularly in rural areas or in distinct neighborhoods (of large East Coast cities, for example) use community-based recruitment. These institutions take a three-to-five-sentence depiction of the open position, point of contact, and salary range, and make copies on their stationary. They post these copies on bulletin boards in five key areas within the community: (1) supermarkets and convenience stores (which have high traffic and prominent bulletin boards); (2) libraries and other community centers (which also have high traffic and common bulletin boards); (3) post offices (which always have bulletin boards or areas for posting notices); (4) places of worship (which commonly have posting areas); and (5) cleaners or uniform stores (an often-overlooked opportunity—health care people wear uniforms!).

When using community-based recruitment, be sure to get permission from the appropriate authority at each posting area. Getting authorities' permission is also an opportunity for you to gain their support and participation in the search effort by having them review the contents of your notice and discussing any potential applicants they might know among their customers or congregation members. Business and religious anchors in the community are almost always willing and positive allies in the health care recruitment process.

Undertaking Application and Screening Procedures

Once the organization has communicated its need to fill positions and applicants have responded, it moves on to screening the applicants to identify those with the requisite KSAOCs.

Employment applications are often the first step in the screening process. Applicants fill out a form asking them to answer a variety of questions. The questions must not violate local, state, or federal employment discrimination laws. The rule followed by the Equal Employment Opportunity Commission, state agencies, and most courts is that if the employer asks a question on an employment application form, it is assumed that the answer is used in the hiring process. If the question does not pertain to the job applicant's qualification for the job in question, the question may be held illegal if it has a disparate impact on a protected group. When developing an application, an organization should refer to the state's fair employment laws to eliminate any potential discriminatory questions. Questions about age, race, gender, and disability are permitted only when responding is voluntary and the information is required for record-keeping purposes. Equal employment opportunity data should be collected by the personnel office and should not be used to screen out applicants.

Most applications are generic and not tailored for any one position. They usually provide limited space for applicants to provide detailed information about relevant work or educational experience. A supplemental questionnaire should be developed that asks questions related to the specific job to facilitate the screening process.

After individuals apply for a position, the applications need to be screened to identify a list of qualified applicants and eliminate unqualified applicants. This process is different for each position. It is not uncommon for a large urban government that is recruiting firefighters to receive hundreds of applications. Positions typically inundated by applicants use multiple screening procedures to pare down the number of candidates. The first screen is to weed out applicants who do not meet the minimum requirements, such as age (for example, law enforcement positions require applicants to be at least twenty-one years old); level of education; or required certification. The second screen might eliminate applicants who lack the requisite experience.

For administrative or professional positions, which usually have more stringent education and experience requirements, there are likely to be fewer applicants. To reduce the number of applicants to the most qualified, it is important to have preestablished criteria to facilitate the screening. Requiring previous experience as a city planner or community development specialist might be one standard. Requiring previous financial management experience with a budget of $2 million might be another. To screen résumés, an instrument, such as a checklist, might be developed to keep track of the relevant experience and education required. Anybody who has spent time reading many résumés knows that after the first ten or so, fatigue sets in. You become less attentive as the review progresses. A checklist keeps you focused on the salient KSAOCs.

Background investigations have become more common, and not only for public safety and homeland security positions: health care is perceived as—and often is—a public trust. Employees and volunteers working with children must undergo a background investigation and have their fingerprints reviewed by law enforcement agencies to screen out pedophiles or individuals with criminal histories. The Internet has created informal means, not necessarily sanctioned by a given agency, to screen applicants. Conducting a Google search may provide news reports, press releases, or even blogs disclosing an applicant's personal characteristics. Visits to social networking sites, such as MySpace, Facebook, and Xanga, have also been used to ascertain if there are pictures of or comments made by the applicant that might embarrass the agency.

Employment screening techniques and tests must comply with the general principles and technical requirements of the Uniform Guidelines on Employee Selection Procedures (1978), which apply to public, for-profit, and nonprofit organizations. Preemployment testing is used to measure the KSAOCs of applicants and predict their ability to perform a job. It is an attempt to standardize the screening process and determine whether applicants possess the characteristics necessary to be successful on the job. Both the Uniform Guidelines and the Principles for the Validation and Use of Personnel Selection Procedures, developed by the American Psychological Association (Society for Industrial and Organizational Psychology, 2003), broadly define tests as a variety of instruments or procedures used in the selection or promotion process.

Following are some of the selection techniques commonly used in employment settings, as well as alternative approaches:

- **Cognitive ability and aptitude tests** are designed to reflect the general and the specific capabilities and potentials of the individual applicant by measuring verbal, quantitative, nonverbal, and oral skills, or motor functions. For example, mechanical ability, numerical aptitude, finger dexterity, or perceptual accuracy could be measured. These tests are used to determine whether applicants possess the aptitude to learn the KSAOCs required in the position.

- **Achievement tests** are designed to measure the degree of mastery of specific material to assess whether an individual has profited from prior experience and gained specific knowledge. Most of the items on achievement tests assess whether the individual possesses specific knowledge of concepts considered critical for a job. Trade tests are an example of this type.

- **Personality inventories** are designed to assess a person's typical behavioral traits and characteristics by measuring such factors as dominance, sociability, self-control, or introversion and extroversion. Some of the more common personality tests used in the public sector are the Minnesota Multiphasic Personality Inventory, the California Psychological Inventory, and the Edwards Personal Preference Schedule. They are used when interpersonal skills are key to successful performance.

- **Interest inventories** are designed to predict job choice behavior rather than job performance by ascertaining the occupational likes and dislikes of the individual and indicating the occupational areas that are most likely to be satisfying to that person. They are used to make a compatible person-job match.

- **Experience and training rating** is a procedure that quantifies the education, experience, training, achievements, and other relevant data that applicants provide on job applications and questionnaires. Points are assigned to applicants based on the number of years of experience, education, and training relevant to the position. Experience and training exams are often referred to as unassembled examinations.

- **Structured oral exams** are used to evaluate job requirements that are not easily assessed by paper-and-pencil measures, such as interpersonal, oral communication, and supervisory skills. Although the specifics of the exams may differ, all structured oral exams share similar components. They are based on a job analysis that captures the critical KSAOCs necessary for the position. The questions are job related, and all applicants are asked the same questions. Rating scales are used to evaluate the responses, and the raters receive training prior to conducting the examination. Structured oral exams are used a great deal in the public sector.

- **Work sample or performance tests** require applicants to demonstrate that they possess the necessary skills needed for successful job performance. Applicants are asked to perform tasks that are representative of actual job activities. For example, applicants applying for the position of editor of a nonprofit newsletter may be asked to write and edit copy, and applicants applying for a training position could be required to prepare and present a training module.

- **In-basket exercises** are written tests designed to simulate administrative tasks. They consist of correspondence designed to be representative of the job's actual tasks. A set of instructions usually states that applicants should imagine that they have been placed in the position and must deal with the memos and other items that have accumulated in their in-basket. The test is used to measure skills pertaining, for example, to task prioritization, written communication, and judgment.

- **Drug testing** has become commonplace for reasons of on-the-job safety. Drug-dependent employees are more likely than nondependent employees to be involved in workplace accidents.

- Decreased productivity, increased absenteeism, and threats to fellow employees' or clients' safety are some of the problems manifested by substance abusers (Office of National Drug Control Policy, 2004). Consequently, many organizations have instituted drug testing as part of preemployment screening. It is important to note that applicants do not have the same rights as employees. Although applicants for a position may be tested for substance abuse at the organization's request, organizations do not necessarily have the right to test employees who are already on the payroll.

- **Lie detector exams** are permitted in certain circumstances. The Employee Polygraph Protection Act of 1988 prevents employers involved in or affecting interstate commerce from using lie detectors. It is unlawful for employers to require prospective employees to take lie detector tests or for employers to use test results or a worker's refusal or failure to take a test as grounds for failure to promote, for discharge, or for discipline. The law does not, however, apply to the federal government, state or local governments, or any political subdivision of a state or local government. Other exemptions include individuals or consultants working under contract for federal intelligence agencies; makers and distributors of controlled substances; and security companies whose business involves the protection of currency, financial instruments, or vital facilities or materials.

- The right of a public employer to require a public employee to take a lie detector test may be limited by state statute. Federal law and most state laws prohibit questions that ask about the applicant's views on religion, politics, race, and unions, or on sexual and marital matters. Subjects must be informed of their rights, and written consent must be obtained before administering the test. The test results must remain confidential, and only licensed, bonded examiners may administer the tests. Polygraph exams are used primarily for law enforcement and public safety positions.

- **Honesty and integrity tests** are lawful under the Employee Polygraph Protection Act of 1988 and most state polygraph laws. There are two kinds of honesty and integrity tests: overt and personality. Overt tests deal with attitudes toward theft or admission of theft or other illegal activities. Personality tests do not look at honesty per se but at a variety of counterproductive work behaviors, such as impulsiveness, nonconformance, and dislike of authority.

- **Physical ability tests** are used when a significant level of physical activity is involved in performing the job. In the public sector, physical ability tests are used most often in the selection of law enforcement and public safety officers, such as police officers, firefighters, corrections officers, and park and conservation safety officials. These tests require applicants to demonstrate their ability to perform actual or simulated job-related tasks. They are not medical examinations, and they do not seek information concerning the existence, nature, or severity of a physical or mental impairment or information concerning an applicant's health. They may be administered at the pre-offer stage.

  Physical ability testing has replaced height and weight requirements, which were often used to screen applicants, resulting in adverse impacts on women and Hispanics, and they were difficult to defend as being job related. Agencies have turned instead to physical ability tests that were developed to replicate the physical tasks necessary to perform specific jobs (Arvey, Nutting, & Landon, 1992; Hughes, Ratliff, Purswell, & Hadwiger, 1989).

- **Psychological examinations,** such as aptitude tests, personality tests, honesty tests, and IQ tests, are intended to measure applicants' capacity and propensity to perform a job successfully and are not considered to be medical examinations. Psychological tests that result in a clinical diagnosis and require interpretation by a health care professional are considered medical examinations and are prohibited at the pre-offer stage.

Reviewing Résumés and Setting an Interviewing Slate

The preselection planning process now continues with the résumé review, in which a slate of candidates from the applicant pool is established for in-person interviews. The main objective in reviewing résumés is to determine which candidates *could* do the job; the purpose of the subsequent interviews is to determine *how* they would do the job by using your wish list, expectations list, and job description to try to establish a match with the résumés. It is important to remember that you will never (or at least very seldom) find a "perfect" match, so avoid being fooled by the product of a good résumé-writing service.

Sort the résumés by your criteria, and organize the candidates into three basic categories as depicted in Figure 8.2. The first category should be individuals who are not qualified because they simply do not have the quantitative skills vital for the job position, such as the required degree(s) or years of experience (or specific experience) required. The second category is made up of possible candidates who definitely have the quantitative skills needed as well as possibly the additional factors that merit consideration. For example, for the position of staff pharmacist, an individual in the "possible" category would have all the necessary degrees, including the specific professional accreditation to prepare for state compliance reviews, and a good range of years of professional experience. Furthermore, this candidate might have good experience working as part of a team, as evidenced by information on the résumé and by the number of employment years at the current or a previous health care organization.

The third category consists of probable candidates, which is likely to be the lightest but most valuable grouping, as it is made up of the individuals who seem most qualified in most aspects of the subject position. Again using the hospital pharmacist example, assume that you have received a résumé from an individual who not only has all the quantitative characteristics but also has completed several successful state reviews, worked as a team leader, participated as part of a quality management process throughout the entire organization and perhaps in several employee relations committees, and currently works at a hospital nearly equal in size and scope to yours. Assume further that the candidate works with youth groups on the weekends (as indicated in the personal interests section of the résumé) and therefore

Figure 8.2   Candidate Evaluation

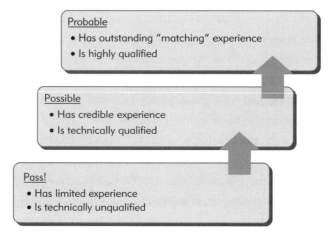

probably has terrific people skills. This candidate goes into your "probable" file and will almost certainly merit interview consideration.

After you have completed this process and sent thank-you letters to the unqualified candidates, establish a "short list" roster of a maximum of seven interview candidates. Beginning with your probable group, rank them in numerical order based on your insight and your summary perception from the preselection process. If you have fewer than seven candidates in this category, go to your possible group to complete your list of seven candidates and keep any remaining candidates from the possible group on file for any future job considerations.

Some salient points to remember at this stage:

- Often the best candidate is not necessarily the one with the best résumé, so don't fall into the seductive trap of reading too much into a résumé.

- Try to take the information at face value—that is, remember that the résumé is simply a summary of qualifications, not an in-depth insight into the applicant's personality.

- A good rule of thumb is to review résumés strictly based on quantitative characteristics, with only an initial thought to qualitative characteristics.

- Usually any résumé that is more than three pages in scope might be a bit too lengthy. This must be taken in context, however. For example, if you are reviewing the curriculum vitae of a research scientist, ten pages might be too short. The best rule of thumb in this case is to consider what is appropriate for the position, based on what your instincts tell you.

- Don't be overwhelmed by the résumé review process or consider its parameters to be absolute. In establishing a list of seven, you are simply coming up with the best seven candidates who will be the first to be interviewed.

- The individual who appears to be the best candidate should be the first one you interview so that he or she sets a basis of comparison throughout the selection process, and should be the first one scheduled for an interview so that he or she can pick the time and location for the interview.

The résumé review process simply helps you establish a pool of qualified candidates who will be interviewed, and in many cases one person will be your candidate of choice. If none of the candidates in this initial pool measures up completely to your satisfaction, you will simply establish another pool. The objective is to strike a balance between the "perfect" candidate and a "somewhat suitable" candidate in a realistic manner. In progressing through the next subsection, you will see more clearly how this process works.

CRITICAL DIMENSIONS OF EXTERNAL RECRUITMENT

External recruitment is the seeking of qualified applicants from outside the organization. The health care organization searches for applicants from the relevant labor market, defined by the skills required for the position and the location (geographical region) in which those skills can be found. For example, local labor markets are neighborhoods, towns, cities, or metropolitan statistical areas. Laborer, office and clerical, technical, and direct service provider positions are often filled from the local labor market, and it is common for health care organizations to recruit clerical and trade employees, such as maintenance or custodial personnel, from this source.

Regional labor markets are larger. They usually comprise a particular county, several areas of a state, or even the entire state. Depending on the skill supply in the region, technical, managerial, and professional workers, as well as scientists and engineers, may be recruited from a regional labor market. Agencies in the metropolitan St. Louis area, Washington DC, Metro New York–New Jersey, and the New England area, for example, can use the regional labor market to recruit applicants for all kinds of positions because of the large number and variety of colleges, universities, and medical facilities located there. Agencies in the federal government, such as the Department of Veterans Affairs, the Centers for Disease Control and Prevention, and the Department of Health and Human Services, may recruit nationally through regional offices for professional positions.

Technology has made information more accessible to job seekers. Personal-computer-based kiosks provide job seekers with current job information at the touch of a finger. At the federal level, job seekers can access USAJOBS, an automated employment information system in which all federal jobs are announced by telephone, fax, personal computer, and touch-screen kiosk. This system includes vacancy announcements and application forms and is available around the clock. Applicants can search for job opportunities using a variety of criteria, such as job title, keyword, agency location, and pay. They can create a federal résumé, store it on the site, and in some instances use it to apply for multiple federal jobs (U.S. Merit Systems Protection Board, 2008). New employees under thirty years of age used to rely on college-related sources, such as job fairs and college placement offices. Now, such job boards as Monster.com, JobsOnline, and Indeed.com allow employers to post jobs or search for candidates.

Many large heath care agencies, such as hospitals or public health departments, post open positions and accept applications on their own Web sites. There are also Web sites tailored for specific types of health care positions, such as Hospital Jobs Online, Physicians Employment, and HEALTHeCAREERS network.

When advertising is part of the recruitment process, advertisements should be written in a manner that will attract responses from qualified individuals and deter responses from those who are not qualified. It is important for an advertisement to focus on the job qualifications required for the position so that only candidates with qualifications matching the requirements of the position desire to apply.

To comply with the Americans with Disabilities Act, employers should inform applicants on an application form or job advertisement that the hiring process includes specific selection procedures (for example, a written test; demonstration of job skills, such as typing, making a presentation, or editing a report; or an interview). Applicants should be asked to inform the employer within a reasonable time period prior to the administration of the selection procedure of any reasonable accommodation needed to take a preemployment examination, participate in an interview, or demonstrate a job skill. Employers may request from the applicant documentation verifying the need for an accommodation.

The Immigration Reform and Control Act of 1986, as revised in 1990, prohibits the initial or continued employment of unauthorized aliens and provides civil and criminal penalties for violations of this law. However, the law also prohibits employment discrimination on the basis of national origin or citizenship status. The purpose of this provision is to discourage employers from attempting to comply with the prohibition against hiring unauthorized aliens by refusing to hire applicants who look foreign or have foreign-sounding names.

In 2007 U.S. Citizenship and Immigration Services revised Form I-9, which is used to verify employment eligibility in the United States. It updated the form in response to the Illegal Immigration Reform and Immigrant Responsibility Act of 1996, which mandated a reduction in the number of documents that employers may accept from newly hired employees. Employers should use the revised form for individuals hired on or after November 7, 2007. Employers may apply for temporary H-1B visas for temporary foreign workers. H-IB visas allow U.S. employers to employ foreign guest workers in specialty occupations. A specialty occupation requires theoretical and practical application of a body of specialized knowledge, and guest workers must hold at least a bachelor's degree or its equivalent. For example, architecture, engineering, mathematics, the physical sciences, the social sciences, medicine and health, education, business specialties, accounting, law, theology, and the arts are specialty occupations.

PREPARING AND PLANNING FOR THE INTERVIEW

The interviewing human resources professional and line manager must comprehensively prepare for the interview by being as thoroughly knowledgeable about the candidate's background as possible so that critical areas targeted for discussion get the most interview time. Proper preparation also shows the candidate that the interviewer is interested enough to take time to learn about the candidate, which will enhance comfort and flow and also indicate to the candidate that the progressive health care organization cares about quality in its process and about people, beyond the usual self-promoting clichés.

Preparation incorporates the processes of reviewing all applications and résumés, targeting several in-depth interviewing dimensions, analyzing a compendium of key factors in each one, and choosing appropriate questions to adjust the scope and maximize the productivity of the session. Important indicators include length of time in school, grade point average, extracurricular activities, and relevant work history. The interviewer should ensure that all relevant factors are considered, including any expertise obtained outside the health care arena that would have value in the field. For example, few guest relations experts have previously worked in health care; their work history usually encompasses work in the resort, restaurant, or hotel and motel fields. However, the skills they need in those fields are not vastly different from what they need in the health care arena, as firms in these fields, such as Marriott, are considered to be exemplary not only in their primary business but also in their forays into health care food management.

Other considerations for bridging résumé review and interview focus include

- The quality of the organization in which the candidate currently works or previously worked

- The scope and responsibilities of the candidate's current job

- The reporting relationships of the candidate's current or last job position, its financial responsibilities, its physical and staff resources, and its teamwork dimensions

- The source of the application (for example, direct, via an agency, from a college placement office) for the position, which should be reviewed and assessed as part of the interview preparation process

When preparing for an interview, be certain to have on hand the candidate's résumé, a notepad, and a set of prepared questions. Use targeted interviewing questions to structure a set of questions appropriate for the interview; you can add a professional touch by using a file folder bearing your organization's logo and placing the résumé and your questions on the right-hand side of the folder. With this folder and notepad, you'll be well organized and convey to each candidate that he or she is interviewing for a position with a well-structured organization that has a high regard for professional conduct.

In preparing the structure of the interview, use targeted selection questions that will give you the maximum information you need to match the candidate's skills and personality to the qualitative criteria that you established on your wish list. Each question will generate at least two to five minutes of response time if asked properly, so ten to fifteen questions should be more than enough for the conduct of a thirty- to forty-five-minute interview. Review the résumé one final time prior to the interview to make certain that you have areas targeted for questioning and that you have a strong grasp of the candidate's background.

CONDUCTING THE INTERVIEW

Several guidelines should be followed throughout the interview to make it an effective tool. The candidate's feelings and self-esteem should be respected above all else at all times; the candidate will make an assessment of the organization based on his or her experience during the interview—and, fundamentally, the candidate is interviewing you and your organization as much as you are interviewing the candidate. Therefore, even if you are having a bad day, it is essential that you maintain professional courtesy and a positive demeanor.

Strive to put the candidate at ease and maintain comfort and candidate flow. Many industrial psychologists debate whether an interviewer should conduct the interview from behind a desk or in a setting in which interviewer and interviewee sit in two chairs facing each other in close proximity. The bottom line in this debate: do whatever is most comfortable for you because any discerning candidate will sense your behavioral cues and react accordingly. So if you appear nervous, the candidate will become edgy; if you appear comfortable, the candidate will be at ease. Candidate comfort is key to garnering candid and extensive information about the candidate's background, so set up the interview forum in the manner that will facilitate maximum comfort for the candidate and interviewer.

An interview should be a pleasant exchange of ideas, not an interrogation. The problem with the so-called stress interviews, so fashionable in the late 1970s, was that they only monitored one psychological reaction—how a candidate handled stress. Interviews using this technique fail to get a good look at the candidate's qualifications for the position. If the interview is a pleasant exchange of ideas—a professional conversation and an opportunity for both the interviewer and interviewee to learn more about their mutual fit—the interview has met its objective. The interview, then, should give you a microcosmic view of the candidate's professional life. There is nothing mystical about the interview, nor is it an in-depth psychological assessment—however, it is your main tool in selecting an important team member.

Begin the interview with a pleasant, professional introduction and initiate some appropriate light conversation. There are three topics you can always discuss with a candidate to begin an interview correctly and to set the stage for a professional conversation. You can always talk about the weather, traffic, and how the candidate traveled to your facility, and about a nonthreatening piece of information from the résumé to help initiate conversation. For example, the fact that the candidate attended the same college as you can provide an opener. At the initial meeting, take note of how the candidate introduces himself or herself. Use whatever title is used in the introduction, such as Dr., Mrs., Ms., Mr., a religious title, or simply a preferred nickname or first name; once again, the key is comfort, so whatever form of address the candidate uses is probably the name or title preferred. Use this title appropriately throughout the interview, as it will increase familiarity and again underscore the fact that this is a professional conversation, not an inquisition. As you open the interview, thank the candidate for coming down, and explain that you will be asking a series of questions concerning his or her background and potential for the job, and that you will be taking notes. Finally, use the outset of the interview to explain to the candidate not only the time parameters of the interview but also that there will be time at the end of the interview to ask questions.

As you begin your questioning, remember to start off with the prototypical "life story" question: "Tell me about yourself, beginning with . . . " The open-ended segment of this question should be filled starting with the point at which the candidate entered the health care workforce, or began secondary education in college or professional school. For example, you might ask the candidate, "Tell me about yourself, starting with your graduation from [name of college]." Usually a candidate is well prepared for this question, and it increases the comfort level following the light conversation. It also signals to the candidate that you have now assumed control of the interview and that it is time for the candidate to start presenting his or her ideas and credentials through a comprehensive overview of his or her background, from which you can begin your specific questioning.

As the interview progresses, remember to ask as many questions as needed to elicit the responses you require to make a clear determination about the candidate's suitability. In addition to asking targeted selection questions, use a rejoining process involving both verbal and nonverbal triggers. For example, follow up with the candidate with such verbal rejoinders as "Tell me more about that," "Give me another example," "What else was involved?" and "Why?" These verbal rejoinders will make the candidate's response fuller in scope, add to the context of the interview, and provide you with specific information essential to your evaluation of the candidate. It is important to use verbal rejoinders whenever the candidate appears to be stalled in a particular area, is hesitant about answers, or has given an abbreviated answer. Use rejoinders freely to trigger new lines of response, to get additional information in a specific area, or to clarify the candidate's response.

Nonverbal rejoinders can be equally important in this regard. Such rejoinders include eye contact, facial gestures, hand gestures, and any other nonverbal communication that might encourage the candidate. It is essential that you not lead the candidate toward a desired end, so do not react emotionally in either a verbal or nonverbal manner. Rather, maintain steady eye contact throughout the course of the interview, and clearly demonstrate that you are vitally interested in what the candidate is saying without rendering immediate judgment.

The key words *pleasant* and *professional* should be your guiding lights in using nonverbal communication throughout the interview. As you conduct the interview, keep in mind your role as the organization's representative—to the candidate, you *are*, in the candidate's perception, the progressive health care organization. In addition, the interview is a public relations tool in health care, as a potential candidate from your health care organization's service area is also a potential customer-patient. Therefore, you want to give the candidate as many opportunities as possible to answer a question fully and be patient in allowing him or her to respond. Let the candidate do most of the talking; a good guideline is to allow the candidate at least 80 to 85 percent of the interview "airtime," with you doing 15 to 20 percent of the talking, as demonstrated in Figure 8.3. On the one hand, a candidate who is talking 90 to 95 percent of the time is probably going into areas from which you do not need information; or you are not guiding him or her strongly enough toward your objectives. On the other hand, if you are talking 30 percent of the time, either the candidate is not seizing the opportunity to present his or her background assertively, or you are not affording the candidate opportunities to do so. Finally, if a candidate cannot convince an interviewer of the value of his or her potential and past background, it is unlikely that the candidate will be a strong communicator and advocate of the health care organization if hired.

In questioning a candidate, try to avoid closed-ended question, case study questions, or legally sensitive questions. Closed-ended questions require a simple yes-or-no response, thus adding little to the interview and

---

Figure 8.3   Interview Dyad Dynamics

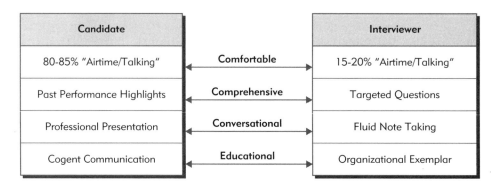

Candidate		Interviewer
80-85% "Airtime/Talking"	Comfortable	15-20% "Airtime/Talking"
Past Performance Highlights	Comprehensive	Targeted Questions
Professional Presentation	Conversational	Fluid Note Taking
Cogent Communication	Educational	Organizational Exemplar

providing you with minimal useful information. In case study questions, you present a situation to a candidate and seek a rhetorical or hypothetical answer rather than a practical insight into his or her problem-solving ability. These questions also have limited value because a candidate merely demonstrates that he or she can resolve a pertinent situation in theory. A better way of getting at this information is to ask a question along the lines of "Tell me about the most difficult operational problem you had to resolve." This forces the candidate to provide his or her own case and gives you a realistic, not a theoretical, perspective on ability.

Direct questions about a candidate's religious beliefs, race, sexual orientation, family status, marital status, or age are strictly prohibited by federal law. However, once a candidate volunteers a certain amount of information, the material becomes open ground if it is relative to job performance, and should be addressed tactfully and effectively. Assume that you are assisting a nursing manager seeking to hire a staff nurse who will work alternately on both the night and day shifts, and one of your more qualified applicants is a young woman who has a family at home, as gleaned from her application or disclosed in the initial stages of her interview. Rather than waiting for this candidate to volunteer information on marital or family status, simply make the following statement: "This particular job requires alternating on the night and day shifts, often with no more than half a day's notice in terms of when you might be working. Does that present any major problems?" This is a legally valid way of asking this question, and the candidate thus has a fair opportunity to alleviate any concerns you had about this bona fide (Latin for "good and true") occupational qualification.

Finally, the interviewer should tell the candidate in appropriate detail the next steps of the organization's recruitment process. If the candidate wants to ask additional questions (which indicates interest and aggressiveness in varying degrees), he or she should be told that perhaps an opportunity to discuss things further will present itself in the future. A candidate may occasionally request immediate feedback on his or her performance and potential for selection; the interviewer should counter this aggressive ploy by tactfully explaining to the candidate that although the interview was enjoyable and enlightening, there are other candidates to be interviewed before a final decision is made. As previously mentioned, in the health care business word of mouth is the most powerful advertising force; to not follow-up appropriately after an interview foolishly risks bad publicity, so the interviewer should in all cases thank the candidate and express appreciation for his or her time and interest.

EVALUATING THE INTERVIEW

Three facets of candidate disclosure are central to evaluating the interview. The first area is interview behavior. For example, if you need a worker who has a high degree of energy, try to gauge the candidate's energy level in the interview process. An individual who has a positive outlook and is somewhat animated and enthusiastic probably would have a suitable energy level for the position that you are trying to fill. The second area is work philosophy and beliefs. Candidates at all levels of a health care organization will state their commitment to the health care mission as well as to the customer-patient. Determine if this has been underscored with action in the past, and also try to note any other beliefs and convictions a candidate holds relevant to the job position at hand. The third area of candidate evidence lies in past performance and accomplishment. Looking beyond the résumé, try to get a complete sense of the candidate's experience and expertise-based accomplishments in previous work roles and of the duration of his or her professional and academic career. A good candidate will cite accomplishments and professional achievements, and give you a wealth of specific episodes of contribution to the good of a health care organization. Use all three areas of evidence in combination; do not appraise any one facet exclusively or delve into one area of evidence at the expense of another. For example, the interviewer who simply looks at candidate behavior in the interview and discounts philosophy and beliefs and achievements and accomplishments risks hiring someone who is a good interviewer but not a particularly strong performer.

Candidate likeability can be a pernicious factor in interview evaluation, and is defined as the interpersonal ability of a candidate to endear himself or herself to the interviewer immediately and thus to sway the interviewer's subjective judgment in the candidate's favor. In the first type of candidate likeability, the candidate couples an engaging personality with requisite knowledge of the subject position, demonstrating an apparent ability to handle its responsibilities flawlessly. The candidate uses the balance of the interview to validate the impression the manager has formed and reinforce his or her suitability for the subject position. The second type of likeability is created when the interviewer uncovers a factor or set of factors in the candidate's background that is similar to the interviewing manager's personal history, and naturally becomes biased in favor of the candidate from the outset of the interview. This is commonly referred to as "hiring in the same image" or the "Halo Effect," an example of which is evident in a health care organization that has a number of managers who graduated from the same college or university. Their alma mater becomes, in essence, a seal of approval, and its new graduates receive preferential treatment in the organization's recruitment process. The obvious fallacy in this approach is that although certain schools may have a curriculum or faculty that makes them a good gamble in recruitment, there are absolutely no guarantees that such schools will produce winners.

A third type of candidate likeability exists when the interviewer believes that the candidate is of the same personality type as him or her and thus arrives at the premature conviction that the candidate is "my type of person." Two problems exist in this case. First, the candidate may be merely playing a role that, simply put, has little or no relationship to his or her real personality, thus leading the interviewing manager to hire an act, not a person. Second, the manager who hires someone solely on the basis of a similar personality is probably overlooking the requirements of the job because the personality factors might be receiving too much consideration in the assessment.

A primary function of the interviewer is to gauge the technical ability that the candidate possesses, specifically the amount of accrued and formal knowledge of the particular area of the business. Obviously this dimension takes on added importance in the health care field, in numerous disciplines of which mastery of key procedures can spell the difference between life and death. Although the résumé or application invariably indicates essentials in this category, it is the responsibility of the interviewer to determine the depth of technical expertise; the breadth of technical knowledge; and, most important, the extent of the candidate's ability to draw from that bank of knowledge and apply it expediently and effectively to the situation at hand. In addition to determining the candidate's expertise in a specific field or discipline, most health care managers want to learn how well versed the candidate is on health care issues and business dynamics in general. A major complaint of many health care executives is that recent college graduates and young managers from other industries, for example, have no idea of the day-to-day nature of the health care sector and the inner workings of a health care organization.

If the candidate does not have any substantial experience in health care, the interviewer should determine initially if this type of experience is essential; in some fields, like accounting and technology, health care experience is not of paramount importance. In these cases the interviewing manger should determine if the candidate has worked successfully in environments similar to that of a health care organization in which high stress is the norm and the quality of customer service is of principal concern. In all cases the candidate should demonstrate proficiency in his or her specialty through the command of technical terms and creditable employment of skills. The candidate should display not only depth of knowledge but also breadth, including an understanding of dynamics in closely related fields and of how the candidate's specific discipline fits into the organization's "big picture." Another factor to be considered is the methods the candidate uses to keep abreast of new developments and significant changes in his or her field, such as active participation in professional and technical societies or regular reading of appropriate publications. The ability to communicate acumen in a clear and cogent manner displays not only technical ability and understanding of the overall organizational mission but also the confidence to share technical ability in the interest of organizational achievement and solid team performance.

SUMMARY

Although selection is by definition a subjective process, its outcomes are perhaps the most important dimension of health care human resources, as they set the foundation for the organization's human capital renewal and growth. Using structured selection in concert with the other techniques and strategies delineated in this chapter helps make this important process as objective as possible, minimizing the bias that some interviewers might bring to the process and ensuring the use of job-related selection and interviewing processes that can differentiate between successful and unsuccessful employees.

Successful interviewing requires planning, strategy, and structure. The components of a structured oral exam should be incorporated into the interview process along with criteria-based questions related to the dimensions of the job. The interviewing human resources professional and line manager should agree in advance what competencies the position requires. The focus should be on the KSAOCs that interviewers can assess most effectively, such as interpersonal or oral communication skills and job knowledge, with the objective of hiring the best possible person for the job at the forefront of the whole process.

KEY TERMS

achievement tests	lie detector exams
cognitive ability and aptitude tests	personality inventories
drug testing	physical ability tests
experience and training rating	psychological examinations
external recruitment	recruitment
honesty and integrity tests	selection
in-basket exercises	structured oral exams
interest inventories	work sample or performance tests
internal recruitment	

DISCUSSION QUESTIONS

1. Define recruitment and selection.

2. Compare internal and external recruitment. What are the benefits of each type of recruitment?

3. Describe at least three employment screening techniques and tests.

4. What are some of the risks associated with not staffing an organization correctly?

5. Discuss the strategic recruiting considerations your organization or an organization you may have worked for in the past should address, and why.

6. Does your organization use Internet recruiting? What are the advantages and disadvantages for a health care organization relative to Internet recruiting?

9

Maximizing Performance Management and Evaluation

LEARNING OBJECTIVES

- Understand the importance of criteria-based performance evaluation in health care
- Incorporate the tenets of performance management systems and strategic human resources management as part of an overall health care human resources strategy
- Identify the major applications of performance evaluation
- Describe the different elements of a sound performance evaluation
- Delineate the components of an effective health care organizational performance evaluation system
- Use a set of management strategies for implementing and delivering a sound performance evaluation

THE DEMANDS FOR accountability made by health care organizations' stakeholders have increasingly focused on performance management. As a result, agencies have begun to reevaluate their performance management systems. Because employees are essential to the delivery of quality services, **performance evaluation** is a critical component of strategic human resources management (SHRM). The information gleaned from an effective evaluation system can be used to assist an agency in accomplishing its mission. The performance evaluation process also provides feedback to the agency about whether the other human resources management (HRM) functions are working in concert to execute the agency's mission.

Performance evaluations provide management with essential information for making strategic decisions about employee advancement, retention, or separation. Evaluation links training and development with career planning and the agency's long-term human resources needs. Used to support job analysis and recruitment efforts, performance evaluations are an important component of evaluating the knowledge, skills, abilities, and other characteristics (KSAOCs) available among the agency's internal supply of labor. Evaluations can be used to assess career advancement opportunities, for succession planning, and to develop compensation and reward systems, as well as to identify deficiencies in incumbents' KSAOCs.

Accurate evaluations provide information and feedback to employees. Employees must be informed about the goals and objectives of the agency and about the role employees play in ensuring the agency's success. They must know what standards will be used to judge their effectiveness. Supervisors must communicate to employees their strengths as well as their deficiencies, thus providing the opportunity for employees to correct their weaknesses before serious problems emerge. Through the evaluation process, training and development needs can be identified and addressed.

DEVELOPING AN EVALUATION PROGRAM

There is little consistency in performance evaluation systems across health care organizations. Some systems tie performance with pay, with yearly evaluations determining pay increases, bonuses, or both. At other agencies formal performance evaluation systems do not even exist. In many health care organizations collective bargaining agreements determine promotions and pay increases. In this environment, if evaluations exist they are used strictly as communication vehicles.

The only commonality often found in performance evaluation systems is that both the raters and ratees typically dislike having to participate in the evaluation process. Yet despite the reservations expressed about performance evaluation systems, most organizations do undertake some form of appraisal. Because performance evaluations are used for different and sometimes multiple purposes, employees and supervisors must understand why evaluations are being conducted. The integrity of a performance appraisal system depends on the raters' and ratees' understanding its objectives.

Individual Performance Appraisal Techniques

There are three general approaches to performance appraisals: absolute methods, comparative methods, and goal setting. Absolute methods evaluate the employee without referring directly to other employees. Employees are instead evaluated against their own standards. For example, John Doe is evaluated in March and then again in September, and his September evaluation is compared to his March evaluation. The strengths identified in March should have been maintained, and any deficiencies or problems identified in March should have been corrected by September. Absolute evaluations are used most frequently for developmental purposes.

Comparative methods evaluate the employees in one unit relative to everyone else in the group. For example, in March all of the juvenile probation officers were evaluated on the same performance dimensions and then compared to one another. Case manager A received the highest ratings in accuracy and timeliness of reports, whereas case manager C received the lowest rating for that dimension. Case manager C, however, received the highest rating for number of clients supervised, whereas case manager B received the lowest rating on that dimension. Comparative evaluations are used to differentiate levels of performance across employees.

Goal setting evaluates whether the ratee attained predetermined goals. For example, the supervisor and employee agree that the employee will prepare seven more grant applications in the next five months to secure a greater percentage of external funding. After five months have passed the supervisor will evaluate whether the employee met this agreed-upon, preestablished goal.

There are differences not only in the format of evaluation but also in the types of data collected and evaluated. Some evaluations rely on direct indexes, or objective data. These indexes can be quantified, such as the number of errors, the number of clients on a caseload, the number of grants that received funding, the number of arrests made, or the number of proposals written. Direct indexes are referred to as objective measures because they do not rely on someone's opinion to be verified. Another type of data commonly used are subjective measures, which depend on human judgment and should be based on a careful analysis of the behaviors viewed as necessary for effective job performance. Decision-making skills, the ability to solve problems, and oral communication skills are examples of subjective measures.

The types of data and the performance standards used should be based on a current job analysis, and performance standards should be developed according to the critical tasks and responsibilities of each position. The standards should be measurable through quantifiable or observable methods. The following subsections provide an overview of some of the most common types of evaluation instruments used in the public and nonprofit sectors.

Trait Rating Scales

Raters are provided with a list of personality characteristics, such as coop-eration, creativity, attitude, and initiative. Raters then assign a number or adjective, such as "unsatisfactory," "improvement needed," "average," "very good," or "outstanding," to indicate the degree to which employees possess those traits. Trait rating scales are difficult to defend in court if challenged. They tend to be subjective, and raters often disagree on the definitions of trait ratings and how they should be measured. Furthermore, trait rating scales are often not related to job performance or relevant behaviors. Someone may have a poor attitude but still be technically proficient. The scales also do not define what is meant by "average" or "superior." Different raters may apply different standards in evaluating the same behaviors. An example of a trait rating scale is presented in Figure 9.1.

Essays

The rater writes a narrative essay describing the employee's performance. The weakness in this method is that the evaluation may depend on the writing skills of the supervisor or the amount of time the supervisor takes to

Figure 9.1   Example Trait Rating Scale

Name/Rank _____ Section _____ Unit/Platoon _____

Outstanding = 1   Very Good = 2   Average = 3   Improvement Needed = 4   Unsatisfactory = 5

Trait	Evaluation				
	1	2	3	4	5
Judgment					
Dependability					
Work Initiative					
Quality of Work					
Appearance					
Cooperation					
Knowledge of Work					
Public Contacts					
Supervisory Ability					
Overall Evaluation					

complete the evaluation. Another problem is that raters and employees do not necessarily use common criteria.

Productivity Data or Work Standards

Raters evaluate employees on expected levels of output and the quality of output. If employees are to believe that the standards are fair, they should understand how the standards were set.

Management by Objectives

Raters and employees together determine goals or objectives and a plan of action for achieving them that the employee is to undertake during the upcoming evaluation cycle. At a scheduled time, the rater and the employee reconvene and determine whether the goals have been met. The effectiveness of management by objectives depends on the skills of supervisors and subordinates in defining appropriate goals and objectives. Often easy objectives are set. Sometimes there is an overemphasis on objectives at the expense of specifying how these objectives are to be obtained. For example, bill collection agents need to retrieve revenue from delinquent clients, but not through illegal or intimidating tactics.

Critical Incident Reports

Raters record actual incidents of successful or unsuccessful performance of work actions. The rater uses these observations to evaluate employee performance. An example of a critical incident report is presented in Figure 9.2.

Behaviorally Anchored Rating Scales

Raters evaluate employees based on a set of behavioral descriptions. The descriptions list various degrees of behavior with regard to a specific performance dimension and identify a range of behaviors from unacceptable performance to outstanding performance. Ratees do not have to actually exhibit the behaviors on the scale; rather, the behaviors serve as a guide to help the rater and ratee understand the level of performance required for an assigned rating. Unlike some of the other instruments, behaviorally anchored rating scales (BARS) rely on employee behaviors—what employees actually do and what is under their direct control.

Figure 9.2   Example Critical Incident Report

Positive:

Date	Employee volunteered for four extra assignments.
Date	Received phone call from professional X commending the assistance given by this employee.
Date	Employee submitted progress report B two weeks ahead of deadline. The report was complete and accurate. Employee exercised independent judgment.

Negative:

Date	Employee failed to submit accurate and complete verification reports. Auditors found deficiencies that warranted a payback.
Date	Employee refused to return phone calls to the patient, resulting in the loss of the patient.
Date	Employee missed the deadline for report submission. This resulted in the loss of reimbursement.

A problem for many health care providers is that despite the proficient performance of staff, unacceptable outcomes often result. For example, a psychiatric client may have a psychotic relapse that requires hospitalization, despite her social worker's best efforts to help the client remain in the community. BARS would evaluate the social worker on his behaviors, not on the number of patients needing hospitalization. An advantage to using BARS is that they reduce ambiguity because employees are provided with descriptions of desired levels of performance. They are also accepted by both raters and ratees because both employees and supervisors participate in their development. A disadvantage to using BARS is that their development is time-consuming and complex in that each dimension requires its own behavioral anchors. An example of a behaviorally anchored rating scale is presented in Figure 9.3.

Behavioral Observation Scales

Behavioral observation scales (BOS) are ratings based on the frequency of critical incidents that are deemed to be important for satisfactory job performance. A BOS provides a list of critical incidents that the supervisor has to rate in terms of frequency. To develop a BOS evaluation instrument, a large number of behavioral statements are compiled, employees are observed and rated on a five-point scale as to the frequency with which they engage in the behaviors, and then a total score for each employee is determined by adding together the rater's responses. Figure 9.4 provides an example of a BOS.

Personnel Data

Raters tabulate such information as the number of absences or the number of times employees report late to work. The data are used to regulate employees' conformance to organizational policies.

360-Degree Evaluations

The typical performance evaluation is a top-down process whereby a supervisor evaluates a subordinate. However, for many jobs employees interact not only with their supervisors but also with coworkers; clients or patients (and other stakeholders, such as their families); subordinates (or direct reports); and individuals from other departments or organizations. Jobs encompass a number of different tasks and responsibilities, and supervisors are often not in the best position to evaluate an employee on tasks or responsibilities that they

Figure 9.3   Example Behaviorally Anchored Rating Scale

Job: Supervisor of therapist outpatient services

Dimension: Assigning and reviewing treatment plans

Superior:	Reviews all treatment plans for compliance with standards. Assigns cases to therapists on a daily basis, giving clear, verbal instructions about what is expected of them in reference to a particular therapy. Makes recommendations or other therapeutic suggestions when necessary. Keeps a case management log of all assigned cases.
Very good:	Reviews all treatment plans submitted by therapists. Assigns cases to therapists. Answers questions when asked. Reviews cases with therapists when necessary.
Satisfactory:	Reviews all treatment plans. Assigns cases to therapists.
Needs improvement:	Takes several days before reviewing cases. Rarely reviews therapists' work. Takes several days to a week to assign cases to therapists.
Unsatisfactory:	Does not review therapists' cases. Does not assign cases in a timely manner.

Comments: _____

_____

_____

Rater's signature: _____

do not observe. To eliminate this dilemma, more and more organizations are implementing appraisals referred to as 360-degree evaluations.

Such performance dimensions as leadership, training and developing employees, communicating agency policies, and delegating and assigning work are responsibilities commonly found in supervisory or management positions. Competence in these dimensions can best be assessed by subordinates who have frequent contact with the supervisor or manager and can observe different aspects of his or her performance.

Figure 9.4   Example Behavioral Observation Scale

Behaviors or Critical Incidents	Almost Never → Almost Always				
	1	2	3	4	5
Influences others in achieving a high level of safety and health training					
Uses slack periods for training, if people are available					
Follows up on training to determine effectiveness of learning					
Develops written safety and health training plans and schedules					

Rating	Percentage of Time Observed
1	0–64
2	65–74
3	75–84
4	85–94
5	95–100

For example, university professors are typically rated on three dimensions: teaching, research, and service. Students can evaluate the professor's teaching, and in fact they do so near the completion of every semester through course evaluations. However, they are not in the position to judge the research or scholarship in which their professors engage, nor are they in a position to evaluate the level and quality of faculty members' community and university service. So although students provide input concerning teaching, other faculty members or the department chairperson evaluates research and service. Figure 9.5 depicts a 360-degree evaluation.

Team-Based Performance Appraisal Techniques

In health care organizations, which are made up of team-based environments that focus on continuous improvement and measuring performance outcomes, traditional performance appraisal techniques are being reexamined, and in some cases there is a movement away from individual appraisals. Many organizations have introduced gainsharing and team-based pay-for-performance systems. In these models, team members share the savings from higher productivity or reduced errors and waste. Although team goals and objectives are becoming more common, however, frequently team members work as individuals collaborating with one another to accomplish the team's goals. Often each team member has fixed tasks that are completed

Figure 9.5   Example 360-Degree Evaluation

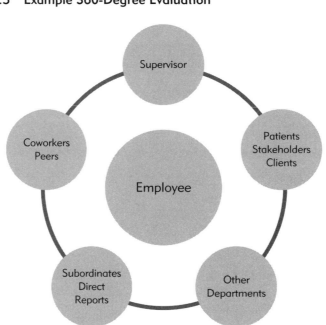

independently but that contribute to the team's objectives. Team members must be aware of their responsibilities and be challenged by their work. Team members decide which measurements set the standards for performance, and teamwork is more productive when each team member is expected to conduct a self-assessment of his or her own achievement level and understand the relationship between individual performance and the team's success.

Individual goals should be set after the team has set its goals. That way employee goals can be directly tied to what the team needs to accomplish. Teams should schedule meetings to discuss their objectives and progress made toward them. The purpose of meeting is to identify and remove any barriers that may exist. This also ensures that individual actions do not interfere with team productivity. Task accomplishment is important to teams, but general competencies are important as well, such as effective communication, demonstrating initiative, volunteering to assist team members, responding to requests for information in a timely manner, and other behaviors and competencies necessary for team success.

For team-based performance systems to work, team objectives need to be identified and agreed on. There must be clear and specific performance objectives. Each team member needs to understand her or his responsibilities in relation to the other team members' responsibilities to eliminate confusion. It is important for team members to document what they have agreed on and follow up with progress meetings. If necessary, training and development should be provided to help individuals contribute to the team's objectives.

Some team-based performance techniques that are becoming more common are gainsharing and goalsharing.

Gainsharing

A **gainsharing** plan is a group incentive plan that distributes gains from improved performance to employees in a department or organization based on an established sharing formula. Participative management and teamwork are used to develop performance techniques and standards that control costs or units of output. All members of the team, department, or agency benefit from the increased cost savings. Lawler (2000) refers to gainsharing as a management style, a technology for organizational development, and an incentive system. Gainsharing and increases in compensation are discussed in greater detail in Chapter Ten.

Goalsharing

Goalsharing plans, like gainsharing plans, pay bonuses when performance is above a standard. The difference is that goalsharing plans seek to leverage an organization's operational strategy by measuring performance on key strategic objectives. Goalsharing plans can reward things that do not have an immediate or direct monetary payoff for an organization, such as quality or customer satisfaction. A specific bonus amount is tied to achieving performance on the goals that were set. At the end of the year, a different set of measures and standards may be established as part of a new plan, or the old plan may continue. Goalsharing plans are typically used when the external environment is rapidly changing and the organization wants to target a particular kind of performance improvement for a limited time period (Lawler, 2000).

Balanced Scorecard Approach

Another strategy that goes beyond financial indicators to evaluate performance and is related to goalsharing is the **balanced scorecard approach** (Kaplan & Norton, 1996). Although no one will dispute the importance of financial measures (and the importance of operating in the black), financial measures are not always the best indicators of effectiveness in health care organizations. These organizations often provide unprofitable services to citizens and clients who need special and often expensive assistance. The balanced scorecard approach to evaluating performance includes such measures as customer satisfaction, employee satisfaction, and quality, in addition to relevant financial indicators.

Gainsharing, goalsharing, a balanced scorecard approach, and other team-based quality improvement processes rely on many of the same principles as individual performance evaluation and are not antithetical to the individual performance evaluation process. If implemented correctly, quality improvement processes require the development of performance standards and measures to determine whether the standards have been achieved; they require feedback from multiple sources and the development of an action plan for reaching future goals. What is key to the success of any of these quality improvement and performance assessment systems is not the name of the process used but the HRM policies and rules that support and enhance quality improvement processes across the entire organization.

Each of the evaluation instruments and systems has advantages and disadvantages and may be appropriate when used in the correct context. It is important that appraisal instruments are congruent with the objective for the evaluation and suitable for the positions being evaluated.

Documentation

During the evaluation period, raters should document both positive and negative aspects of job performance. One way to do this is by maintaining employee performance logs. Raters note in the logs any critical behaviors (positive and negative) that employees exhibit. Recording when an employee volunteered for difficult assignments or received letters of commendation is an example of documenting positive aspects of performance. An employee's failure to submit an assignment by its deadline or submission of inaccurate and incomplete reports is an example of unacceptable performance that should be recorded. By documenting performance throughout the evaluation cycle, raters are able to provide specific feedback and minimize their susceptibility to committing rating errors.

It is important that employees receive feedback throughout the evaluation cycle, not only when it is time to review the formal evaluation. Employees who receive feedback from their raters on a regular basis know how well they are performing their job and what improvements might be needed. Poor performers should be receiving feedback on what they can do to improve their performance, and excellent employees should receive positive recognition for performing well. For many employees positive reinforcement is a powerful motivator that encourages them to sustain excellent performance.

Prior to completing the formal evaluation instrument, raters should retrieve the employee performance logs for inclusion in the evaluation. Raters should be required to justify each rating they give with explicit examples. This corroborates the job relatedness of the evaluation and diffuses allegations of unfairness, prejudice, favoritism, and so on. For employees who must improve their performance, supervisors should recommend some potential strategies for employee development. Raters should provide clear, descriptive, job-related, constructive, frequent, timely, and realistic feedback.

Evaluation Review

It is not enough for raters to complete performance appraisal instruments; they must also review the evaluation with their employees. Employees should play a critical role in the process, and they should be given advance notice of when the review is scheduled so that they too can prepare. Employees should be encouraged to bring to the review any documentation they feel is relevant, such as letters of commendation or records of accomplished objectives of which their raters may not be aware. Some raters ask their employees to complete a self-evaluation, including relevant documentation, prior to the scheduled review. This puts employees at ease, making them feel that they are part of the process, not just its victims. By asking employees to complete self-evaluations, raters can elicit input from employees about how they rated themselves and why, what accomplishments they are most proud of, and in what areas they believe they need to improve performance.

In many health care organizations supervisors lack the authority to determine the purpose of an evaluation. As noted earlier, promotions may be based on competitive examinations and seniority, and pay-for-performance may not exist. In such cases, however, supervisors can use the evaluation process to develop their employees. The evaluation process should open up communication between supervisors and employees and allow supervisors to discuss with employees areas for development and the best ways to achieve their goals. A systematic approach to performance appraisals will help employers make sure that they and their employees have the same understanding of the expectations for satisfactory performance.

Rater Training

Training is essential for both ratees and raters if performance evaluation systems are to be used in the strategic human resources planning process. Ratees who receive training and understand the evaluation system tend to be more committed to its goals. They should understand why the evaluation is being conducted, how it will be used, and what their role is in the process. Through training they become aware of the difficulty that raters face in evaluating performance. Training also informs ratees of the levels of performance expected of them.

For evaluations to be as accurate as possible, raters should receive training in the development of performance standards and objectives, goal setting, observation, and recall and documentation skills; they should also learn how to complete the evaluation instruments, how to give performance feedback, and how to avoid rating errors. Because performance appraisals rely on human judgment, which is subject to error, personal biases need to be removed from the rating process. Employees must be rated on the basis of job-related, nondiscriminatory criteria, and the appraisals must accurately reflect job performance. Because of the sensitive nature of performance evaluations, agencies have a responsibility to train their raters. Training can improve raters' documentation and counseling skills, thereby not only reducing their discomfort but also enabling them to help employees clearly understand what the employees' strengths are and what areas need improvement. Training can teach raters how to describe job-related behaviors and develop performance standards, emphasize the importance of accuracy and consistency in the appraisal process, and provide constructive feedback. The agency can offer training through a variety of methods: in workshops conducted in-house by the HRM department or off-site by trainers from universities or consulting firms, or through video packages tailored to the performance evaluation process.

Executive Evaluation

The evaluation of executive directors of health care organizations is typically performed by the board of directors or by subcommittees of the board. Again, there is little consistency in evaluation procedures. BoardSource recognizes that there is not one best technique for evaluating chief executives. Instead, each board must decide which procedures best serve the agency. Nason (1993) has identified four general methods of assessment:

1. *Intermittent or continuous observation of the chief executive by board members, especially the chairperson.* This method is used mostly in small organizations in which the board works closely with the chief executive. If problems arise, it is easy to identify the cause and provide remedies. Nason notes, however, that as an organization expands and board members become less involved in the agency's operations, this method may no longer be effective. Should this become the case, the board will have to reanalyze its oversight role and restructure its own performance.

2. *Periodic assessment of the chief executive by the board's chairperson or other board members.* This assessment should reflect the chief executive's performance over the previous year. The evaluation should consider the assessments of other board members, especially those of the chairs of standing committees. Nason believes that board members should not discuss the chief executive's performance with the staff. He claims that "to do so is to risk good morale within the organization and to distort proper lines of responsibility" (p. 5). That statement needs further consideration. Some aspects of the chief executive's performance, such as communicating agency policies, informing employees about changes, and delegating tasks and responsibilities—and the chief executive's leadership characteristics—are best evaluated by subordinates. Should subordinate evaluations be used, it is important that employees receive training and be asked to evaluate only relevant dimensions. Information from proximate sources is important because council and board members spend most of their time away from the organization. For evaluating such responsibilities as maintaining council and board relations and communication, board members are the most appropriate source. But for other dimensions, such as fiscal management, they may need to rely on an audit prepared by an outside accounting firm or government regulators to verify that the chief executive's performance in regard to fiscal management was satisfactory.

3. *Annual board committee review designed to assess the state of the agency and the chief executive's performance.* This is a formal review of the chief executive's goals and accomplishments and is conducted by the executive committee, the personnel committee, or another committee. The standard procedure is for the chief executive to review the accomplishments of the previous year in relation to the goals set and to propose goals for the next year. During the evaluation, the chief executive's strengths and weaknesses are identified and discussed, and the evaluation concludes with an agreement about the next year's goals.

4. *Full-dress public assessment of the chief executive, including formal hearings and survey data from an extensive variety of interested parties.* Only a few nonprofit organizations use this approach because it is time-consuming, often requires an outside consultant to administer the process, and can be an emotionally charged procedure.

Regardless of the type of assessment, chief executives must have advance notice of the board's expectations and the criteria used for the evaluation. Self-assessments by chief executives are recommended because they permit them to review how they have met the responsibilities, expectations, and objectives of the position. Opportunities are provided for chief executives and boards to resolve any differences they might have in their perspectives concerning the requirements of the chief executive's position and the role of the board in its governance and management functions.

The strategic purpose of evaluating the chief executive is to strengthen the agency by improving its management. The board's evaluation of the chief executive should assist in improving his or her performance by identifying the executive's strengths and the areas in which improvement is needed. Boards should also support and encourage executives' participation in professional development activities (Nason, 1993; Pierson & Mintz, 1995).

Nonprofit executives are often evaluated on the following competencies:

- Accomplishment of management objectives
- Program management
- Fiscal management
- Effectiveness in fundraising

- Maintaining board relations
- Maintaining the agency's public image and external relations

Fundamental Elements of a Sound Performance Evaluation

There are essential elements of a performance evaluation that must be incorporated as intrinsic parts of the process. A review of all of the factors and their value is presented in this section for implementation by human resources managers and for use by health care line managers.

Validity

The evaluation must be based on performance data that are as objective as possible, and it must use performance measures that are directly related to the specific job scope and set of responsibilities.

Viability

The performance evaluation system is practically based, using a format and data that are easily understood by the employee and reviewing manager; in addition, the system works fluidly with the wage and compensation system, and helps in setting pay increases and other performance incentives.

Relevance

The evaluation reviews specific, individual job accountabilities, and is an exclusive interaction between the employee and the manager concerning particular assignments and responsibilities; the employee's career and professional aspirations, education and development needs, and unique contributions are all considered.

Completeness

The performance evaluation examines not only the job description components but also the attitude, people skills, professional responsibility, and team orientation of the employee, as well as the employees' critical contributions and management of significant incidents.

Continuity

The performance evaluation cycle is not a once-a-year report card exercise; rather, the process begins on the employee's first day on the job, and continues with meetings, checkpoints, and other methods of monitoring and discussing performance throughout the work year in the interest of maintaining dialogue and work focus.

Participation

Both the employee and manager maintain responsibility in the performance evaluation process to communicate key information, work achievement, significant accomplishments, and new work direction; major changes in the scope of work should also be efficiently communicated.

Progressiveness

The evaluation should not only act as a review of past performance but also provide meaningful insight into future performance expectations and emergent needs relative to the position; it should facilitate a discussion of the employee's individual career development and educational needs as they relate to his or her responsibilities.

Components of an Effective Performance Evaluation Form

Not only is it critically important for the health care manager to use an effective method of collecting performance data, setting goals, and communicating performance feedback to the employee but also it is vital to have a good, workable performance evaluation form. Several appraisal forms have been used successfully by numerous leading health care organizations, and have been validated by research, quantitative measurement, and, perhaps most important, practical use by thousands of health care managers who know that a comprehensive form is vital to making the evaluation process a reality-based function of daily management. By examining these forms and reviewing their components, the health care manager will be able to present to the individual employee all critical elements of performance in a cogent, direct manner.

Administrative Data

The administrative data section of the performance evaluation form must supply several important facets. These include the date on which the appraisal is actually conducted, and the employee's legal name as it appears on all documents in the employee file, accompanied by an organizational ID number or Social Security number.

Furthermore, the job title as it appears on the job description and all other significant organizational records should be in this administrative section, as well as the departmental designation of the work group to which the employee is assigned on a regular basis. If the employee is on loan to another department for a significant time that should also be noted, particularly if his or her performance in that department is being assessed in this appraisal. The reviewing manager or supervisor's name and organizational ID number are also needed in this section. The date on which the employee started work in the organization, along with the employee's current position and the date on which the employee started in the job he or she currently holds are also part of the needed performance evaluation administrative data. The occasion for the appraisal—usually the normal annual or semiannual review, or perhaps a disciplinary or other special reason—should also be in the opening administrative section.

Job Description

The second section of a performance appraisal form should be the job description. This can be taken verbatim from the job description on file, or it can be an abbreviated version of that description. The job description portion of the appraisal form must be criteria based to conform with the guidelines of The Joint Commission, as well as a plethora of federal and state employee statutes. As described in Chapter Seven, the job description should include the overall scope of the current position, replete with a delineation of its major responsibilities. It should be tailored to the individual employee's actual duties as much as possible, rather than being an outdated, generic overview of the position. In this regard, the employee should have been given a copy of the job description on the first day of the job, and this, along with the supervisor's direction, should continue to be the employee's general guide to job performance.

Review of the Past Year's Expectations and Objectives

A good performance appraisal should list all of the major expectations and objectives that the employee was to have met in the past grading period. These goals should have been set by the reviewing manager and understood and agreed to by the employee. In each case the manager should rate the individual employee's accomplishment of each goal. Similar to when rating candidates in an interview, the manager should use a three-tier grading system, using one grade for poor performance, a second for satisfactory performance, and a third for stellar achievement. This system discourages the manager from rating everyone in the organization as a six or seven on a scale of one to ten, or a little higher than satisfactory. This also encourages the manager to grade each goal individually and critically, rather than giving the employee one blanket, general rating.

By listing each objective, the manager provides continuity and consistency in the assessment and appraisal process. This also simplifies the review for the manager because he or she merely has to check the roster of objectives against actual performance. It further helps to show the employee clearly what is needed on the job, how a given objective was achieved, and what should be accomplished from this point forward.

Work Characteristic Ratings

This section is an essential part of the performance appraisal form, as it provides an assessment of employees' work-related personality attributes. In essence, this section rates *how* employees do their job, in concert with the first section, which rates *what* they do in their job. This provides continuity starting with the selection interview and continuing constructively to the compilation of the performance evaluation. In the case of a supervisor who is being reviewed by a manager, the managerial attitude category will have particular application.

The manager should review the employee's performance and determine how the various work characteristics affected the employee's scope of performance. For example, if an employee was particularly adaptable in successfully handling a unique situation, adaptability should be cited as the stellar commodity and the manager should appropriately note evidence of the characteristic's positive application on the job. Conversely, if the employee was inflexible in most work situations, the manager should grade the employee accordingly and provide constructive insight on how the employee can improve his or her adaptability rating. Average or satisfactory application of these characteristics does not particularly need to be cited, because it does not greatly affect performance in an overtly negative or positive manner.

Objectives and Expectations Adjustment

Because goals change, employees come and go, and circumstances of the workplace fluctuate, a good performance appraisal form will have a section in which the employee and manager can jointly review new or amended goals that arose throughout the completed grading period but were not part of the original roster of job components. The manager should select goals that are current, that are maximally applicable to current business desires and objectives, and that spark the employee's interest by presenting new and significant job challenges. The concepts of job enrichment and job enhancement are both vital to this process. The manager can also discuss at this time a list of any new goals that are needed to meet emerging business demands as well as amend any current goals according to what is needed in the future.

Development Plan

A good performance appraisal is also a good development tool. The performance appraisal form should have a section that acts as a plan, or prescriptive prognosis, for useful development activities, and that identifies and discusses opportunities for the employee's development, including any objectives for educational accomplishment. By making this a required part of the performance evaluation form, the manager formalizes the organization's commitment to fostering employee development. Furthermore, the employee now has a formal plan for development that he or she has helped construct—one that he or she is committed to completing for personal growth. As with the entire assessment process, the two-way planning of a development activity elicits a commitment from each side and demonstrates the organization's true interest in employee growth. Chapter Twelve will provide an overview and compendium of development strategies that line managers can use to get the most from health care staff members.

Employee Comments

On all performance appraisal forms employees must be given the opportunity to rebut the appraisal informally and submit their own impressions of their performance. Some organizations use a binary form, allowing the employee to review a supervisor on another appraisal form. Most organizations, however, simply have a section on the appraisal form in which the employee has the opportunity to provide commentary on managerial direction and guidance. As is the case in many dimensions of performance evaluation design, the effectiveness of the approach depends on the individual organization and its philosophy in this regard. Most state labor statutes require, however, that the appraisal form have some sort of accommodation for employee commentary on organizational and managerial performance.

If the manager has allowed the employee ample opportunity for feedback on a daily basis, the employee section does not need to be very lengthy. However, on every appraisal form there should be a dedicated section for employee comments, whether or not the employee decides to use it in the performance evaluation process.

Overall Rating

Finally, the manager must attach an overall rating to the employee's performance. If the manager has used a three-tier system in rating each objective component and has rated all of the work characteristics that might apply, the overall rating can be an easy summation process. In fact, if any numerical sequence has been used in the appraisal, it is simply a mathematical process to attach an overall rating number. The best guideline is for the manager to review the content of the appraisal form and try to quantify the entire appraisal with an overall evaluation rating that can be applied to compensation, as per the organization's particular policies and structure. Because there seem to be as many rating systems as there are appraisal forms, readers might want to really understand the intricacies and nuances of their own organizational system while employing the three-tier system advocated in this text.

Signatures

At the conclusion of the performance appraisal form there should be space for both manager and employee to sign the form, with the date of the appraisal. This is a simple legal requirement, and in some cases, especially with a negative review, the employee might refuse to sign the appraisal form. In this instance the manager should note on the form that the employee refused to sign the evaluation, then initial and date the document. This should be done so that the employee cannot contest the date or the validity of the appraisal form in any litigation that might arise from a deserved termination.

In all health care organizations the appraisal form should be easily understood, easily read, and easily acted on in planning for future performance. Unfortunately, many existing forms are either too simplistic to be useful, too full of psychobabble and corporate jargon to be understood, or too full of specious "quality indicators" to be relevant to individual performance. Appraisal forms of this nature not only are a potential legal risk but also give employees no true indication of their performance and can invite objections from employees because of their lack of pertinent details. It is therefore vital to use a reality-based, field-proven instrument, containing the elements delineated in this chapter, that will portray performance accurately and provide direction for development.

Format for an Appraisal Discussion

In order to conduct the actual performance appraisal expeditiously and effectively, the health care manager should use a proven, simple, five-step method of organizing and delivering the performance evaluation.

Step 1: Opening Overview

In the first five minutes of the performance appraisal discussion the reviewing manager should explain to the employee in general terms what he wishes to accomplish during the meeting. To get the employee involved in the discussion, the manager should provide the employee with a basic overview of the points covered in the review. If this is the employee's first exposure to the organization's performance appraisal process, the manager should also explain the basics of the appraisal form. If the employee is an hourly worker, the manager should explain that the session will take about a half an hour; in the case of a supervisor, the manager should dedicate a full hour to the process. While reviewing the appraisal form with the employee, the manager should emphasize that the employee's active participation is needed for both parties to get the most from the appraisal discussion, as well as for the manager to understand all significant input from the employee. This will assure the employee that her input is valued, and also will take some of the "report card" flavor out of the process.

Prior to the review the manager might ask the employee to make some general notes about her performance. In a well-managed unit, the employee will naturally have a list of objectives established for her position, and will have those ready for easy reference for the session. This helps the employee reflect on her own performance and come to the appraisal session ready to discuss performance constructively.

Because of the performance evaluation's legal function as a critical source of evidence in cases of potential probation or termination, it becomes particularly important for the manager to direct the employee to prepare for the review session by reflecting on her performance. With this accomplished, both manager and employee have in essence done their homework, and will be fully prepared to address the core of the appraisal.

Step 2: Key Goal Attainment

After the opening of the appraisal session the manager should focus the discussion on goal attainment and performance output. This should begin with the manager and the employee jointly reviewing the job description as it appears on the appraisal. The manager should also be prepared to review goals not contained in the job description but essential to job conduct at this time. The manager can then review each goal that was set, replete with his ratings for each goal and accomplishment.

The manager should provide some insight into how each rating was determined by citing the objective performance evidence in each case. If the communication was evident between employee and manager throughout the year, there should be very little surprise on the part of the employee concerning the relevance and rationale of the ratings. The manager should get understanding—but not necessarily agreement—from the employee for each rating before moving on to the next one. The manager might also discuss how the importance of each goal and its relevance to the overall organizational mission were weighed in his estimation. Only the prior period's goals should be reviewed at this time; that is, there should be no discussion at this point of new goals or amended objectives for the coming grading period.

Step 3: Work Personality Assessment

The third phase of the performance evaluation discussion focuses on the work characteristics that pertain to employee performance. Simply put, in this stage the manager discusses the criteria-based, established characteristics that affected work performance in either a positive or a negative fashion. The manager should cite appropriately as much objective evidence as possible to support his ratings.

If an established work characteristic was evidenced in the employee's performance in a negative fashion—through a consistently poor attitude or an inability to work effectively with colleagues, for example—it is particularly important for the manager to offer an explanation of why this characteristic is important to the conduct of the job, augmented by suggestions of positive use of the characteristic in the employee's work situation.

Because interpersonal characteristics are more subjectively perceived than goal achievement, it is necessary for the reviewing manager to use as many objective examples and illustrations of desired behavior as possible to keep the discourse focused on the business of health care delivery, as opposed to creating a potentially injurious perception of character assassination.

Step 4: Developmental Direction

Providing developmental direction in the appraisal discussion should consist of establishing new or amended work goals as part of the planning of training and development activities for the employee for the coming evaluation period. It is essential for the manager and employee to agree on specific goals to be established for the upcoming evaluation cycle, although the manager should have the last word on these goals.

Likewise, the manager and employee should reach an agreement on a solid plan of development activities. A good rule of thumb in this case is for the manager to designate a third of the goals and development activities and the employee to suggest another third, with the two jointly designating the final third. In the case of an hourly employee, one development activity is probably sufficient; with a reporting supervisor, three is a good number. Chapter Twelve offers further insight into development activities.

Step 5: Constructive Consensus

In the final stage of a performance evaluation discussion the manager and the employee should endeavor to come to a strong agreement about the appraisal and, more important, about future work direction. Achieving such a consensus is infinitely easier when steady communication has always been present. If this has not been the case, the manager should use the appraisal as a new beginning and follow the appraisal session with a rededication to solid, hands-on management.

Managing Potential Employee Reactions in the Review Session

In the consulting role that human resources professionals fill in helping health care line managers deliver performance assessments, there are ten common employee reactions to the performance evaluation session. The following subsections identify each of these reactions, explain the root of the problem in each instance, and provide a remedy that the manager can use to get the discussion back on track.

Complete Surprise

Perhaps the most telling of all reactions to a performance appraisal is complete surprise at the content of the appraisal form and the ensuing dialogue that takes place in the review. The employee might register surprise in regard to a particular segment of the performance evaluation discussion or from the outset of the appraisal, and continue to demonstrate this reaction through to a negative conclusion of the review discussion. On the one hand, when an employee is truly surprised by the content of the performance appraisal, he usually spends the entire session dealing with his emotional reaction and thus misses much of the objective content of the session itself. On the other hand, an employee given an accurate review might feign surprise to communicate to the reviewing manager that he has a radically different opinion about his performance.

The reason for genuine surprise is usually found in a lack of communication, which probably stemmed from a dearth of feedback or direction from the manager to the employee. If the employee has not been told previously that his performance was lacking, he will assume naturally that his performance was at least satisfactory. Hence, at the appraisal itself when the reviewing manager presents a litany of missed objectives, examples of substandard output, and other work-related problems, the employee will be genuinely shocked. In this case, the fault lies primarily with the reviewing manager who has not used solid communication techniques in supervising the employee. Because the manager is at fault, the best remedy is for the manager to continue with the review such as it is, and state a sincere commitment to the employee to provide feedback on a more timely basis. Specifically, the two parties should set a schedule of regular meetings between the two of them on a monthly basis—at a minimum—so that a lack of communication will not reoccur as a problem. This problem is common among new managers, so it is important for more senior managers in the organization to guide the novices toward making the review process a continuous and meaningful one.

When the employee feigns surprise, the remedy is somewhat different. In this instance, the employee is using surprise as a ploy to deflect criticism or other negative feedback, and to lend credibility to his own point of view. It therefore becomes imperative for the manager to provide several pieces of concrete evidence that clearly show the employee's shortcomings on the job. They should be reinforced by references to any conversation the manager might have had with the employee in which the employee's poor performance was discussed. When faced with examples of poor performance and reminders of corrective discussion, the manipulative employee's case loses most of its veracity. The manager should seriously question the employee's loyalty and dedication to the job, as well as his basic desire to perform at a satisfactory level. If the employee subsequently attempts to improve his performance, the manager's actions will be rewarded. If the employee continues to perform poorly, the manager's next discussion about performance will be centered on putting the employee on probation with an eye toward termination.

Misunderstanding of Objectives

Another common reaction that seems particularly to affect novice managers is the employee's misunderstanding as to what was expected on the job on a daily basis. This problem usually occurs when the manager has not set meaningful, clear-cut expectations and objectives for the employee's performance from the outset. This problem can also result when the employee has been provided with objectives that he did not fully understand at the time of establishment. For example, the employee might not have been provided with a time frame for completion of a set objective, or might not have understood the importance of a specific deadline.

In these situations the fundamental problem is communication. By constructing clear objectives and goals and, whenever possible, providing a written outline of what is expected on the job, the health care manager eliminates the problem of misunderstood objectives. Then, during the performance review session, the outline of objectives—which has been reviewed informally but regularly by both the manager and employee—can be a constructive focal point.

Expected Praise

Some managers in the health care industry, because of their own enthusiasm and energy on the job, have a propensity to appear overly positive about everything. They tend to praise employees throughout the year to avoid situations in which they should provide corrective feedback. This is particularly true of managers who are excessively concerned with being liked by their employees. Thus the expectation of undue praise is present in the performance evaluation session, as the employee comes into the session expecting a stellar review when in reality his overall performance has been lackluster.

As is always the case in the health care labor market, there are more jobs for skilled people than there are skilled people to fill those jobs. Health care managers, therefore, take every opportunity they can to convey to employees a sense of appreciation for their efforts and talents. However, if the appraisal process is to be truly constructive, it should not be reduced to a "stroking session" that the employee attends just to hear how terrific and invaluable he is to the organization. The employee who comes into the performance evaluation session expecting a review to be 100 percent positive might be disappointed even if the review is 95 percent praise and 5 percent constructive criticism. The employee who has been unduly spoiled by too much positive reinforcement throughout the rating period will then focus on the 5 percent that is constructive criticism—to the extent that the employee perceives the entire process as a negative one. If this is not resolved, it can lead to poor performance and a lack of desire on the job in the future.

In this sensitive situation the manager should emphasize the fact that the individual is a valued and productive employee. The manager should make it clear that the organization therefore has a vital interest in the employee's further development so that he can become an even greater resource. The manager should convey that she and the employee must address aspects of the employee's overall performance that are not outstanding and discuss ways in which they might be improved. In taking this approach the reviewing manager assuages the ego of the employee without sacrificing the critical core of the performance appraisal. This also lessens the probability of damaging the employee's motivation, as the employee is still given credit for solid achievement.

In the case of employees who have performed at a substandard level in the past grading period, managers should use the review to provide performance assessments that are more accurate than the misguided perceptions the employees hold. This is a clearer problem to deal with, and considerably more challenging than the case of a good performer.

Immediate Blame

A favorite offensive tactic of employees who are aware that they have performed poorly is that of passing immediate blame. This is the practice of blaming another person, a lack of resources, unusual circumstances, or anything else other than their own performance as the root of poor productivity. New supervisors are usually the prime targets for this strategy.

An employee might have several reasons for using this strategy. If the employee has received clear and timely feedback about his poor performance, he will have a feeling that a negative review is in the offing. He will then prepare a suitable roster of alibis to deflect the blame to another party or work factor. Another reason might be that the employee is simply a classic "blamer" who rarely takes responsibility for his own actions and blames others out of habit. Because many health care organizations are overworked and understaffed, there are an infinite number of targets for the blame of the negatively oriented, sneaky nonplayer. People like this have spent most of their lives blaming others, and they should have been weeded out during the interviewing process by the use of artful targeted questions.

In any case, it is vital for the health care manager to keep the emphasis of the appraisal directly on the employee's work objectives. It must be stressed to the employee that he alone is responsible for his actions; if a problem exists that prevents him from performing adequately, that problem should be identified and brought to the attention of the supervisor immediately, not six months later in the review.

Some vainglorious nonplayers believe they are indispensable. The reviewing manager must stress that no employee is indispensable and that each employee is getting paid to produce results, not to create excuses. The reviewing manager herself should consider whether the blaming employee is really worth the paycheck. Of the ten possible reactions to a performance evaluation, this one in of itself is an indicator of a person who would rather apply his energies to negative ends than to positive ones. A blamer in the review session is most likely a blamer in all aspects of the job. If such a blamer is allowed to continue his behavior, other workers will believe that such bad behavior is acceptable to the manager and the organization. It is therefore essential for the manager to use the review session to stop the problem before it spreads. If the manager does not subsequently witness a drastic change in this behavior, termination based on poor performance and insubordination becomes a logical remedy.

Charge of Personal Bias

"You just don't like me"; this statement is usually the answer from an employee to a manager when the employee wishes to make personal bias or prejudice an issue in the performance review. Many nonplayers enjoy using this cheap tactic to avoid discussing the essence of the bad results and lack of work output. The alleged bias is always subjective and difficult either to disprove or discuss objectively, and is thus problematic to resolve effectively.

This type of behavior is a symptom of a larger illness; the employee probably uses this argument whenever things get difficult on the job. When the employee is simply using a charge of personal bias to shift blame and accountability, the manager must address this in no uncertain terms in the appraisal, with the promise that it will not be tolerated as an excuse for poor performance in the future.

Strong Verbal Reaction

Another frequent response to a performance appraisal discussion is a strong verbal reaction. The employee may raise his voice, use profanity, or otherwise verbally register disagreement with the appraisal. The manager must first find the root of the disagreement by asking the employee why his reaction is so strong. The manager should then calmly explain that nothing constructive will come from shouting and hollering, and that the difference in opinion about the appraisal should be discussed in a regular, conversational fashion. Furthermore, the manager should emphasize that the health care organization is a professional setting and that she must insist on professional employee conduct, no matter how angry the employee might be. If the reaction is extremely intense, the reviewer should use one of the Return to Objectivity strategies discussed in the next section of this chapter.

Strong verbal reactions can be expected from employees whose overall performance has been poor. If they have a notion that the process will be negative, they will probably prepare a tirade that will both express their displeasure and shift the focus of the session from objective performance to subjective emotionalism. It is essential in these cases that the manager keep the performance appraisal process on an even keel.

Strong Nonverbal Reaction

Like a strong verbal reaction, a strong nonverbal reaction conveys an employee's bitter disagreement with the performance appraisal. The employee decides to smolder, stare, or steam, in all cases intending to express displeasure to the manager rather than pay attention to the context and conduct of the review. In this case, the possibility of conducting a constructive performance evaluation is remote.

The remedy is somewhat similar to the previous one. The manager should tell the employee that she can easily discern, from the employee's expressions and emotions, that he does not agree with the substance of the review. The manager should indicate, however, that although the employee obviously disagrees with the appraisal, the manager believes that it is indeed a valid assessment and will continue with its conduct. She should then give the employee a printed copy of the completed review form and suggest that he review it himself for a couple days, and prepare to objectively rebut the review in writing or at another scheduled discussion. This gives the employee the chance to read the review—which is in fact a formal record of assessed performance—and to come to the realization in his own way that whether he agrees or not, this is how he is being appraised, and he must improve his performance quickly to remain employed.

Complacency

Certain employees are naturally complacent about their job as well as about life in general. This attitude, unfortunately, will insinuate itself into their performance and the performance appraisal session. Complacency might be expressed by a marginal employee, or perhaps by one who is a satisfactory worker but who is just not interested in being a top performer. The manager then undertakes the delicate task of trying to motivate an employee whose performance is acceptable to improve without alienating or disenchanting him. After all, as the employee might reason, what is wrong with being graded at a satisfactory level?

In this case, the manager must weigh the complacency against what is desired and needed in the position and decide how much that complacency affects the job performance. The very complacency that the employee exhibits during the appraisal session becomes another piece of evidence of undesired on-the-job conduct. In citing situations in which the employee's complacency produces negative results, the manager can add the observation that the employee seems uninterested in his own performance appraisal. With a marginal employee, the manager should seize the opportunity to take corrective action. With the average or above-average employee who just seems to have a temporary lapse of motivation, the manager should explore with the employee the aspects of the job that are of greater interest to him and that might help restore his motivation.

Contradiction

Contradiction is present in the performance evaluation session when the employee takes exception to certain segments of the review, or to the entire appraisal. The employee may contradict the reviewing manager when she is discussing what the established performance goals were, what performance was achieved as evidenced by work output, or any other aspect of the job. This obviously can diminish the effectiveness of the performance appraisal session, and can greatly hinder the chances of the employee and manager's coming to an agreement on future goals and objectives at the conclusion of the session.

The first remedy for contradiction is setting clear-cut goals from the outset of the grading period, along the parameters discussed throughout this chapter. The second is to provide the employee with objective examples to support each negative rating. For every goal that was not met according to expectations, the manager must have a related illustration showing why the goal was not achieved satisfactorily. Ideally the manager should have two examples to discuss in order to present a negative pattern of performance. When compared to the overall assessment of performance, the trivial disagreements from the employee concerning minor issues should pale quickly. If the employee contradicts the overall appraisal and his current level of performance is not acceptable, the employee should be counseled strongly and directly on the possibility of seeking other employment.

It is truly amazing how many examples there are of health care employees who are contradictory, disloyal, and more than willing to spend precious time and energy spouting opinions about their boss and the organization to anyone who will listen. Unfortunately, this malady is not unique to hourly employees; countless executives and managers have been the greatest proponents of badmouthing, contradiction, and disloyalty. This behavior undermines the authority and credibility of the organization, and its attendant game playing stirs up problems and can easily become an undermining contagion in the workplace if reviewing managers do not handle it forcefully and resolutely.

Taken Initiative

This is the least harmful of the ten reactions discussed in this section. Employees who take the initiative are usually highly motivated and have performed well during the current rating period. They are so enthusiastic that they are eminently agreeable to anything the manager says, and to each and every performance evaluation section and its outcomes.

The problem with these well-intentioned employees is that in their enthusiasm they do not listen closely to new dimensions of performance. Accordingly, they're liable to miss the point of any substantial feedback provided by the manager as they try to make the performance evaluation discussion as fluid as possible. The only remedy needed in this case is for the manager set a slower pace in the evaluation, so that the employee takes the time to understand the information. The manager must do this to make sure that the stellar employee gets as much from the appraisal session as does the marginal employee—a common mistake is for health care managers to spend more time in trying to redirect nonplayers with little effect than in encouraging their superstars.

USING DEFUSERS—THE RETURN TO OBJECTIVITY FORMULA

As is clear from the previous section, there is a range of possible reactions to the performance evaluation process. In some situations the remedies just covered might be inappropriate or ineffective. This section, therefore, provides four basic defusing strategies that a reviewing manager can use to return a highly emotional performance appraisal to its objective and constructive tone.

A defuser is a communication technique that eliminates emotionalism from a work-related conversation. Defusing an emotional conversation is like defusing an explosion by either extinguishing or cutting off its fuse. The health care manager can use the four techniques described here to eliminate argument and disagreement immediately and efficaciously. These techniques also allow the employee to come to a less emotional, more objective frame of mind before continuing with the substance of the performance review.

Pacification

Pacification is the practice of allowing the employee to display her anger immediately so that the rest of the performance appraisal can continue constructively. If the first reaction of an employee, for example, is a strong verbal reaction in the initial stages of the performance evaluation, the reviewing manager might tell the employee that he understands that the employee is upset. After then letting the employee make her "point" to her satisfaction, the manager redirects the conversation toward the appraisal itself. If he thinks the employee's point of contention is substantial, the manager might include a commitment to discuss that issue more deeply and specifically in another separate conversation.

Pacification is a good technique if the employee has just one specific argument that is not particularly consequential and that is known to the manager at the outset of the performance evaluation discussion. General or partial agreement with the employee's point satisfies the employee, who is usually responsive to the rest of the appraisal. However, if an employee wishes to contest every segment of the performance evaluation, pacification will merely encourage her to turn the appraisal session into a debate. The other risk with this approach is that the employee, having attained agreement on one argument, might get the false impression that the manager will be agreeable to other issues of interest to the employee. Again, however, if it is a minor issue at stake and the employee is sincerely interested in making her feelings known without any underlining motives—as is the case with a steady employee—this technique is usually very effective.

Facilitation

Facilitation encourages the employee to discuss any meaningful contentions in the context of the performance appraisal session. This is an extremely effective method if the employee's points of contention are related to a performance issue covered in the performance appraisal and if the employee is interested in making realistic suggestions for solutions to problems, as opposed to merely reiterating existent problems in an ignorant fashion. In fact, the intent of a performance appraisal session is to discuss critical dimensions of performance and developmental direction. It is therefore entirely appropriate for the manager to use facilitation to encourage the employee to discuss more specifically her concerns and her potential solutions to stated problems, and then to come jointly to an agreement with the employee on how the problem might be better addressed in future circumstances.

Facilitation may not be accomplished with a malevolent employee who has major problems on the job and wishes to provide a full-scale diatribe on "why things go wrong all the time." Facilitation also may not work well with employees who are overly conversational and will seize the opportunity to present a dissertation on the organization, their department, and, of course, their job. Managers must call on their independent judgment to decide when to employ facilitation, and to what degree to allow facilitation to become an integral part of the performance appraisal process. The manager must be mindful that the performance appraisal is vital to individual employees and their compensation, and that the dialogue that takes place in this forum is a very serious and sensitive issue for them. Accordingly, employees will remember and mark well the manager's response to the presentation of their concerns.

When using facilitation, the reviewing manager must also keep in mind the time parameters allocated to each employee's appraisal. The employee who receives less time in the appraisal session than average—usually because there is no need for facilitation or extended discussion—might feel cheated of the time discussing critical performance with the manager. Therefore, the manager must remember that facilitation is a good practical tool that should be applied intelligently and appropriately, and in accordance with the requirements of each employee's individual work situation. If major issues cannot be resolved within the time allotted for the appraisal session, the manager might wish to schedule a specific time for the employee to discuss the significant work situations in more detail.

Suspension

In some appraisal sessions, the employee becomes so highly charged that it is virtually impossible for the manager to discuss the completed review. Employees can become distraught or angry, and demonstrate other emotions that prohibit sound conduct of the appraisal. In such cases it is imperative that the manager employ a strategy of suspension. Suspension is the practice of putting off the performance evaluation discussion for a set period of time, during which the employee can cool off, collect her thoughts about the appraisal, and prepare to approach the next appraisal session more objectively.

During an appraisal session on a Thursday afternoon, for example, the manager might tell an overwrought employee to forget about the appraisal until Tuesday morning at 10 o'clock. In doing this the manager gives the employee the opportunity to spend the rest of the workweek and a weekend reflecting on the performance appraisal. He should give the employee a copy of the appraisal itself so the employee can study it and reconcile its contents with her own perceptions. The employee will usually approach the situation with a cooler head on Tuesday morning and, ideally, will have a more educated perspective. An obvious proviso is that if the manager uses suspension, he must ensure that on Tuesday morning the scheduled meeting is conducted without fail. If it is not, the employee can easily get the impression that the appraisal must not have been that important to the manager, and that the employee was merely being " put off " as the manager clearly must have "more important" things to do than discuss the employee's performance. This can violate the intent of the performance evaluation as a constructive leadership tool.

A potential pitfall of suspension is that the employee might become even angrier or more distraught between sessions. If that occurs, the manager must distinguish between the employee's emotionalism and the reasons for that emotionalism, and then decide whether or not the employee's points are valid. If they are not valid, the manager should determine whether the employee's emotional outburst was done purposefully for dramatic effect. In either case the use of suspension will probably give the manager sound insight into the employee's current motivation and desire to work hard for the organization.

Cancellation

The final defusing strategy, both in terms of the Return to Objectivity formula and because of its "last resort" nature, is cancellation. Cancellation is the abrupt halting of a performance appraisal session in which a negatively assessed employee counters the conduct of the session with negative emotionalism that is typical of her overall work behavior. By "blowing up" in the appraisal, the employee is providing the manager with a perfect example of unacceptable behavior. The manager should then get a third party to be present in the discussion—perhaps his own boss or a representative from human resources—and use the session to either put the employee on probation or terminate the employee from the organization. This approach is used primarily with an employee whose continued employment is somewhat doubtful at best. This approach gives the manager a critical opportunity to dismiss the employee from the organization, because the employee is in essence terminating herself with her reaction (and with her poor prior performance). The manager might simply stop the appraisal and ask for a resignation. If the employee is reluctant to resign at that point, the manager should just terminate the employee. Although this at first might seem to be a hard-line approach, a major problem in health care organizations today is the "softness" of line managers toward employees who do not merit employment and who probably should not have been hired at all in a people-oriented health care organization. In these days of diminishing operating revenue and high competition, the organization's all-important bottom line can be severely hampered by the behavior of loudly contentious, unproductive employees. The manager is doing himself, his motivated and productive employees, and his organization a major disservice by sheltering poor employees in the false hope that they might someday "turn things around." If the manager believes that the employee who has demonstrated poor work consistently for at least two years will suddenly turn into a solid performer, he simply lacks the independent judgment and accountability to be a leader in the modern health care organization. Obviously, all terminations and probations must be performed with the professional guidance of a trustworthy human resources professional or legal counsel.

SUMMARY

Performance management and evaluation are line management accountabilities that are monitored and in many cases led by human resources professionals. The implementation of the processes and strategies delineated in this chapter can help you in making this essential process an organizational mainstay as opposed to just a superfluous paper chase.

KEY TERMS

balanced scorecard approach   goalsharing

gainsharing   performance evaluation

DISCUSSION QUESTIONS

1. How are performance evaluations used to support strategic human resources management?

2. What are common points of ineffective performance evaluation in health care?

3. List and discuss at least five common errors made by managers in performance evaluation.

4. When should positive and negative aspects of job performance be documented?

5. A common lament in health care management is that performance evaluation ratings tend to be inflated in the same manner that grades in the college classroom are sometimes "too generous." Can you suggest three factors that might make this perception valid?

6. Identify and discuss team-based performance appraisal techniques.

10

Compensation Strategies

LEARNING OBJECTIVES

- Understand the importance of compensation to strategic human resources management
- Understand basic theories underlying pay systems
- Explain external, internal, and employee equity
- Understand the role that labor markets play in determining compensation
- Explain how to determine the relevant labor market for a specific job
- Discuss what compensable factors are and how they relate to job evaluation

EMPLOYEES ARE COMPLEX and motivated by many factors. An employee's performance is often determined by the levels and interaction of ability and motivation. Motivation is the desire within a person to act in a particular way. Employees are motivated by both intrinsic and extrinsic rewards. Intrinsic rewards are part of the job itself, such as having challenging job tasks, learning new skills and developing additional job knowledge, and assuming increased levels of responsibility. Extrinsic rewards are a part of the job situation, provided by others. Extrinsic rewards may include the salary and benefits or status one receives from being employed. For individuals with a routine job, the job itself may not lead to these employees' motivation, but they may be motivated by the compensation and benefits they receive.

MOTIVATION

According to Rainey (2003), work motivation refers to a person's desire to work hard and work well—to the arousal, direction, and persistence of effort in work settings. He notes that the definition is far too simple and leaves many questions about what it means to work hard and well, what determines a person's desire to do so, and how one measures such behavior. He states that motivation is an umbrella concept that serves as an overarching theme for research on a variety of related topics, including organizational identification and commitment, leadership practices, job involvement, and characteristics of work goals. He further notes that there are a variety of words used to describe motivation. *Needs, values, motives, incentives, objectives,* and *goals* are often used and frequently overlap. According to Rainey, a need is a resource or condition required for the well-being of an individual. A motive is a force within an individual that causes him or her to seek to obtain or avoid some external object or condition. An incentive is an external object or condition that evokes behaviors aimed at attaining or avoiding it. A goal is a future state that one strives to achieve, and an objective is a more specific short-term goal, a step toward a more general, longer-term goal.

Content Theories of Motivation

Content theories of motivation refer to the needs, motives, and rewards that people are attempting to satisfy. They are often referred to as *need* theories of motivation. These theories use personal characteristics or attributes of the individual to explain motivation. Needs are latent internal characteristics activated by stimuli or objects a person encounters. The person tries to behave in a way that satisfies an activated need.

Hierarchy of Needs

Abraham Maslow's **hierarchy of needs** (1954) is one theory suggesting that needs can be reduced into five groups of basic human needs whose satisfaction is sought by adults. The lowest-level needs are *physiological needs*. These include food, water, sleep, and sex. *Safety needs* come next. They are the desires of a person to be protected from physical or economic harm. *Belongingness and love needs* include the desire to give and receive affection and to be in the company of others. *Esteem needs* address a person's self-confidence and sense of self-worth. The highest-level need is *self-actualization*. This need describes the desire for self-fulfillment. As each of these needs becomes satisfied, the next need becomes dominant. Physiological and safety needs are referred to as lower-order needs, and social needs, esteem needs, and self-actualization are categorized as higher-order needs. According to this theory people must satisfy needs at the bottom of the hierarchy before high-level needs emerge as important.

ERG Theory

Clayton P. Alderfer (1972) proposed a modification of Maslow's hierarchy of needs. Alderfer reduced the five need levels into three more general levels: *existence needs, relatedness needs,* and *growth needs* (ERG). According to **ERG theory,** existence needs are those required to sustain human existence, including both physiological and safety needs. Relatedness needs are needs concerning how people relate to their surrounding social environment, including the need for meaningful social and interpersonal relationships. Growth needs pertain to the development of human potential, including the needs for self-esteem and self-actualization. This is the highest need category. Alderfer's model is similar to Maslow's in that in both models individuals move up the hierarchy one step at a time as a need is met. An unmet need is a motivator. If both lower-order and higher-order needs are unsatisfied, then the lower-order needs will be the most important motivators of behavior. Where the theories differ is in that according to Maslow, individuals progress up the hierarchy as a result of the satisfaction of lower-order needs. In contrast, Alderfer suggests that in addition to this satisfaction progression process there is also a frustration regression process. When individuals are continually frustrated in their attempts to satisfy growth needs, relatedness needs will reemerge as a primary motivating force and the individuals are likely to redirect their efforts toward lower-level needs.

Theory of Needs

According to David McClelland's **theory of needs** (1961), individuals have three primary needs: *achievement, affiliation,* and *power*. A strong need for achievement is characterized by a strong desire to assume personal responsibility for finding solutions to problems, a tendency to set moderately difficult achievement goals and take calculated risks, a strong desire for concrete feedback on task performance, and a preoccupation with tasks and task accomplishment. A low need for achievement is typically characterized by a preference for low risk levels on tasks and for shared responsibility on tasks. When an employee or manager with high achievement is placed on a difficult job, the challenging nature of the task serves to cue the achievement motive, which in turn activates achievement-oriented behavior. However, if high-need achievers are placed in routine or unchallenging jobs the achievement motive will probably not be activated. Hence there would be little reason to expect them to perform in a superior fashion under such conditions. This concept is important for understanding how people respond to the work environment. It has implications for job design in that high achievers prefer autonomy and willingly assume responsibilities, whereas low achievers may withdraw from challenging situations.

A strong need for affiliation is characterized by a desire for human companionship and reassurance. People with a high need for affiliation typically possess a strong desire for approval and reassurance from others, a tendency to conform to the wishes and norms of others when pressured by people whose friendship they value, and a sincere interest in the feelings of others.

A strong need for power is characterized by a desire to influence others and to control one's environment. Employees with a power need will try to control or lead those around them. They tend to influence others directly by making suggestions, giving their opinions, and using persuasion. They seek positions of leadership in group activities, and are usually verbally fluent, often talkative, and sometimes argumentative. Employees with a strong need for power tend to be superior performers and tend to be in supervisory positions. They are often rated by others as having good leadership abilities.

Motivator-Hygiene Theory

Frederick Herzberg, in his **motivator-hygiene theory** (1964, 1968), concluded that people have two different categories of needs that are essentially independent of each other and affect behavior in different ways. On the one hand, when people are dissatisfied with their job they are concerned about the environment in which they are working. On the other hand, when people feel good about their job this has to do with the work itself.

Herzberg referred to the first category of needs as being made up of environment, hygiene, or maintenance factors. *Hygiene* because they describe people's *environment* and serve the primary functions of preventing job dissatisfaction, *maintenance* because employees are never completely satisfied. They have to be maintained. Agency policies, supervision, working conditions, interpersonal relations, money, status, and security are referred to as hygiene factors because they are not an intrinsic part of the job but are related to the conditions under which a job is performed. These factors do not contribute to productivity; they only prevent losses in worker performance due to work restrictions—which is why they are also called maintenance factors. When maintenance factors are adequate, people will not be dissatisfied but neither will they be satisfied. According to this theory, to motivate people on the job, factors associated with the work itself or with outcomes directly related to it, such as promotional opportunities and opportunities for personal growth, recognition, responsibility, and achievement, should be emphasized.

Herzberg referred to the second category of needs as *motivators.* These factors involve feelings of achievement, professional growth, and recognition that one can experience in a job. They are called motivators because these factors appear to have a positive effect on job satisfaction and drive people to superior performance.

Process Theories of Motivation

Process theories of motivation concentrate more on the cognitive and behavioral processes behind motivation. They suggest that a variety of factors may serve as motivators, depending on the needs of the individual, the situation the individual is in, and the rewards the individual expects for the work done.

Expectancy Theory

Victor H. Vroom (1964) developed an early model of **expectancy theory,** which holds that the force to act in a certain way results from a conscious decision-making process undertaken by an individual. The decision to act rests on three kinds of perceptions: *expectancy, instrumentality,* and *valence.* Expectancy is the individual's perception that a certain level of effort is required to achieve a certain level of performance. Instrumentality is the strength of the belief that a certain level of performance will be associated with various outcomes, such as a promotion, a pay increase, or the opportunity to telecommute. Valence is the attractiveness of the outcomes. In making the decision to act, it is assumed, an employee takes account of all three of these perceptions.

The theory focuses on the following relationships:

- *Effort-to-performance relationship,* referring to the probability perceived by the individual that exerting a given amount of effort will lead to the desired performance

- *Performance-reward relationship,* referring to the degree to which the individual believes performing at a particular level will lead to the attainment of a desired outcome

- *Rewards–personal goals relationship,* referring to the degree to which rewards satisfy the individual's personal goals or needs and the attractiveness of those rewards for the individual.

Equity Theory

Equity theory is often referred to as a social comparison theory (Adams, 1965). Employers and employees enter into an exchange relationship. The employer provides outcomes, such as pay, praise, promotions, and benefits, and the employee provides inputs, which is his or her performance.

When the employee perceives that the ratios of outcomes to inputs are about equal, the employee is likely to be satisfied with the exchange relationship. The balance of outcomes to inputs is the goal that employees are motivated to achieve. Employees compare themselves to other employees both within and outside of the organization. If the employee perceives that the ratio of his or her outcomes to inputs is less than the ratio of outcomes to inputs for others, then the employee may feel underrewarded. Rarely do employees feel overrewarded. Positive outcomes are pay, fringe benefits, a pleasant work environment, friendly coworkers, and intrinsic outcomes of the job itself. Negative outcomes include unpleasant or hazardous working conditions, a monotonous job, and controlling supervision. The perception of inequity creates an internal state of tension. The tension motivates the individual to reduce the tension. This can be done by changing the inputs.

The employee may reduce his or her inputs or efforts or, under conditions of positive outcomes, may increase those inputs.

Goal-Setting Theory

Goals that are specific, challenging, reachable, and acceptable to employees lead to higher performance than goals that are unclear, unchallenging, or unattainable (Locke, 1968). High performance results from clear expectations. Employees who are told to do their best do not do as well as those who have specific task goals to reach. **Goal-setting theory** does not view goals as static. Instead, goals are based on the past and some predictions for the future. As circumstances change, goals may need to change. An important consideration is the ability to change goals after they have been set because circumstances surrounding the goals may have changed.

An analysis of motivational theories has led researchers to conclude that many of the theories are difficult to test. In a health care context, goals are not always clear; there are not necessarily reward-performance contingencies; rewards may be scarce; and motivational situations or contexts are often dictated by institutions and embedded in laws, rules, and external expectations (Perry, 2000).

EQUITY

To develop **compensation** systems, employers rely on three types of equity: external, internal, and employee.

External Equity

External equity is the standard that compares an employer's wages with the rates prevailing in external markets for the employee's position. What do other health care organizations pay employees who perform similar tasks and have similar responsibilities? For example, what do other counties pay entry-level registered nurses? What do program directors at mental health nonprofits that provide services to substance abusers get paid? The federal government and state governments that hire pharmacists to work in their hospitals (that is, public health departments, veterans affairs facilities) want to know the salary range for pharmacists working in private for-profit and nonprofit hospitals. External equity is determined by surveying the competitive labor market. Labor markets are identified and defined by some combination of the following factors: education and technical background requirements; licensing or certification requirements; experience required by the job; and geographical location, such as a local, regional, or national labor market (Wallace & Fay, 1988). The labor market reflects the forces of supply and demand for qualified labor within an area. These forces influence the wages required to recruit or retain qualified employees. If employees do not see their pay as equitable compared to what other organizations pay for similar work, they are likely to leave if they have an opportunity.

If an organization cannot conduct a survey itself or hire consultants to do so, various government agencies, such as the state or federal Department of Labor, or firms associated with commerce, such as the Bureau of Labor Statistics, the Bureau of National Affairs, and the Commerce Clearing House, publish area wage surveys and industry wage surveys, as well as professional, administrative, technical, and clerical surveys. Professional associations and consulting firms also publish salary data.

Internal Equity

Internal equity is the standard that requires employers to set wages for jobs within their organization that correspond to the relative internal value of each job. Positions that are determined to be more valuable to the organization receive higher wages. High-level employees typically receive greater compensation than low-level employees.

The internal value of each position to the organization is determined by a procedure known as job evaluation, which determines the worth of one job relative to another. To institute internal equity into its compensation structure, Congress passed the Classification Act of 1923. Prior to the establishment of the system, federal employees were paid according to which agency they worked for, and wages were determined at the discretion of agency management. The lack of standardization permitted disparities among employees performing the same type of work. Different positions were often given the same title, and similar positions were often given different titles. Pay was not necessarily related to the work performed. The act created the Personnel Classification Board, which mandated that positions be grouped according to similar responsibilities and duties and that employees be compensated accordingly. Employees would be paid in keeping with the value of their work, to be determined by the job's compensable factors, such as the level of education and amount of experience required, the amount of responsibility, and job hazards. Table 10.1 lists some of the most common compensable factors.

A variety of factor comparison systems are used to determine job value. Compensable factors are identified, weighed, and assigned point values that reflect their weight. Jobs are broken down into their compensable factors and rated along a continuum of points or rank-ordered. After the compensable factors have been rated or ranked, they are summed to derive a total point value for the job. Positions with higher point values are considered more valuable to the agency.

In 1949 Congress passed the Classification Act of 1949, which established the General Schedule (GS) system. The GS system defines the basic compensation system for nonmanagerial, white-collar positions. There are fifteen grade levels, with ranges of pay within each grade. There are approximately 450 job categories in the GS, sorted into such specialized groups as finance and accounting, social science, psychology and welfare, engineering and architecture, and physical science. Each grade contains examples of the kind of work performed in jobs that would be assigned to that grade on the basis of their duties, their responsibilities, and the qualifications required to perform them. These examples are referred to as **benchmark positions**. Benchmark positions are jobs with characteristics similar enough to jobs performed in other organizations that they can serve as market anchor points when using a factor comparison system. Nine factors with different levels and different point values are used to evaluate jobs: knowledge required by the position, supervisory controls, guidelines, complexity, scope and effect, personal contacts, purpose of contacts, physical demands, and work environment. After all nine factors have been evaluated and levels have been established for the position, the points are summed across each factor to derive an aggregate total. The total points are then compared to a chart, and the position is assigned to a grade.

A problem with this job evaluation system is that the duties and responsibilities of a specific job do not always neatly fit into one grade or job class. The GS has been criticized for its lack of flexibility in supporting individual agency missions, structures, and cultures and for its inability

Table 10.1   Typical Compensable Factors

Compensable Factor	Description	Question(s) Addressed in Job Specifications
Experience	Experience encompasses the training and development acquired from previous work that are necessary to qualify for a position, plus the training and development on the job that are necessary for proficiency. The requirement for this factor is usually expressed in terms of the time necessary to acquire the experience.	How long should the incumbent have worked in this job or in a closely related job?
Education	Education refers to the basic abilities, skills, and intellectual requirements the position demands, normally assumed to have been acquired by attending high school, business school, trade school, college, or graduate school. Referring to periods of formal schooling is convenient when comparing positions; however, the phrase ''or its equivalent'' should usually form a part of the educational specifications when such reference is made.	What does the job require in terms of formal schooling, training, or knowledge of a specialized field?
Complexity of duties	This factor is a measure of the variety and difficulty of the work performed and the degree of skill and judgment necessary in performing it. Complexity is found to some extent in all positions.	Does the job require the incumbent to show judgment and initiative and to make independent decisions?

Table 10.1   Typical Compensable Factors (*Continued*)

Compensable Factor	Description	Question(s) Addressed in Job Specifications
Supervision received	This refers to the degree to which the work is supervised, guided by practice or precedent, and the requirements of the position in regard to problem solving and decision making.	How closely does the incumbent's supervisor check his or her work and outline specific methods or work procedures?
Supervision exercised	This factor measures the responsibility for directing the work of others. Its value is determined by the nature and complexity of the work supervised, the degree of responsibility for attaining desired results, and the number of persons supervised.	How many people does the incumbent supervise directly or indirectly?
Mental demands	This factor appraises the amount and continuity of mental demands required to perform the job. It is a compensable factor in positions requiring a degree of concentrated mental effort or constant attention to detail.	What degree of concentration does this job require?
Physical demands	This factor appraises the amount and continuity of physical effort required to perform the job. It is a compensable factor in jobs that require the employee to stand, lift, carry, bend, or walk for extended periods.	Are there special physical demands of this job?
Working conditions	This factor has value for positions in which excessive heat and noise, use of chemicals, poor ventilation, and so forth are elements in the job environment.	Is there anything in the work environment that is unusually hazardous or uncomfortable? If so, what percentage of the time is the incumbent exposed to this?

to respond to rapidly changing external conditions. As a result, some federal agencies have received permission to modify the GS by reducing the number of occupational categories and to establish broadbanding systems (Thompson, 2007). (Broadbanding is described later in this chapter.)

Employee Equity

Employee equity is the comparison of pay across employees performing the same or similar work. It focuses on the contributions of an individual worker within a job classification. At issue is what coworkers performing the same job are paid. Are differences in levels of proficiency or contribution reflected in compensation?

Most compensation structures include pay ranges. A pay range exists when one or more rates are paid to employees in the same job. The range permits organizations to pay different wages for differences in experience or differences in performance. A pay range reflects the minimum and maximum that the employer will pay for the position.

Table 10.2 presents the general salary pay scale for federal employees. Each grade has ten pay-level increments. New college graduates usually begin at the base pay for the grade, but the Office of Personnel Management may authorize recruitment at rates above the minimum for jobs in which there are shortages, such as engineers, chemists, and architects. There is, however, a different pay scale for the Department of Veterans Affairs.

To design pay ranges, employers need to establish the current market rates for benchmark jobs. After the data have been compiled, organizations develop salary ranges to fit their structure. Each salary range should have a midpoint, a minimum, and a maximum. The distance separating a grade's minimum and maximum salaries is the grade's range. The midpoint for each range is usually set to correspond to the external labor market. It specifies the pay objectives for employees performing at satisfactory levels. The minimums and maximums are usually based on a combination of the size of the range identified in survey data and judgments about how the range fits the organization. These judgments are based on a variety of factors, such as salaries paid by the organization's competition, the organization's culture, and standard salaries across an occupational classification. For example, production and maintenance positions typically have ranges of 20 to 25 percent, whereas professional, administrative, and managerial personnel

Table 10.2 Salary Table 2010-GS Incorporating the 1.50 Percent General Schedule Increase (Annual Rates by Grade and Step)

Source: U.S. Office of Personnel Management, 2010.

Grade	1	2	3	4	5	6	7	8	9	10	Within Grade Amounts
1	17,803	18,398	18,990	19,579	20,171	20,519	21,104	21,694	21,717	22,269	Varies
2	20,017	20,493	21,155	21,717	21,961	22,607	23,253	23,899	24,545	25,191	Varies
3	21,840	22,568	23,296	24,024	24,752	25,480	26,208	26,939	27,664	28,392	728
4	24,518	25,335	26,152	26,969	27,786	28,603	29,420	30,237	31,054	31,871	817
5	27,431	28,345	29,259	30,173	31,087	32,001	32,915	33,829	34,743	35,657	914
6	30,577	31,596	32,615	33,634	34,653	35,672	36,691	37,710	38,729	39,748	1,019
7	33,979	35,112	36,245	37,378	38,511	39,644	40,777	41,910	43,043	44,176	1,133
8	37,631	38,885	40,139	41,393	42,646	43,901	45,155	46,409	47,663	48,917	1,254
9	41,563	42,948	44,333	45,718	47,103	48,488	49,873	51,258	52,643	54,028	1,385
10	45,771	47,297	48,823	50,349	51,875	53,401	54,927	56,453	57,979	59,505	1,526
11	50,287	51,963	53,639	55,315	56,991	58,667	60,343	62,019	63,695	65,371	1,676
12	60,274	62,283	64,292	66,301	68,310	70,319	72,328	74,337	76,346	78,355	2,009
13	71,674	74,063	76,452	78,841	81,230	83,619	86,008	88,397	90,786	93,175	2,389
14	84,697	87,520	90,343	93,166	95,989	98,812	101,635	104,458	107,281	110,104	2,823
15	99,628	102,949	106,270	109,591	112,912	116,233	119,554	122,875	126,196	129,517	3,321

might have ranges of 40 to 50 percent under certain circumstances. Wider ranges are designed to reflect greater discretion, responsibility, and variations in performance. Pay ranges are useful because they allow an organization to provide a competitive salary and recognize individual differences among employees.

When establishing pay ranges, employers must look at the degree of overlap in adjacent pay ranges. Overlap is the amount of comparability of pay between pay grades. The amount of overlap between pay grades signifies the similarities in the responsibilities; duties; and knowledge, skills, abilities, and other characteristics (KSAOCs) of the jobs whose pay ranges overlap. Overlap between pay ranges permits more valuable senior employees in lower-paying jobs to be paid more than new employees in higher-level jobs who have not yet begun to make significant contributions to the organization (Henderson, 2000).

When developing a salary structure, you may find that certain jobs in the organization have been underpaid or overpaid. Underpaid positions are referred to as "green-circled," and overpaid positions as "red-circled." To bring these wages in line with market rates and internal equity standards, underpaid employees should be given pay increases that raise their rates to at least the minimum of the range for their pay grade. The salaries of overpaid employees may need to be frozen until other jobs are brought into line with them. Other options include cutting the wages to the maximum in the pay range for the pay grade, increasing the employees' responsibilities, or transferring or promoting them to positions in which they can be paid their current rate.

Employee equity addresses **pay differentials** within the same position. It recognizes that employees who possess the same job title and responsibilities often perform at different levels of productivity or proficiency, making different contributions to the agency's mission.

In many organizations seniority is frequently used to differentiate pay. More senior employees receive higher wages regardless of their performance. For each year of service, an employee's salary is automatically increased to the next grade step to reward his or her years of service to the organization. The problem with seniority-based differentials is that longer tenure does not necessarily translate into more effective performance. If seniority is the only system in place to differentiate pay, organizations may find it hard to attract and retain competent employees. Employees who believe that their pay is low after comparing their inputs and level of pay to those of other employees in similar positions will become less motivated over time. Dissatisfied employees are prone to file more grievances, to be absent more frequently, and to search for higher-paying positions elsewhere. Employers must have in place different strategies to address employee equity concerns.

The following subsections provide brief descriptions of alternative pay systems that are used to enhance traditional pay systems.

Longevity Pay

Longevity pay rewards employees who have reached pay-grade maximums and are not likely to move into higher grades. Its purpose is to reduce turnover as well as reward employees for continuous years of service. It may be a percentage of the employee's base pay, a flat dollar amount, or a special step increase based on the number of years the employee has spent with the organization.

Broadbanding or Paybanding

There has been a movement away from using a system of many pay grades. Instead, salary grades are being collapsed into broader bands with wider ranges. The use of broadbands, also referred to as paybands, eliminates having to maintain many narrow salary grades. Broadbanding grants managers the discretion to offer a variety of starting salaries and reward employees with pay increases or different job assignments as needed to fulfill the agency's mission. Advocates of broadbanding claim that it simplifies pay administration, helps facilitate career development, creates a performance-driven culture, and links compensation with strategic human resources management.

Skill-Based Pay or Pay for Knowledge

In skill-based or pay-for-knowledge pay plans, pay is determined by the number of tasks or jobs or the amount of knowledge an employee masters. It is a compensation system based on paying for what employees can do, for the knowledge or skills they possess. Under skill-based pay, employees can be expected to perform a broad range of duties. Benefits attributed to skill-based pay from an organizational standpoint include developing a cross-trained and more flexible workforce, improving the flow of information throughout the organization, placing an emphasis on the work to be done rather than on the job itself, encouraging the acquisition of skills needed to perform a variety of jobs, and increasing employees' interest in and commitment to their work. Benefits from the employees' perspective include higher motivation, increased job satisfaction, and greater opportunities for increased pay (Feuer, 1987; Gupta, Jenkins, & Curington, 1986; Shareef, 1994, 1998; Thompson & Lehew, 2000; Towers Perrin, 1992). The implementation of skill-based pay is not without problems. Changing a compensation system in the public sector typically requires obtaining the approval of multiple external stakeholders, such as legislative bodies and union representatives, as well as the managers or supervisors and employees who will be affected. Employees may be reluctant to give up annual step or cost-of-living increases while developing new competencies (Gupta, 1997; Shareef, 1998, 2002; Thompson & Lehew, 2000).

Organizations that implement skill-based pay need to be aware that wages and salaries will increase as employees learn new skills. And despite the strategic focus of skill-based training, all other human resources management systems must be aligned. Performance evaluation systems, training and development systems, communication systems, and record-keeping systems all must change and reinforce the implementation of skill-based pay systems, or the implementation will not be successful (Shareef, 2002).

Merit Pay or Pay for Performance

Merit pay, also known as pay for performance, is grounded in the belief that individuals should be paid according to their contributions. Increases are awarded on the basis of performance rather than seniority, equality, or need (Heneman, 1992). As logical as that may sound, research over the years has indicated that merit pay systems have not achieved the expected and desired results (Heneman; Kellough & Nigro, 2002; Kellough & Lu, 1993; Perry, 1995; Risher, Fay, & Perry, 1997; U.S. Merit Systems Protection Board, 2006).

Pay-for-performance systems fall victim to much of the same criticism that surrounds performance evaluations as noted in Chapter Nine. Critics claim that the pay-for-performance evaluation process is subjective, that employees are rated by instruments that do not reflect their actual job competencies, that supervisors lack skills to develop performance standards and provide feedback, and that comparing individuals to one another sets up a competitive environment that can be destructive to the cohesion of an organization, department, or unit. An additional criticism is that adequate financial resources are not always allocated (U.S. Merit Systems Protection Board, 2006). Even when pay rewards are not restricted, the small percentage of difference between high and low performers typically found in merit systems does not encourage improved performance or reward outstanding employees (Heneman, 1992).

Merit pay systems have been condemned for focusing on compensation rather than improved performance. Research has found that when pay and performance are discussed, employees fail to address the developmental issues and instead focus on not receiving a pay increase or on receiving an increase lower than expected. When provided with constructive feedback in a training-and-development context, employees are likely to accept the information. When feedback is tied to pay increases, however, employees process the information differently. They tend to get defensive, believing that the rater is taking something away from them by not granting a pay increase. Other research indicates that when performance appraisal results determine pay, employees often set lower goals so that they can achieve them (Cascio, 1991; Lawler, 1989).

The concepts of procedural justice and distributive justice must be considered when developing and administering pay-for-performance systems. **Procedural justice** focuses on the perceived fairness of the evaluation procedures used to determine performance ratings or merit increases. For example, what procedures or instruments are used to guarantee a link between pay and performance? **Distributive justice** focuses on the perceived fairness of the ratings or increases received relative to the work performed (Greenberg, 1986, 1996). For example, is the rating or increase congruent with the performance inputs? Merit systems that are not developed with these principles in mind will lack the integrity and credibility necessary for employees to believe that the system can discern and will reward differences in performance.

Heneman (1992) found that for employees to perceive the process as just, five components must exist: performance must be clearly defined, rewards must be communicated to employees, rewards must be made contingent on desired performance, opportunities to improve performance must exist, and the perceived relationship between rewards and performance should be considered to be as important as the actual relationship.

To be successful, a pay-for-performance system must be linked to the strategic mission of the organization, and upper-level management must support the plan. Employees should participate in the development of the plan, which increases their understanding of, commitment to, and trust in the plan. Organizations must provide training to the raters and hold them accountable for the accuracy of their ratings, and a system of checks and balances is necessary (Healy & Southard, 1994; Heneman, 1992; Newlin & Meng, 1991; Perry, 1995; Risher, 2002; U.S. Merit Systems Protection Board, 2006).

Gainsharing

Gainsharing is a team bonus program that measures controllable costs, such as improved safety records, decreases in waste, or increased units of output. Teamwork is encouraged, and all team members are rewarded for controlling costs or improving productivity. Formulas are used to measure costs that are controllable, and these costs are then compared to the costs of a historical base period. When performance improves relative to the base period, a bonus pool is funded. When performance falls short, no bonus pool is created. Employees keep a percentage of the bonus pool, and the organization keeps the rest.

Not all gainsharing plans are the same. The formulas and participative management features need to fit each other as well as the organization, and different situations require different designs. However, some common critical elements are necessary for any plan to succeed:

- There must be a credible and trusted plan development process.

- Employees must believe that improved performance and decreased costs will lead to a bonus, the bonus must be understandable and large enough to influence performance, and employees must recognize how their behavior can influence the size of the bonus.

- Employees need to be involved in the process; they must have influence over the measures used to calculate the bonus.

- There must be appropriate measures of productivity. Such measures as units of output, materials, and supplies must be addressed; otherwise, employees may focus on one cost, leading to its reduction but also to increases in other costs. For example, data processing clerks may produce a greater number of records, but if the number of errors on the records has increased, the effort has been counterproductive. Or public works employees may be able to maintain and landscape more of the city's property in less time, but if the increased productivity results in equipment breakdowns and expensive repairs, then that is counterproductive. The program must be maintained; because missions and environments change, gainsharing formulas and programs must change as well to stay relevant (Lawler, 1989, 2000).

Closing Thoughts on Equity

Despite an organization's best efforts to ensure equity, a number of factors that affect compensation are outside an agency's control. For example, as positions demand higher skill requirements, organizations can expect to pay more for those skills. If skills are in abundance, then employers can offer less, even if those skills are critical to the organization. Or jobs with unpleasant or hazardous working conditions, such as in sanitation or public works, might demand higher salaries because these are necessary to attract individuals to those positions.

Developing a compensation system that meets employee and organizational goals requires fine-tuning. Not all employees have the same priorities. Today applicants and employees consider quality-of-life issues also to be important. To attract and retain employees, organizations need to offer either competitive wages or other benefits deemed important to employees and applicants, such as flexible work schedules, career mobility, a sense of purpose and the opportunity to use their skills, and child care or educational reimbursement programs. Some of these topics will be discussed in Chapter Eleven.

EXECUTIVE COMPENSATION AND BENEFITS

The compensation and benefits provided to executives in health care organizations are often different from the compensation and benefits other employees receive. In most private for-profit and nonprofit organizations, executives serve at the discretion of the board of directors. Because the positions lack security, executives are likely to have negotiated employment contracts that specify the level of compensation and benefits they will receive. Some common benefits found in executive employment contracts are severance protection; moving expenses; health, retirement, and disability insurance; professional association memberships and dues; and paid conference registration and associated expenses, such as for travel and accommodations.

Executives are hired for their professional experience and expertise. They must often make hard choices and unpopular decisions that run counter to the wishes of the policymaking and governing body. Severance protection allows executives to be free to make those decisions without having to worry about their financial situation if they are terminated. Severance protection usually includes a fixed amount of the executive's salary and the continuance of insurance benefits for a predetermined period of time.

Executives are typically recruited from the national labor market and often relocate to accept a position. Organizations that pay for moving expenses and in some cases provide a housing allowance, in jurisdictions where housing is expensive, have an easier time attracting key executives. Executives will be less likely to relocate if they will continue to lose equity in their home or if the costs associated with moving are prohibitive.

Because it is the responsibility of executives to guide as well as manage the organization, it is imperative that they have access to training and development opportunities, such as attending conferences and belonging to professional associations. Organizations benefit when their executives are aware of the external forces affecting their agency and of changes in industry standards and practices. Agencies that maintain their competitive posture are led by proactive executives.

Health care organizations determine salaries by surveying what relevant organizations in the external labor market pay for executive positions (Albert, 2000). Albert recommends that executive salaries should be at the median or above the median of comparable organizations in the area. Board members should assess the agency's resources and offer the best salary and benefits package they can afford.

Concerns about some of the high salaries paid to nonprofit health care executives have been raised in light of the financial difficulties many nonprofits face. However, nonprofit officials and consultants believe that although boards must be sensitive to public perception, they have an obligation to pay salaries high enough to allow them to recruit and retain talented executives who will help an organization operate its programs effectively. Manzo (2004) notes that the real salary scandal is not that executives of nonprofits are paid too much but that most nonprofit employees are paid too little.

Deciding what the compensation of executives should be is difficult. Executives in public, nonprofit, and for-profit organizations may possess the same levels of responsibilities, administer similar-size budgets, and supervise similar-size staffs (public, nonprofit, and for-profit hospitals, for example).

Health care organizations must be careful that their executive salaries do not come at the expense of adequately paying lower-level employees. All employees should be paid fair wages. Paying low salaries can be self-defeating—after two or three years employees leave, and agencies need to recruit and train new staff, incurring significant costs.

FEDERAL LAWS GOVERNING COMPENSATION

All employers are required to comply with two federal laws, the Fair Labor Standards Act and the Equal Pay Act.

The Fair Labor Standards Act

The main provisions of the **Fair Labor Standards Act (FLSA),** enacted in 1938, are minimum wage, overtime pay, equal pay, and child labor rules. The FLSA requires that employers keep records of the hours that employees have worked. Its overtime provision requires that employers pay one-and-a-half the regular rate of hourly pay for each hour worked that exceeds forty hours per week.

The FLSA divides employees into exempt and nonexempt workers. Exempt employees are not covered by the overtime provisions. They can be expected to work more than forty hours per week without additional compensation. In 1993 Title 29, Chapter V, Part 541 of the Code of Federal Regulations defined exempt employees as those who spend 80 percent of their work time performing administrative, executive, or professional duties. In 1985 the Supreme Court ruled in *Garcia v. San Antonio Metropolitan Transit Authority* that the FLSA could be applied to state, county, and municipal employees. This meant that public employers could no longer use compensatory time in lieu of dollars and would have to pay overtime. Because of the financial burden this would cause, public agencies petitioned Congress for relief. Congress reacted by amending the FLSA with the Fair Labor Standards Amendments of 1985. Section 7(o) of the FLSA authorizes compensatory time off as a form of overtime. It applies only to public sector agencies. To be legal under the FLSA, compensatory time must be one-and-a-half hours for each hour worked; personnel who are not sworn (that is, public employees other than sworn officers, such as police, fire, and corrections officers) may have no more than 240 hours of compensatory time on the books at any one time, and sworn personnel can accrue no more than 480 hours of compensatory time at any one time. Nonsworn and sworn personnel who reach the limits of 240 and 480 hours, respectively, must receive cash for additional hours of overtime worked or use some compensatory time off before accruing further overtime compensation in the form of compensatory time off.

The 1985 amendment also has special provisions for hospital employees and police and fire officials who typically work nontraditional shifts. Section 7(j) permits the use of a fourteen-day work period (instead of the usual seven-day workweek) in the computation of overtime provisions. An employee must be paid overtime only if he or she works more than eighty hours during the fourteen-day period.

Section 7(k) provides work periods up to twenty-eight days for public safety officials. These officials do not have to be paid overtime until they work more than 212 hours.

Nonprofit employers must comply with the FLSA overtime provision of one-and-a-half times an employee's normal hourly rate of pay for each hour that exceeds forty hours per week. Employees may elect to receive compensatory time in lieu of overtime, but it must be their choice and not imposed by the employer.

Equal Pay Act of 1963

The FLSA was amended by the **Equal Pay Act of 1963,** which prohibits unequal pay differences for men and women who are performing equal work in jobs requiring equal skill, effort, and responsibility and performed in the same establishment under similar working conditions. Pay differences between equal jobs can, however, be justified when that differential is based on a seniority system, a merit system, a piece-rate payment system that measures earnings by quality or quantity of production, or any factor other than gender (for example, different levels of experience or different work shifts).

SUMMARY

Compensation systems should be designed with the intent to attract, motivate, and retain proficient employees. A number of factors determine the salaries paid to employees: the salaries paid in the external labor market; federal laws, such as the FLSA and the Equal Pay Act; and the responsibilities and KSAOCs required to perform a given job, as well as an agency's ability to pay competitive wages.

Equity refers to the perception by employees that they are being paid fairly. External, internal, and employee equity influence compensation systems. Market factors influence external equity, job evaluation or job worth influences internal equity, and employee equity is said to exist when employees performing similar jobs are compensated based on their individual contributions. Longevity pay, broadbanding or paybanding, skill-based pay or pay for knowledge, merit pay or pay for performance, and gainsharing are examples of some of the innovations in compensation systems.

KEY TERMS

benchmark positions	Fair Labor Standards Act (FLSA)
compensation	goal-setting theory
distributive justice	hierarchy of needs
employee equity	internal equity
Equal Pay Act of 1963	motivator-hygiene theory
equity theory	pay differentials
ERG theory	procedural justice
expectancy theory	theory of needs
external equity	

DISCUSSION QUESTIONS

1. Describe four content theories of motivation: hierarchy of needs, ERG theory, theory of needs, and motivator-hygiene theory.

2. Describe three process theories of motivation: expectancy theory, equity theory, and goal-setting theory.

3. Identify and discuss at least five compensable factors.

4. Discuss three alternative pay systems and describe how they are used to enhance traditional pay systems.

5. What are the main provisions enacted by the Fair Labor Standards Act?

6. What type of equity is determined by surveying competitive employers?

11

Benefits

LEARNING OBJECTIVES

- Understand and explain how employee benefits are an important component of strategic human resources management

- Distinguish between government required benefits and discretionary benefits.

- Describe strategies to improve the quality of work and quality of life in health care organizations

THE PRECEDING CHAPTER on compensation provided an overview of salaries and wages, the direct financial compensation provided to employees for their contributions to the organization. But wages constitute only part of the compensation package. This chapter addresses indirect compensation, more commonly referred to as **benefits**.

The emphasis in compensating employees should be on the total compensation package, not just on direct wages or salary. Benefits are a critical ingredient in creating an accurate compensation picture, and the importance of benefits should not be underestimated; an attractive benefits package can assist in the recruitment and retention of qualified employees. Traditional benefits, such as health insurance, retirement pensions, and paid time away from work, combined with less-traditional benefits, such as child and elder care, flexible scheduling, and educational assistance, are critical for attracting qualified applicants, encouraging loyalty and long-term employment, and motivating and rewarding incumbent employees.

Employee benefits often reach 40 percent of total compensation costs. Medical insurance premiums are the highest-cost single benefit. Research conducted by the Kaiser Family Foundation and the Health Research and Educational Trust found that premiums for employer-sponsored health coverage rose $13,770 on average in 2010, with workers paying an average of nearly $4,000 toward those premiums (Kaiser Family Foundation, 2010). Paid time off, vacations, holidays, and sick leave combined account for about one-third of all benefits.

Employees often think of benefits as entitlements and not as compensation. In reality, the only entitlements are those benefits that are required by federal or state laws. Aside from these, employers have tremendous discretion in deciding what types of benefits to provide. This chapter discusses the variety of benefits that organizations may choose to offer, as well as the quality-of-life and quality-of-work issues that are becoming more prevalent in today's workplaces.

GOVERNMENT REQUIRED BENEFITS

All employers have to provide **government required benefits:** they must contribute to contribute to Social Security, Medicare, unemployment compensation, and workers' compensation, and provide for military leave. Public employers may be required by federal or state statutes to offer additional benefits, such as retirement or disability. The benefits a private health care organization provides are determined and approved by the board of directors.

Social Security

Social Security provides retirement, disability, death, survivor, and Medicare benefits for those beyond age sixty-five. The Social Security system was established in 1935; however, public and nonprofit employers and employees could decline to pay Social Security taxes and earn no credit toward Social Security benefits. The Social Security Amendments of 1983 made Social Security coverage mandatory for all employees of nonprofit organizations as of January 1, 1984. Coverage was extended to nonprofit employees working for organizations that had previously terminated coverage, as well as to employees who had never been covered by Social Security. The 1983 amendments included a special section that provided for nonprofit employees fifty-five years and older to be considered fully insured for benefits after acquiring at least twenty quarters of coverage.

The Social Security Act of 1935 originally excluded state and local governments from coverage because of the concern that taxation of state and local governments by the federal government might be unconstitutional. The act was subsequently amended in the 1950s to permit state and local governments to choose coverage for employees not already covered under a retirement system. After five years of participating in the Social Security system, state and local governments could choose to repeal their action and terminate coverage of their employees. This was changed in 1983 by the Social Security Amendments, which eliminated the right of state and local government employers to withdraw from the system. Another change came in 1986, when the Budget Reconciliation Act amended the Social Security Act and required all individuals hired by a state or local government to be covered by the Medicare segment of the program and subject to employer and employee payroll taxes. As of July 2, 1991, all state and local government employees (except police officers) not covered by a retirement program are required to participate in the full Social Security program. Federal employees hired on or after January 1, 1984, are covered by Social Security and are subject to full Social Security taxation.

Social Security provides four kinds of benefits: old-age or disability benefits, benefits for the dependents of retired or disabled workers, benefits for the survivors of a worker who dies, and the lump-sum death benefit.

Medicare

Funding for **Medicare**, a federal program that pays for certain health care expenses for individuals sixty-five years of age or older, comes partially from payroll taxes, known as Federal Insurance Contributions Act (FICA) taxes. FICA taxes comprise Social Security and Medicare taxes. The rate of the Medicare tax is 2.9 percent. Employers withhold 1.45 percent from their employees and match it with another 1.45 percent. There is no wage base for the Medicare portion of the FICA tax. Both the employer and the employee continue to pay Medicare taxes, no matter how much is earned.

Unemployment Compensation

Unemployment compensation, established as part of the Social Security Act of 1935, was designed to provide a portion of wages to employees who have been laid off until they obtain another job. The employer pays into the unemployment compensation fund at a rate based on the average number of former employees who have drawn benefits from the fund. The fund is primarily financed through a payroll tax paid to the state and federal governments based on employees' wages. The employer pays state and federal unemployment taxes. Each state determines its own waiting period for eligibility, the level of benefits provided, and for how long benefits are paid. Some states even impose unemployment taxes on employees.

Workers' Compensation

Workers' compensation is an employer-financed insurance program that provides compensation to employees who are unable to work because of job-related injury or illness. Most states have their own workers' compensation laws and are responsible for administering their own programs. For this reason the levels of protection and the costs of administering the programs vary from state to state. Some features that all of the programs have in common are the following (Commerce Clearing House Business Law Editors, 1992, p. 8):

- Workers receive benefits for accidental injury; wage-loss, medical, and death benefits are provided.

- Fault is not an issue; if the employee was somewhat or entirely at fault in the injury, the employee still has the right to receive workers' compensation benefits.

- In exchange for the assurance of benefits, the employee (and the employee's dependent family members) gives up the right to sue the employer for damages for any injury covered by a workers' compensation law.

- Responsibility for administering the system usually resides with a state board or commission. Employers are generally required to insure their workers' compensation liability through private insurance, state insurance funds, or self-insurance.

Independent contractors are not considered to be employees and do not have to be covered under the workers' compensation policy of the organization that hired them. Most state workers' compensation agencies apply the same test as the Internal Revenue Service (IRS) for determining whether a contractor is truly independent and not just called so by an employer who does not want to match the contractor's Social Security contributions or deduct and withhold income taxes. To decide whether a contractor is "independent," the IRS examines the relationship between the worker and the organization. Evidence of behavioral control, financial control, and the type of relationship are considered. *Behavioral control* covers facts that show whether the business has a right to direct and control how the work is done, through instructions, training, or other means. *Financial control* covers facts that show whether the organization has a right to control the business aspects of the worker's job. This includes the extent to which the worker has unreimbursed business expenses, the extent of the worker's investment in the business, the extent to which the worker makes services available to the relevant market, how the organization pays the worker, and the extent to which the worker can realize a profit or incur a loss. *Type of relationship* covers facts that show written contracts describing the relationship the parties intended to create; the extent to which the worker is available to perform services for other, similar businesses; whether the business provides the worker with employee benefits, such as insurance, a pension plan, vacation pay, or sick pay; and the permanence or impermanence of the relationship.

The contractor should probably be covered under the organization's workers' compensation policy if the contractor can be fired or quit without any contractual liability; the contractor is reimbursed for business and travel expenses; the contractor performs the task in person, on company property, and during set hours; the contractor is paid by the hour, week, or month rather than by the job; and the organization provides the contractor with tools or equipment. The state's workers' compensation agency should be contacted for verification.

In most states unpaid volunteers are not considered to be employees and are typically not covered by workers' compensation. But in some states there are exceptions for police and fire volunteers, and other volunteers may be covered under special circumstances.

Military Leave

Reserve and National Guard units called to active duty have rights with respect to retirement and health benefits provided by their employers. The Uniformed Services Employment and Reemployment Rights Act of 1994 strengthens and clarifies the Veterans' Reemployment Rights Statute. The Department of Labor's Veterans' Employment and Training Service developed a fact sheet to provide information as to the rights and responsibilities of individuals and their employers under the act (www.dol.gov/vets/programs/userra/userra_fs.htm).

DISCRETIONARY BENEFITS

Health care employers recognize that to be competitive they need to offer **discretionary benefits**—additional benefits beyond those mandated by law. Research indicates that integrated benefits programs lead to increased productivity, decrease turnover, increase the effectiveness of recruitment and retention programs, and assist in developing employees' loyalty to the organization (Cayer, 2003; Cayer & Roach, 2008; Champion-Hughes, 2001; Coggburn & Reddick, 2007; Daley, 2008; Durst, 1999; McCurdy, Newman, & Lovrich, 2002; Reddick & Coggburn, 2007; Roberts, 2000, 2002, 2004). Table 11.1 provides a list of some common benefits.

Pensions

Pensions provide retired or permanently disabled employees with income throughout the remainder of their lives. Two types of pension plans are commonly found in health care organizations: defined-benefit and defined-contribution pension plans.

Defined-Benefit Pension Plans

Defined-benefit pension plans specify the benefits or the methods of determining the benefits to be supplied at the time of retirement. The benefit amounts to be paid are determined by a formula that weighs the retiree's years of service, age, and salary history. Advantages of defined-benefit pension plans are that employees and employers can estimate the probable size of pension benefits by assuming retirement dates and salary histories.

Vesting occurs when contributions made to a retirement plan belong to the employee. For most defined-benefit pension plans, if you leave the

Table 11.1   Employee Benefits

Government Required Benefits	Discretionary Benefits
• Social Security • Medicare • Unemployment compensation • Workers' compensation • Military leave	• Pensions • Health insurance • Disability insurance • Paid time away from work • Education programs • Flexible benefits • Employee assistance programs • Outplacement assistance • Flexible job environment

organization you retain the nonforfeitable right to those benefits when you retire. However, you may be required to wait until you actually retire before receiving the benefits. Most defined-contribution pension plans allow you to take the accrued amount when you depart in a lump-sum payment that is taxable.

Vesting standards for private organizations were amended as part of the Tax Reform Act of 1986. New minimum standards went into effect in 1989 that enable employees to become fully vested in their pension plan after five years of service, or they may be 20 percent vested after three years of service, 20 percent more vested for each year thereafter, and 100 percent vested after seven years of service.

Defined-Contribution Pension Plans

In **defined-contribution pension plans,** employers guarantee that specified contributions, usually a percentage of annual salary, will be deposited to employees' accounts every year that they work. These accounts are invested. Employees are provided with a variety of investment options from which to choose. When employees retire, they receive lifetime payments or an annuity, the size of which is determined by the amount on deposit, the interest rate earned on funds in the account, and the length of time during which the annuity is expected to be paid. The employee, the employer, or both may contribute to the pension plan.

Defined-contribution pension plans are becoming more popular as more employers have realized the expense and long-term liabilities associated with funding defined-benefit pension plans. An advantage of defined-contribution pension plans is that the money is portable if employees change jobs because there are no vesting requirements. In today's economy workers tend to be more transient, moving among different organizations and even between the public, nonprofit, and private sectors. One disadvantage of defined-contribution pension plans is that employees tend to be more conservative in selecting their investment options than professional investors would be. Conservative investment plans will lead to lower interest rates and fewer funds for retirement. Another potential disadvantage is that the money available at retirement is tied to the stock market. Employers who offer defined-contribution pension plans need to provide training and offer their employees information on how to invest their money and plan for retirement.

Health Insurance

Health insurance, life insurance, and long-term sickness and accident and disability insurance are some of the benefits provided to employees. Health insurance is the most frequently provided benefit and the benefit that receives the most attention, with good reason. The number of people without health insurance was 50.7 million in 2009 (DeNavas-Walt, Proctor, & Smith, 2010). In California a quarter of the state's population is now uninsured. The number of uninsured adults and children in California increased from 6.4 million in 2007 to 8.2 million in 2009 (Lavarreda, Brown, Cabezas, & Roby, 2010). The future looks worse. A study funded by the Robert Wood Johnson Foundation and the Urban Institute projects that without health care reform the number of uninsured Americans could grow by almost 10 million people in five years, and that by 2015 there could be 59.7 million uninsured, to be followed by 67.6 million by 2020 (Garrett, Buettgens, Doan, Headen, & Holahan, 2010).

Given that the costs of health insurance continue to rise at more than twice the rate of employees' wages and overall inflation, several managed-care plans have been designed to focus on controlling costs. The most common are health maintenance organization (HMO) plans, preferred provider organization (PPO) plans, point of service (POS) plans, and high-deductible health plans (HDHPs). Each style of plan has its advantages and disadvantages. Employees with an HMO plan must receive their health care from an HMO physician. If they do, then their expenses are typically covered in full. Employees with a PPO plan have lower deductibles and coinsurance if they use physicians or hospitals in the preferred provider network. Employees with a POS plan are reimbursed at a lower rate for services received outside the network; they also have a primary care physician who must approve visits to specialists and hospitals. It is typical for an HDHP to have a single deductible of at least $1,000 and a family deductible of at least $2,000 annually (Reddick & Coggburn, 2007). Some employers offer health savings accounts (HSAs). HSAs allow employees to have a savings and investment account for money put aside to cover health care costs. The money is excluded from taxable income. If the money is withdrawn and used for health expenses, it is never taxed.

The types of health insurance programs and the amounts that employees and employers contribute to the plans vary. Keeping track of them and figuring out the best plan takes some research and asking questions. The **Consolidated Omnibus Budget Reconciliation Act (COBRA)** of 1986 was enacted to provide employees with the opportunity to temporarily continue receiving their employer-sponsored health insurance under the employer's plan if their coverage otherwise would cease due to termination, a layoff, or other changes in employment status. COBRA covers employers of twenty or more employees, except for federal government and religious organizations. Many states have their own versions of COBRA to cover small employers. COBRA enables former employees, spouses, and dependents to purchase insurance coverage for a limited amount of time after leaving the organization. COBRA also applies to divorced, separated, or widowed spouses. Furthermore, COBRA extends Medicare coverage to state and local government employees.

The Health Insurance Portability and Accountability Act (HIPAA) of 1996 allows employees to switch their health insurance plan from one organization to another to get new health coverage, regardless of preexisting health conditions. The legislation also prohibits group insurance plans from dropping coverage for a sick employee and requires employers to make individual coverage available to people who leave group plans.

Mental Health Parity Act

In an effort to encourage individuals to seek mental health treatment, the Mental Health Parity Act was passed into law in 1996. The act stated that beginning in January 1998, health insurance plans must provide the same coverage for mental illness as for physical disorders. It required that employer-provided plans provide parity for treatment of mental illness.

Congress passed the Paul Wellstone and Pete Domenici Mental Health Parity and Addiction Equity Act of 2008 as part of the $700 billion financial rescue package in October 2008. The measure requires employers that provide health plans to cover mental illness and substance use disorders on the same basis as physical conditions. It prohibits employers' health plans from imposing any caps or limitations on mental health treatment or substance use disorder benefits that aren't applied to medical and surgical benefits. The Mental Health Parity Act does not require health insurance plans to provide mental health or substance use disorder benefits. However, for group health plans covering fifty or more employees that provide mental health and substance use disorder treatment benefits, the act does require parity with medical and surgical benefits.

Additional Benefits

More insurance programs are also beginning to offer dental, optical, and prescription drug benefits in addition to traditional medical coverage.

Disability Insurance

Disability benefits are paid to employees who become disabled before qualifying for regular or early retirement benefits. In general, disability insurance provides monthly benefits to employees who cannot work for an extended period of time due to injury or illness. Some employees, however, are not insured for long-term disability but are eligible for an immediate disability pension through their retirement plan. In most instances long-term disability payments are a fixed percentage of predisability earnings. Most plans distinguish between disability attributed to an accident on the job, which entails higher benefits and fewer requirements with respect to years of service, and disability that is not job related.

Paid Time Away from Work

Most employers grant employees paid sick leave, vacation days, holidays, and personal days. Employers are not obligated to grant these benefits, and they vary across organizations.

In many public organizations employees who accumulate their sick and vacation days are able to exchange them for cash compensation when they retire. This policy is meant to discourage capricious time away from work and to reward employees for their commitment to the organization. However, many organizations are rethinking this policy because accrued time becomes an unfunded liability for the agency.

Education Programs

The Council for Adult and Experiential Learning (2004) surveyed human resources management professionals across the United States about the educational assistance benefits available at their respective organizations. Results were obtained from 1,304 organizations, nearly 86 percent of which agreed that education and tuition benefits are important as a strategic investment. The respondents cited increases in employee retention and productivity as the two most important reasons for offering education and tuition benefits.

Many public and nonprofit organizations provide tuition reimbursement to employees for additional education if the employee receives a B or better grade for the course. Although some smaller or undercapitalized organizations may not be able to afford to offer tuition and education benefits to its employees, most employers are able to assist their employees in other ways. Employers have the discretion to establish flexible work schedules to accommodate an employee's class schedule. For example, if an employee is attending classes at night, the employer might allow the employee to leave earlier in the day to travel to class. Some employers may not be able to afford college tuition; however, they may be able to afford to purchase textbooks that can become the property of the organization once a class is completed. When appropriate, an employer can pay for an employee's tuition instead of funding the employee to attend conferences out of town. Often the cost of a college class for a semester of learning is less than a conference registration fee and the hotel, dining, and transportation expenses—not to mention the employee's time away from work.

Employers can provide information to their employees on the tax credits and deductions sanctioned by the IRS that are available to help offset the cost of higher education. The Hope Credit is available until the first two years of postsecondary education are completed. The Lifetime Learning Credit is available for all years of postsecondary education and for courses taken to acquire or improve job skills. It is available for an unlimited number of years, and students do not need to be pursuing a degree or other recognized educational credential; it is available for one or more courses, and the felony drug conviction rule does not apply. The Lifetime Learning Credit may be limited by the amount of a student's income and the student's tax liability (www.irs.gov/publications/p970/).

QUALITY-OF-WORK AND QUALITY-OF-LIFE ISSUES

Changes in family structures and employee priorities have encouraged the evolution of a variety of employer-provided benefits. Employers wishing to compete for highly skilled employees believe that considering issues of **quality of work** and **quality of life** can give them a competitive edge.

Flexible Benefits

As early as the 1970s, private sector organizations recognized that different family structures necessitate different employee benefits (Johnson, 1988; Wallace & Fay, 1988). Conventional employee benefits plans were designed to serve the needs of the family structure that was dominant during the 1940s and 1950s: a working father and his dependents (namely, a wife who stayed at home with small children). Today families have changed, and so have their needs. Current family structures often include a single parent, multiple generations, and domestic partnerships.

Some solutions have been employer-sponsored group insurance plans that provide lower premiums, or flexible spending accounts that enable greater flexibility in the types of services that benefits will cover (Daley, 1998; Kossek, DeMarr, Backman, & Kolar, 1993).

In the past wives often took care of elderly parents or in-laws and children. Today there are more single-parent families or families in which both spouses work full-time and are unable to care for their children, their parents, or both. Thus many benefits plans now have provisions for elder and child care. Employees with small children may need child care, employees with elderly or infirm parents may prefer elder care, and employees without any dependents might opt for a variety of other benefits, such as dental care.

Child and elder care responsibilities have an impact on job performance as well as having financial costs. Research has found that caregiver responsibilities result in the excessive use of the phone at work, lateness, and unscheduled time off. Employee time spent on caregiver responsibilities affects productivity, absenteeism, turnover, and morale (Nelson-Horchler, 1989). A survey conducted by the National Alliance for Caregiving and Evercare, a division of UnitedHealth Group, found that family members responsible for caregiving often spend on average about $5,500 a year in caregiving expenses, in addition to the physical and emotional stress they already experience (Evercare and National Alliance of Caregiving, 2007). An analysis of over 2,100 lawsuits found that litigation claiming bias against workers who care for children or aging parents has increased 400 percent in the past decade. The report *Family Responsibilities Discrimination: Litigation Update 2010* noted that most of the lawsuits were related to pregnancy and maternity leave (67 percent), followed by elder care (9.6 percent), care for sick children (7 percent), care for ill spouses (4 percent), time off for newborn care by fathers or adoptive parents (3 percent), and care for a family member with a disability (2.4 percent) Eighty-eight percent of the lawsuits were filed by women, and 12 percent were filed by men (Calvert, 2010).

An emerging issue is the provision of domestic partnership benefits to employees. Such benefits extend coverage to unmarried heterosexual or gay couples. One way to support employees and make them feel part of the organization is to recognize and respect alternative families. Health insurance, sick leave, bereavement leave, pension plans, life insurance, and access to employee assistance programs are some of the benefits that have been extended to domestic partners. Couples typically qualify if they are living together and are jointly responsible for their financial well-being (Gossett & Ng, 2008).

Employee Assistance Programs

An **employee assistance program (EAP)** is another important type of employer-provided benefit. Marital conflicts, alcohol and substance abuse, family stresses, AIDS, and other health-related concerns are some of the problems that come to work with employees. These problems often result in lower employee productivity and morale, and may also lead to legal liabilities and high financial costs for the employer. EAPs provide counseling services for employees and their families. In the past the focus of EAPs was on alcoholism and drug-related problems. The services of EAPs have since expanded to include counseling for marital problems, drug abuse, mental illness, and financial stress, and for the improvement of employer-employee communication.

EAPs also address such issues as strategies for maintaining health and wellness. Employees with stressful lives are absent more often, resulting in lost productivity. Wellness programs are designed to improve employees' physical and psychological health, thus decreasing the occurrence and severity of medical problems and lowering the costs and number of medical claims (Hyland, 1990). Accident prevention classes, smoking cessation seminars, weight control and nutrition programs, stress management workshops, and on-site exercise programs are also outgrowths of EAPs. The largest use of EAPs, however, is still for addressing drug or alcohol addiction.

Outplacement Assistance

Layoffs due to economic hardship, consolidations, mergers, reorganizations, changes in management, and the relocation or elimination of specific positions or programs have resulted in agencies' offering outplacement assistance as a benefit. Some of the outplacement assistance benefits include assistance in developing résumés, referrals to employment agencies, and skills and aptitude testing.

Flexible Job Environment

Changing family structures have focused attention not only on the need for variety in employer-provided benefits but also on the need for more flexible workplace policies. Employers must acknowledge that family and work dynamics have changed, leading to increased stress on employees as they strive to balance the demands of both work and family life. Employees who cannot manage these conflicting demands are often less productive and, as noted earlier, are absent more often and have lower morale.

To better meet the needs of their employees, many organizations have developed flexible work structures. Flextime, voluntary shifts to part-time work, job sharing, flexible leaves, compressed workweeks, and work-at-home or telecommuting opportunities are some of the strategies used to alleviate work and family conflicts.

Another issue affecting morale and motivation at work is career plateau-ing. As public and nonprofit agencies are confronted with fewer promotional opportunities, more employees have reached career plateaus. Career plateau-ing is the inability to move upward in the organization. To keep employees motivated, organizations must institute human resources management poli-cies that focus on the contributions employees can make to the organization without being promoted. Such techniques as job rotation, job enlargement, skill-based pay, and midcareer breaks have been used to maintain employee motivation.

Job rotation allows workers to diversify their activities. Employees perform a variety of tasks by moving to a new activity when their current tasks are no longer challenging or when the work schedule dictates it. They are thus provided with a range of experience that broadens their skills, provides them with a greater understanding of other activities within the agency, and prepares them to assume more responsibility. Job enlargement expands the scope of a job by increasing the number of different operations required in it. The job becomes more diverse and challenging because more tasks must be completed. Pay for knowledge or skill-based pay can be used to keep employees motivated by engaging them in learning new skills. Employees are not promoted to a higher-level position, but they are still able to perform new skills and assume new responsibilities.

Midcareer breaks or sabbaticals have typically been considered to be among the benefits of academia. However, many organizations have begun to realize the benefits of time spent away from work, and some foundations are willing to provide support for sabbaticals. Not all organizations can afford to give paid leave to employees, so some have developed alternatives, such as unpaid leave with a guarantee of a job upon return, or unpaid leave but with tuition reimbursement to defray the costs of schooling.

SUMMARY

Employer-provided benefits play an important role in strategic human resources management. Most organizations offer a variety of benefits, ranging from those mandated by law, such as Social Security, unemployment compensation, and workers' compensation, to those that are optional, such as pensions, health insurance, paid time away from work, education programs, and a variety of quality-of-life and quality-of-work programs.

The types of benefits employers provide are key to attracting quality applicants, to encouraging loyalty and long-term employment, and to motivating and rewarding incumbent employees. The literature on organizational culture and employee retention indicates that different human resources strategies result in different psychological climates that foster varying levels of commitment and retention among employees. Flexible and competitive benefits are one way of attracting candidates and retaining workers (Reddick & Coggburn, 2007). Flexible benefits that are sensitive to employee needs have the advantage of creating a work climate that is conducive to high levels of employee commitment, satisfaction, and morale.

KEY TERMS

benefits

Consolidated Omnibus Budget
   Reconciliation Act (COBRA)

defined-benefit pension plans

defined-contribution pension plans

discretionary benefits

employee assistance program (EAP)

government required benefits

Medicare

quality of life

quality of work

Social Security

unemployment compensation

vesting

workers' compensation

DISCUSSION QUESTIONS

1. Identify and describe government required benefits.

2. Which discretionary benefits do you believe are the greatest enhancements to compensation?

3. List and discuss the most common types of health insurance plans.

4. What types of quality-of-life and quality-of-work benefits have been implemented to enhance work environments?

This chapter was adapted and updated from Pynes, 1997, 2004a, 2009a.

Maximizing Health Care Human Resources

12

Training and Development

LEARNING OBJECTIVES

- Define training and development and discuss why a strategic human resources management approach is important in today's environment
- Describe different training delivery methods specific to health care human resources
- Explain the different methods used to evaluate training and development activities in a progressive health care organization
- Explain the role of health care human resources professionals in designing and implementing career development programs
- Understand why it is important to integrate career development programs with other health care human resources programs, such as performance management, training, selection, and compensation

O **F ALL OF** the responsibilities of a health care human resources component, **training and development** are the most important activities in enabling a progressive health care organization to attain future goals and objectives. Training and development encompass the education that provides skills, competencies, and knowledge in every organizational sector. Although many health care organizations will curtail revenue dollars expended on training and development during times of fiscal uncertainty—which, given the reality of health care organizations, is usually a commonplace rather than a rare occurrence—health care organizations should maintain a dedicated sense of continuity in training and development. Especially during times of change, chaos, and crisis, it is imperative for a health care organization to continually and purposefully escalate its efficacy to meet constantly changing and increasing demands for high-quality health care.

Health care organizations are made up of individuals who bring a unique set of skills to clinically and commercially specialized areas. It is therefore vital for a health care organization to provide munificent opportunities for all employees, volunteers, and other constituents to improve their skills in their respective technical areas in the interest of maximizing their contribution to the organization as well as optimizing their sense of job satisfaction.

As has been stated throughout this text, the health care industry is extremely vigilant in its commitment to the delivery of high-quality services. This commitment begins with individual action and achievement, and training and development centered on enhancing the individual competencies of highly skilled personnel is an essential building block of organizational excellence. Knowledge that not only encompasses particular technical proficiencies but also extends to education on customer-patient expectations, emerging trends in community health care, national and regional sociopolitical impact factors, and other pertinent dynamics should also be part of a progressive health care organization's training and development strategy. The focus on skills, competencies, and knowledge ensures positive performance and gives the organization the best chance of success moving forward into the turbulent future.

The shrinking of reimbursement and revenue dollars requires an organization to be enlightened and purposeful in its human resources strategy, an imperative that is particularly important in training and development. Providing sound training and development eliminates mistakes made in the care delivery process; raises sensitivity in key human relations dynamics, such as customer-patient and employee relationships; and increases the everyday professional capabilities of staff members and managers—all of which results in greater effectiveness and efficiency across the organization, leading to a stronger financial profile.

In a similar vein, training and development can be a catalytic factor in curtailing unwanted employee turnover and retaining strong, high-potential employees among the ranks of staff and management. Health care professionals are motivated by an intrinsic desire to learn more about their craft, the provision of health care, and new methods and techniques in pursuing their profession. When an organization provides opportunities to enhance education, it motivates and gives positive reinforcement to the cadre of high-performing employees who are its bedrock. If a talented and motivated employee is not provided with opportunities to learn and grow both on the job as well as through dedicated educational events under the aegis of the training and development function, this shortfall is likely to work in confluence with other negative workplace dynamics, resulting in laggard performance and, ultimately, a good employee leaving the organization for new opportunities.

Key organizational dynamics relative to strategic objectives, the tactical positioning of the organization, and the unique demands on the organization from the customer-patient community are all important topics to be included as part of health care organizational training and development. Furthermore, the organization must make every conceivable effort to provide all employees with education that is relevant and training that is specific to the needs of individual job roles. As is the case with many successful organizations outside of health care, stellar training and development that provide meaningful education can give the organization a true competitive edge. Such great American organizations as IBM, Ford Motor Company, and the United States Marine Corps have all historically made a commitment to providing training and development that are meaningful, relevant, and resonant, and that always reflect the best traditions of selfless service, individual development, and the organization's purposeful progress.

NEEDS ASSESSMENT

The first step in the training process is to determine the specific training needs. A need can be defined simply as the difference between what is currently being done and what should be done. This difference can be determined by conducting a **needs assessment** of the skills and knowledge currently required by a given position and those anticipated as necessary for the future. A needs assessment is critical to discerning whether training can eliminate performance deficiencies. Without a needs assessment, it is possible to design and implement a training program as the solution to a problem that is not actually related to a training deficiency.

For example, it comes to the attention of higher management that one supervisor rates women and minorities lower than he rates white males, and the ratings are not based on job-related performance criteria. The supervisor is sent to performance evaluation training, where he is exposed to common rating errors and the need for unambiguous performance standards, timely feedback, and so on. Despite the training, the supervisor refuses to use job-related performance criteria when he evaluates his female and minority staff. Performance evaluation training did not resolve the problem; the ratings were deliberately lowered because of prejudice and not because the supervisor lacked knowledge of performance evaluation techniques. A true needs assessment would have discovered that the problem was different than originally thought and that the solution would have to involve a different kind of training. In this case the supervisor was not deficient in skills; rather, it was his attitude and behaviors that needed to be modified. Multicultural diversity training or training on employment discrimination would have been more appropriate. A needs assessment must be accurate if training is to be successful.

Organizations can determine training needs through a variety of techniques. A strategic job analysis performed prior to the needs assessment is useful. The job analysis should identify the knowledge, skills, abilities, and other characteristics (KSAOCs) that incumbents need to effectively perform their job today and identify the KSAOCs that will be needed in the future. Surveys and interviews with incumbents and supervisors; performance evaluations that identify performance deficiencies; criticisms or complaints from clients, staff, or personnel in agencies working with your employees; changes in pending laws or regulations or operating procedures; and requests for additional training by incumbents can all provide clues as to what training is needed.

The training required to provide the needed KSAOCs should be divided into training that can be learned on the job and training that requires formal instruction. For example, some jobs require certification or licenses mandated by state or federal regulations. More and more states are requiring, for instance, that substance abuse counselors be state certified. In Missouri, paramedics are required to pass a state written exam and attend refresher courses every three years. In New York State, nonprofit residential facilities for delinquent or status offender youths have to comply with a regulation that new employees must receive training on HIV/AIDS within fifteen days of being hired. In these examples training is provided by experts outside the agency. Training to acquire other KSAOCs can be provided on the job. Having supervisors explain new policies and procedures or train employees on how to use new equipment can be part of any training plan.

DEVELOPING TRAINING OBJECTIVES

Training objectives are statements that specify the desired KSAOCs that employees will possess at the end of training. Training objectives do not include the things the trainee is expected to know or be able to do before the training. These objectives need only describe the KSAOCs that can be expected at the end of a training program. The objectives provide the standards for measuring what has been accomplished and for determining the level of accomplishment. For training objectives to be useful, they should be stated as specifically as possible. For example:

- Clinical nurse specialists will be able to perform discharge planning for patients.

- Medical records technicians will be able to identify, compile, abstract, and code patient data, using standard classification systems.

- Supervisors will be able to explain the agency's sexual harassment policy to employees.

- Receptionists will be able to transfer and route calls on the new telephone communication system without disconnecting callers.

The development of training objectives should be a collaborative process incorporating input from managers, supervisors, workers, and trainers to ensure that the objectives are reasonable and realistic. Three determinants to account for proficiency in any performance component are declarative knowledge or factual knowledge, which is the understanding of things one must do; procedural knowledge, or skill in knowing how to do them; and motivation, or the direction, degree, and persistence of effort in doing them (Guion and Highhouse, 2006).

DEVELOPING THE CURRICULUM

After assessing the training needs and establishing objectives, a training **curriculum** must be developed. Before determining the content and the manner of presenting the information, however, trainers must first conduct an analysis of the trainees. This step is critical because the needs and characteristics of the trainees often determine the kind of training that is likely to be effective. Some of the relevant issues to examine include the following:

- What are the participants' levels of education? For example, classroom instruction may be intimidating for employees with limited formal education.

- What are participants' expectations? Will all participants come to training with the same concerns?

- What are participants' knowledge levels, attitudes, and relationships with one another?

- Are participants prepared to receive technical instruction?

- Is the training voluntary or imposed from above?

- If the training is mandatory, will the participants be threatened by it?

The answers to these questions will provide some guidance to the trainers when developing the curriculum. The curriculum should provide information and be developed to maximize the imparting of KSAOCs. A number of training techniques can facilitate learning: informal, on-the-job, and formal training are typically used in health care organizations. Other-directed training refers to training methods in which one or more trainers assume responsibility for all instruction processes. Self-directed training refers to training methods whereby the trainees use workbooks, CD-ROMs, or other methods to target specific skills or acquire knowledge relevant to the job, but the individual is responsible for completing the instruction. Technology-assisted training can include elements of both other-directed and self-directed training.

One of the first decisions that needs to be made is whether to provide on-the-job instruction or off-the-job classroom instruction, or a combination of the two. On-the-job instruction takes place while the employee is actually working at the jobsite. It is usually provided by supervisors, who instruct subordinates in the correct way to perform a task, such as filling out new purchase order requisitions. As another example, on-the-job instruction is taking place when a representative from the information technology department demonstrates how to load and set up a new software package. On-the-job training is useful when employees are expected to become proficient in performing certain tasks or using equipment found at their workstations. Because the training is directly related to the requirements of the job, transferring skills is easier. Employees learn by actually doing the job, and they get immediate feedback as to their proficiency. Job rotation is another example of on-the-job training, whereby employees move from job to job at planned intervals, either within their department or across the organization. For example, many organizations train managers by placing them in different positions across the agency so that they are provided with a comprehensive perspective of its operation. To retain the knowledge and skills of retiring workers, some organizations have developed mentoring and shadowing programs to allow younger workers to see the more experienced workers in action. Another strategy is to encourage older workers to discuss how past projects were carried out and what they learned from their successes and failures. Some organizations have created blogging forums that employees can use to share knowledge, and others have developed communities of practice. A community of practice is a group that comes together to share information about a common problem, issue, or topic. It is a means of storing and transmitting knowledge from one person or group to another. Another method, discussed in Chapter Seven on job analysis and Chapter Nine on performance management, is using critical incident interviews or questionnaires to document how difficult cases were handled, which helps to create an institutional memory.

Some KSAOCs are difficult to teach at the worksite, necessitating off-site training. For example, training case workers in counseling and listening skills would be difficult to do at their desks because other employees not involved in the training would be distracted by the instruction. Off-site training provides an alternative to on-the-job training; employees receive training away from their workstations. In addition to avoiding disruptions to the normal routine at the jobsite, off-site training also permits the use of a greater variety of training techniques. Discussion of some other common training techniques follows.

Lecture

In a **lecture** format a trainer presents material to a group of trainees. Lectures have been criticized because the information in them flows in only one direction—from trainer to trainees. The trainees tend to be passive participants. Differences in the trainees' experiences, interests, expertise, and personalities are ignored. Lectures are limited to the transfer of cognitive material. Wexley and Latham (1991) report that lectures are beneficial when they are used to introduce new information or provide oral directions for learning tasks that eventually will be developed through other techniques. Lectures are readily adaptable for use with other training methods.

Role Playing

Role playing gives trainees the opportunity to practice interpersonal and communication skills by applying them to lifelike situations. Participants are expected to act out the roles they would play in responding to specific problems that they may encounter on the job. Role playing can be used in a variety of contexts. Law enforcement academies use it when training officers how to interview crime victims, such as sexually abused children, or witnesses to a crime. Role playing is frequently used in supervisory training in which, for example, participants are asked to counsel a problem subordinate suspected of having a substance abuse problem.

Case Studies

The use of **case studies** in training involves having participants analyze situations, identify problems, and offer solutions. Trainees are presented with a written description of a problem. After reading the case, they diagnose the underlying issues and decide what should be done. Then as a group the trainees discuss their interpretations and understanding of the issues and the proposed solutions.

Experiential Exercises

Experiential exercises attempt to simulate actual job or work experiences. Learning can be facilitated without the costs and risks of making mistakes while actually on the job. For example, health and safety agencies use experiential exercises to train employees in disaster and emergency planning.

Audiovisual Methods

Audiovisual methods are often used for training in a variety of contexts. There are videos to educate employees on such legal topics as avoiding sexual harassment, hiring applicants with disabilities, and using progressive discipline; videos that focus on interpersonal and communication skills; and videos that simulate a grievance arbitration hearing, permitting trainees to view the process, hear witnesses testify, see the behavior of management and union representatives, and learn how arbitrators conduct proceedings. Videos can be used to demonstrate particular tasks, such as the procedures to follow when apprehending a suspect or extinguishing a chemical fire. Videos are often used in orientation sessions to present background information on the agency's history, purpose, and goals, thus eliminating the need for trainers or supervisors to repeat themselves for all new employees and ensuring that the same information is always presented.

Trainees may also be videotaped. They may be asked to make a presentation or to provide performance feedback to colleagues. They may then view the videotape to identify their strengths and weaknesses related to the topic. An advantage of using videos is that trainers can slow down, speed up, or stop the video to review specific activities and enable questions to be asked and answered. A disadvantage of using videos is that they can be expensive to purchase or make.

Videos may also be used to disseminate information to a large number of people. Public Health Seattle and King County have launched *Business Not As Usual: Preparing for Pandemic Flu,* a twenty-minute training video to help advance local preparedness efforts. It was created to assist workplace leaders and staff in their pandemic flu planning efforts, describing the threat of pandemic flu and what life might look like during an outbreak. It also shows the benefits of preparedness, and provides practical tips for creating a plan.

The video profiles community leaders who share their experience in preparedness. Featured in the video are local leaders from Washington Mutual, Food Lifeline, Puget Sound Energy, Harborview Medical Center, Chinese Information and Service Center, and the Seattle Fire Department. King County executive Ron Sims and public health experts also offer their expertise in disaster preparation. The video is available online at www .metrokc.gov/health/pandemicflu/video. A free DVD can also be ordered, which includes helpful planning materials ("Washington Counties," 2008).

Programmed Instruction and Computer-Based Training

Programmed instruction and **computer-based training** are self-teaching methods designed to enable trainees to learn at their own pace. Training materials are developed concerning a specific content area, such as grant writing, and learning objectives and instructional goals are delineated. Information and training materials are assembled for the employees to read and use for practice. At their own pace, employees read the materials or practice the competencies required by the training objectives. The employees are then asked to demonstrate what they have learned.

Computer-based training involves the use of interactive exercises on computers to impart job skills. Training materials are on the Web or compact discs. Employees view information, instructions, and diagrams or other graphics on the computer screen and then respond accordingly. For example, computer-assisted technology has been used for nursing education, and drills and practice exercises are used to enhance clinical instruction (Tanner, 2002).

Community Resources

Nonprofit and public agencies should be aware of the many **community resources** that are often available to provide training at nominal cost or even for free. Many health care facilities offer workshops on topics that are targeted to specific clientele groups, such as adolescent or elderly depression, sexual abuse, or substance abuse. Chapters of Planned Parenthood offer seminars on boosting self-esteem and preventing teenage pregnancies. Hospice associations offer training on the issues associated with death and dying, and various professional associations also sponsor training classes. Managers and human resources management (HRM) departments need to be on the lookout for relevant community-based training opportunities.

E-Learning and Technology

New technologies have made it possible to reduce the costs associated with delivering training to employees. New training, delivery, and instruction methods include distance learning, streaming media, simulators, virtual reality, expert systems, electronic support systems, and learning management systems. Digital collaboration involves the use of technology to enhance and extend employees' ability to work together regardless of their geographic proximity. It can include using electronic messaging systems; electronic meeting systems; online communities of learning organized by subject, through which employees can access interactive discussion areas and share training content; and document handling systems that allow interpersonal interaction. Other technology-based training techniques involve the use of streaming media, simulators, and virtual reality. The following subsections address some of the most advanced technologies being used.

Streaming Media

Improvements in streaming media technology have made videoconferencing and webcasting—two possible training methods—less expensive and more accessible to an increasing number of public and nonprofit organizations. **Streaming media** refers to multimedia distributed over telecommunication networks. Teleconferencing refers to the synchronous exchange of audio, video, or text, or a combination of these, between two or more individuals, or between groups at two or more locations. Two-way video cameras and fiber-optic networks are able to transport interactive live images across large geographic distances.

Webcasting can involve broadcasting classroom instruction online. Webcasting can be either live or delayed, depending on individuals' access to computers with streaming video capabilities.

Advantages of this training method include reduced time lost in travel to training sites and increased uniformity of training. The number of individuals who can join in webcasts is limited only to the size of the room in which individuals can view the videos.

Simulators

Anybody who has taken a driver's education course probably remembers the driving simulator that replicated a car's dashboard and gas and brake pedals. Simulators are used to bring realism to training situations. For example, simulation technology is increasingly being used in medical education.

Laparoscopic techniques are used to provide surgeons with opportunities to enhance their motor skills without risk to patients, and there is a cardiovascular disease simulator that is used to simulate cardiac conditions, as well as anesthesia simulators that have controlled responses that vary according to numerous scenarios (Issenberg et al., 1999).

Virtual Reality

Virtual reality is a computer-based technology that provides trainees with a three-dimensional learning experience. Using specialized equipment or viewing the virtual model on a computer screen, trainees move through simulated environments and interact with their components. It allows the trainees to experience the perception of actually being in a particular environment.

For example, some police officers in Memphis, Tennessee, are part of the Crisis Intervention Team (CIT), which is trained to interact with mentally ill citizens who may pose a risk to themselves, a police officer, or the community. The CIT members receive training through "virtual hallucination software" that lets trainees step inside the world of mentally ill persons, giving police officers insight into their state of mind. Through earphones and special viewing goggles connected to software, the officer can see and feel what a mentally ill person might experience during an emergency situation. During training the officers are asked to perform a task while wearing the earphones and peering into the apparatus. The commands are hardly distinguishable amid various voices and virtual images with which the software bombards the officer. This helps officers realize that when dealing with someone with a mental illness of that nature, the person might not hear their commands. According to Major Sam Cochran of the Memphis Police Department, the coordinator of the CIT,

> It's one thing for a person to articulate that he's hearing voices and maybe seeing things, but if you don't really understand what that means, or experience what that means, you don't really understand the complexities of trying to interact with an individual who may be experiencing that. (quoted in McKay, 2007, p. 38)

Training for public safety is not the only use of virtual reality. Lowes Hotels uses Virtual Leaders, a program that helps participants learn how to be effective in meetings, such as in building alliances or getting a meeting agenda approved. As trainees attend the simulated meetings, what they say or do not say results in scores that relate to their influence in the meetings (Borzo, 2004; Hoff, 2006).

Multimedia training combines audiovisual training methods with computer-based training, CD-ROM software, e-interactive video, the Internet, virtual reality, and simulators. It integrates text, graphics, animation, video, and audio, and often the trainee can interact with the content as in virtual reality experiences. Some of the advantages of multimedia training are that it is self-paced and interactive, has consistency in regard to content and delivery, offers unlimited geographic accessibility, can provide immediate feedback, and appeals to multiple senses. It can also be used to test and certify mastery, and provides privacy to the trainee.

Some agencies use blended learning. Blended learning combines face-to-face instruction with technology-based methods of delivery and instruction. An advantage to blended learning is that it provides more social interaction, allowing learners to learn together and discuss and share insights. Live feedback from peers is often preferable to feedback received online.

An advantage of technology-based training is the cost savings due to the reduced number of trainers needed; also, because employees can access the training at their home or office, they avoid expenditures associated with traveling to a training location. Some of the disadvantages are that technology-based training is expensive to develop, it may be ineffective for certain training content, and in some cases it can be difficult and expensive to quickly update.

The different training methods used will often depend on what KSAOCs need to be learned or practiced. Another consideration is the best way for the participants to absorb the information. Millennials are likely to be the most comfortable with technology-based training. Many of their college courses were probably taught online or in a blended format. To them a computer is an assumed part of life. Their learning preferences tend toward teamwork, experiential activities, structure, and the use of technology (Oblinger, 2003). Each of the training methods discussed here has its own advantages and disadvantages that need to be weighed in relation to time constraints, staff resources, the agency's budget, the target audience, and desired outcomes.

DELIVERING TRAINING

Other issues in addition to the training curriculum must be addressed. Should the training take place for short periods of time spread over many days, or should it encompass long periods over fewer days? This is referred to as distributed practice versus massed sessions, respectively. The answer depends on the tasks the training covers. What time of day should the training take place? What size group should be involved? No one right answer exists. It depends on the information being presented or the skills that need to be taught, as well as the aptitudes of the participants and the techniques that are used. Failing to consider any of these factors can negatively influence the results of training efforts. Most health care employers cannot afford such waste.

In order to arrange the training program to facilitate learning, the following variables need to be taken into account: What are the content and amount of information to be learned? Does there need to be sequencing for the training sessions? Will participants need to practice what they have learned? What about the retention and transfer of skills or knowledge? Do trainees need the opportunity to practice the trained tasks on the job?

The delivery of the training program is the stage at which the trainers and the participants converge. At a well-organized worksite the employees selected for training understand what the objectives of the training are and what they can expect, as well as what is in the training for them. Training can be connected to the job or it can be connected to personal life—adults value personal relevance. Trainers need to be able to incorporate the group members' experience into the training. A useful model to consider is that of Kolb (1984), which is based on adults' learning from their own experience. It is up to the trainers to create a climate in which individual learning styles are recognized and considered in the delivery of the content. This is especially important for employees who resist training or perceive it as a punishment and not as an opportunity.

Research on successful training programs shows that training programs should be designed to address not only substantive content or material but also how people learn, and therefore incorporate different learning strategies (Agochiya, 2002). Affective learning results in changes in attitudes, feelings, or emotions. Skill-based learning is the development of procedural knowledge (such as how to make a pizza) that enables effective performance. Cognitive learning involves the acquisition of different types of knowledge, including declarative knowledge, structural knowledge, and cognitive strategies.

As the workforce becomes more diverse there will be more variation in employees' ability to learn, in their learning styles, in their basic literacy skills, and in their functional life skills. It will be even more important for training to take into account individual backgrounds and needs. Adult learners see themselves as self-directed and expect to be able to answer part of their questions on the basis of their own experience. Instruction tailored to adult learners affords the trainees the opportunity to participate in the process of delivering training. The role of the training instructors is to facilitate learning; they use lots of questions, guide the trainees, and encourage two-way communication between the instructor and the class, as well as communication among class participants.

EVALUATING TRAINING

An evaluation of the training program is necessary to determine whether the training accomplished its objectives. Unfortunately this is often the most neglected aspect of training, especially in the public sector (Bramley, 1996; Sims, 1998). Evaluation improves training programs by providing feedback to the trainers, participants, and managers, and it assesses employee skill levels. Evaluations can be used to measure changes in knowledge, changes in levels of skills, changes in attitudes and behavior, and changes in levels of effectiveness at both the individual level and the agency level.

Kirkpatrick (1994, 1998) suggests that there are four primary levels at which training programs can be evaluated. The first level of evaluation gauges the participants' reactions to the training program. He refers to this step as a measure of customer satisfaction. Participants are asked to answer such questions as Was the trainer knowledgeable? Were the material and information relevant? and Will the information we learned assist us in performing our job? Data on the training program's content and the trainer's skill are gathered through the use of surveys distributed at the conclusion of the training session.

According to Kirkpatrick (1998), learning has taken place when one or more of the following occurs: attitudes are changed, knowledge is increased, or skills are improved. The second level of evaluation measures whether learning has occurred as a result of attending the training. Did the participants acquire the skills or knowledge embodied in the objectives? Did the training impart the KSAOCs that were deemed important? To determine whether learning took place, participants can be tested on the information presented, follow-up interviews can be conducted, skill demonstrations can be required, or case studies can be developed to assess the competencies that were intended to be taught. It is important to note that the methods used should be selected on the basis of the level of mastery desired.

The third level of evaluation attempts to measure the extent to which on-the-job behavioral change has occurred due to the participants' having attended the training program. Evaluation activities are aimed at determining whether the participants have been able to transfer to their job the KSAOCs they learned in training. Measurement at this stage is more difficult; it requires supervisors to collect work samples or observe employees' performance. Another technique is to use performance evaluations designed to measure the new competencies.

Kirkpatrick (1998) acknowledges that for change to occur, four conditions must be met: the employee must have a desire to change, must know what to do and how to do it, must work in the right climate, and must be rewarded for changing. Kirkpatrick notes that a training program can accomplish the first two requirements, but the right climate is dependent on the employee's immediate supervisor. Some supervisors may prevent their employees from doing what was taught in the training program; others may not model the behaviors taught in the training program, which discourages the employees from changing. Some supervisors may ignore the fact that employees have attended the training program, and thereby not support employees' efforts to change; others may encourage employees to learn and apply their learning on the job. And finally, some supervisors may know what the employees learned in the training and make sure that the learning transfers to the job. To assist in creating a positive climate so that learning transfers to the job, it is recommended that supervisors be involved in developing the training program.

The fourth condition required for change to occur, that the employee must be rewarded for changing, can include the feelings of satisfaction, achievement, proficiency, and pride that often accompany successful change.

Such extrinsic rewards as praise from the supervisor, recognition from others, and possible merit rewards or promotions can also result from change.

If the training did not accomplish what it was intended to, the HRM department should assess the conditions the trainee has returned to by trying to determine where the problems lie, and then work with the line managers to make the necessary changes. Such an assessment could begin with the following questions: What gets in the way? Does the employee who just received training on a new computer system have to go back to the same old equipment? Does the employee reenter a crisis situation and have to revert to the way things were always done? Often so-called training problems are not training problems at all—they are environmental problems. Some of the most common constraints that can hinder the transfer of training to the job include a lack of job-related information provided in the training, inappropriate tools and equipment in the workplace, a lack of needed materials and supplies, and the absence of job-relevant authority. For training to be most effective, the organization's culture must support training and hold its supervisors accountable for providing a climate in which employees can transfer what they have learned to their job.

The fourth level of evaluation attempts to measure the final results that occurred because employees attended the training. Ideally training is linked to improved organizational performance. At this level evaluation is concerned with determining what impact the training has had on the agency. Satisfactory final results can include, for example, fewer grievances filed against supervisors, greater employee productivity, a reduction in the number of client complaints, a decrease in workplace accidents, increased dollars raised through fundraising, improved board relations, and less discrimination in the workplace. Some final results will be easier to measure than others. For example, the dollars accrued from fundraising activities, the number of workplace accidents, or the number of grievances filed can be easily quantified and compared to times before the training. Other final results, like eliminating discrimination, changing attitudes and behaviors, and improving leadership and communication are less tangible and more difficult to measure. Such results will have to be evaluated in terms of improved morale and attitudes. Although Kirkpatrick (1998) identifies only four levels of analysis, he emphasizes that as a final step organizations must determine whether the benefits of the training outweigh its direct and indirect costs. Phillips and Stone (2002), in their book *How to Measure Training Results,* refer to this as level five, evaluating return on investment. The results from training programs should be converted to monetary values so cost-benefit analyses can be conducted to determine if a training program should be continued. Examples of direct costs include expenses for instructor fees, facilities, printed materials, and meals. Indirect costs include the salaries of participants who are away from their regular job. Has there been a reasonable return on this investment? Was the training worth its costs? Did it accomplish what it was designed to accomplish? Training evaluation reports should present a balance of financial and nonfinancial data.

The potential benefits from evaluating training programs include improved accountability and cost-effectiveness for training programs; improved program effectiveness (Are programs producing the intended results?); improved efficiency (Are they producing the intended results with a minimum waste of resources?); and information on how to redesign current or future programs. Training must be tied to the strategic objectives of the organization. With today's emphasis on outcome measurement it is critical that training programs be designed to enhance individual, unit, and organizational performance.

CAREER DEVELOPMENT

Fitzgerald (1992) defines training as "the acquisition of knowledge and skills for present tasks, which help individuals contribute to the organization in their current positions" (p. 81). **Career development,** however, provides the employee with knowledge and skills that are intended to be used in the future. The purpose of career development is to prepare employees to meet future agency needs, thereby ensuring the organization's survival (Fitzgerald).

Career development is used to improve the skill levels of and provide long-term opportunities for the organization's present workforce. Career development programs provide incumbents with advancement opportunities within the organization so that they will not have to look elsewhere. Taking the time and spending resources to develop employees signals to them that they are valued by the agency. As a result, they become motivated and assume responsibility for developing their career path (Fitz-enz, 1996, 2000).

The focus of a career development plan is where the agency is headed and where in the agency incumbents can find future job opportunities. Employees and supervisors should produce a plan that focuses on employee growth and development. The plan should have measurable development objectives and a designated course of action. For example, supervisors should review their employees' skills in relation to the job descriptions of higher-level positions within the same job family or positions within the organization to which the employee might be able to cross over. By comparing employees' skills with the skill requirements of other positions, employees and supervisors can determine what experience and training might still be needed for advancement or lateral movement. Supervisors should direct employees to relevant training opportunities and, when possible, delegate additional tasks and responsibilities to employees so that they may develop new competencies.

A number of career development programs can be found in the public and nonprofit sectors. Some of them focus on moving employees from clerical or paraprofessional positions into higher-paying administrative jobs. Others focus on developing supervisory and management skills. An example of a program follows.

Many years ago the state of Illinois instituted a career development program called the Upward Mobility Program as part of a master agreement between the American Federation of State, County, and Municipal Employees and the state. Employees can work toward advancement in five major career paths: data processing, office services, accounting, human services, and medical. Employees receive individual counseling to inform them of the career opportunities available and to guide them in developing their career plans. Participants take proficiency exams, complete required education and training programs designed to provide the skills and knowledge needed for advancement, or both. The program covers all tuition costs and most mandatory registration fees for classes taken at public institutions, and up to $400 a credit hour for undergraduate courses and $450 for master's courses at private schools. When all necessary training and education has been completed, employees are given special consideration when bidding on targeted titles (Illinois Department of Central Management Services, n.d.).

HEALTH CARE TRAINING AND DEVELOPMENT IN APPLICATION

Health care training and development objectives must focus on four essential, interdependent elements, as illustrated in Figure 12.1. In fact, these dynamics should act as performance assessment criteria when designing a training and development curriculum, delivering the content to intended audiences, and evaluating the effectiveness of all health care training and development programs.

Relevance

Training and development must take into account all current external dynamics that the organization confronts as well as circumstances within and across the organization. Although training and development programs should not be strictly reactionary, the content, construct, and educational value of any program should be directly related to current and emergent dynamics. Most health care professionals, who are all working at a fast pace and are under considerable pressure to complete their normal job activities, will tune out and are likely to depart from the training forum if the program

---

Figure 12.1   Critical Dimensions of Health Care Training and Development

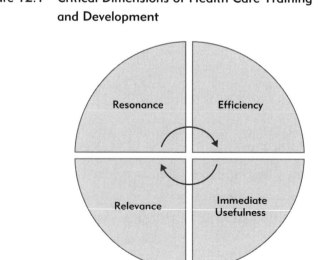

does not incorporate an immediately recognizable and relevant agenda and purpose.

Resonance

Training and development must have an "echo effect" across a certain number of participants to be successful. The immediate reaction in the first hour of the training activity, whether it is online, in person, or in any other delivery format, should be "This not only makes sense to me but also would make sense to most people in my job." Resonance works in concert with relevance. The training should make sense to the individual in its quality and intent, and it also should be validated by clear applicability across the span of its target audience. When this concept is espoused in training, each individual participant receives a worthwhile educational experience and there is also a better chance that the program will generate great word-of-mouth advertising throughout the organization. This bolsters the credibility not only of the specific program but also of the entire training and development effort and the sponsoring health care human resources component.

Immediate Usefulness

Given the paucity of time that health care employees have to do their job, let alone attend a training and development program, it is critical that the value of the program be evident and the content be accessible and readily applicable. To the high-potential health care professional, the overarching determinate of successful training is its "take-away value"—the amount of material that is immediately useful, combined with how swiftly applying this material will result in positive workplace outcomes.

Efficiency

One of the major assets available to any training and development professional is a wide array of possible topic areas and delivery methods. For example, a training program on cross-cultural communication could have an educational focus extending from ethnic nuances in a particular customer-patient community to the behavioral proclivities of part-time interns in the transportation department from the local high school. Likewise, the program can be delivered online, in person, through a manual to be used at the participants' own pace, in a group of five, or in a town hall setting on a Friday afternoon for the entire nursing corps of a community hospital. Accordingly, one of the major considerations in developing training objectives is to determine what is the fastest and most user-friendly method to provide three to five educational delivery objectives to a specific audience.

RELEVANT AND RESONANT HEALTH CARE ORGANIZATIONAL TRAINING AND DEVELOPMENT

This section explores nine essential topics in training and development for progressive health care organizations. All of these subject areas can be covered in a timely fashion by using some of the structural dynamics that have been discussed in this chapter. With thoughtful planning on the part of the training and development or education office, these topics can be presented in such a way as to maximize the impact of training and development on organizational growth and progress.

Strategies for Managing Change in Today's Health Care Business Environment

With change being the only constant dynamic in the health care business environment, it is logical that seminars and other forms of education that provide insight and practical strategies for coping with—and thriving in—change are particularly useful in a progressive health care organization. However, many organizations overlook the need to provide such training, and instead often make the mistake of presenting practicums on performance improvement and quality control. Meaningful education relative to change management can help ensure an escalation of performance improvement and quality control. This is especially true when the organization presents information that increases staff members' awareness of and appreciation for the need to adapt positively to change and to renew, reenergize, and reengineer processes that heighten the effectiveness of patient care. Moreover, strategies provided in these forums should help staff and managers alike adopt communication strategies that encourage and enlighten all members of the progressive health care organization in dealing with change. Finally, strategies that help redirect the focus and outcomes of meetings, instances of departmental communication, and critical conversations should also be infused as part of a comprehensive effort to make positive change management the norm.

Essential Management and Leadership Strategies

Education on management and leadership that is provided in a health care organization should not embrace the latest trends, clichés, and bromides, such as "who took whose cheese," regardless of their popularity, as industry-specific remedies and stratagems are needed in the health care business arena. The most successful management and leadership education in progressive health care organizations usually features several components, starting with a discussion of the Performance Matrix of superstars, studies, and nonplayers. A particular focus should be on strategies for dealing with "difficult personalities"—the nonplayers at every health care organization who present the largest and most formidable challenges for new managers and seasoned leaders alike.

Strategies concerning how to resolve performance problems in redirecting nonplayers—including the eventuality of sending them out the door to other employment after performance improvement is exhausted and after completing the proper documentation—should be offered in training and development programs. These programs should also be diligent in providing instruction on team building, with a particular emphasis on encouraging and empowering the steady advocates who make up the silent majority of a health care manager's staff. Finally, programs should include extensive instruction on how to keep superstars and action agents fully motivated and persistent in any progressive growth pattern relative to their career development and performance within the organization, and should offer specific, proven management and leadership strategies.

Leading Through Change, Crisis, and Conflict

Programs that assist managers and staff in resolving change, crisis, and conflict dynamics should be featured as part of training and development. For example, specific instruction on how to employ a time line system for proactive communication could be featured. In addition, direct approaches for properly managing conflict and reinforcing team orientation can also be central program components. Illustrations are particularly useful teaching tools, and in either in-person or online programs on resolving change, crisis, and conflict situations, trainers can employ examples of time line models as well as communication scripts for both group and individual conversations intended to remedy conflict and plan for action during times of change and crisis. Furthermore, participants' creation of a time line review and role playing of work discussions that resolve conflict should be staples in programs of this kind, as these help to improve participants' confidence, increase their willingness to try techniques in the field at the conclusion of the program, and give the instructor the opportunity to monitor and modify the material as needed.

Team Building

Real-world strategies for building pride, accountability, commitment, and trust among staff members can be very useful components of programs focused on team building. Virtually every segment of the health care organization, regardless of size, scope, and objective, relies on the use of teams to be successful. No meaningful outcome in the delivery of health care is achieved independently of some sort of support system or ancillary supplemental action. Centering on pragmatic approaches for building pride, empowering and encouraging accountability, regenerating commitment, and establishing trust can help frame specific strategies for building a strong work team. Such strategies can be of significant value to new managers, as well as to managers who have recently inherited a new department or have had a new unit added to their ongoing responsibilities. Point-specific strategies for developing interdependence among team members can also be incorporated into programs of this ilk.

Strategic Analysis and Planning

Gathering the right data within the right time parameters, establishing major strategic themes, and then innovating specific tactical actions are all integral components of a strategic plan. Although strategic planning from a larger perspective is the domain of the executive suite, the constant demand for health care services from organizations with limited resources makes strategic planning a necessity at the unit and department levels as well. Methods for making the process continuous and meaningful, from the outset of needs analysis through preparation and planning and into the innovation of a viable strategic plan, should be the subject matter for this training imperative. The ability to "plan your work, and then work your plan" is paramount for all health care leaders. Being able to use methods and executive communication strategies for planning, such as SWOT (strengths, weaknesses, opportunities, and threats), and then translating and presenting technical and pertinent information in a user-friendly fashion within the architecture of a sound strategic plan, can be eminently useful to the individual participant, his or her work unit, and the entire organization.

Encouraging Workplace Innovation and Progressive Creativity

The ability to tap into the innovative and inventive traits of staff members is not only a management technique but also a motivational factor that needs to be mastered by all health care line managers. Education on encouraging workplace innovation and creativity can help transform managers' routine scheduled staff meetings into problem-solving sessions in which new innovations are discussed, designed, and implemented. Again, field-proven techniques can be used in these training and development programs to ensure participants' confidence and capability (for example, participants might work with scripts for a problem-solving meeting). These programs might also include learning games that help participants develop their own individual strategies, which they can then share with the larger learning group and in turn apply directly to the workplace. An example of that is to use the alliteration of the letter "I" as presented in Figure 12.2 to understand a sequential way to engender a spirit of workplace innovation.

Managing Stress, Time, e-Waves, and Administrivia

Every health care manager is overwhelmed by e-mails, time constraints, and inordinate stress, all of which lead to job dissatisfaction at a personal level and potential derailment across the health care organization—resulting in a regressive rather than a progressive organization. For example, fifteen years ago when e-mail became a new management tool, many people "wished that they could have it"; now, with the typical health care manager handling between 75 and 125 e-mails a day not only at his or her desk but also on handheld communication devices, many health care managers now "wish they had never heard of e-mail!". Using such techniques as

Figure 12.2   The "I" Formula

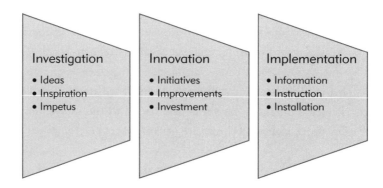

a spotlight method of time management and prioritization methods for balancing e-mail and other forms of communication can lead to increased satisfaction, greater productivity, and a stronger, healthier organization. There is a close relationship among time management, communication management, and stress management, and all three must be fused astutely, artfully, and intelligently into training and development programs to help participants manage stress better and achieve a more balanced leadership perspective. Without question, programs of this type are not merely useful; rather they should be requisites in the training and development curriculum of any health care organization that is truly dedicated to the wellness of its workforce.

Presentation Skills

One of the biggest fears within the frail human psyche is that of speaking in public, or, in health care organizational terms, having to give a management presentation or deliver an in-service educational presentation. Preparation is the key to overcoming this fear, so the opening component of a presentation skills program should be on conducting a comprehensive needs analysis (and an audience analysis), identifying three to five major themes, and crafting an interesting and informative message. PowerPoint has become a wonderful tool that is standard in any communication activity, and using PowerPoint certainly is a skill that a human resources professional can teach as part of a program on presentation skills. Outlining and construction principles should also be incorporated in this program and are best conveyed with instructional pedagogy plans for individual instruction and tailored mentoring for the participants. The process of segmenting and sequencing message components also needs to be part of the curriculum, and these skills are best taught with the presentation of several examples to help participants determine the strategies with which they are the most comfortable. A smaller learning group is preferable for this topic area, as it helps maximize comfort and participation, which in turn will help participants arrive at winning strategies for discerning what needs to be included in a presentation, developing an effective presentation, having good delivery when giving a presentation, and evaluating the effectiveness and impact of the presentation so that it can be refined further.

Strategic Communication and Leadership

For advanced team leaders in a progressive health care organization, such as critical care supervisors in the nursing arena, as well as for new managers who have participated in previous programs on supervisory and management techniques, the emerging educational sector of strategic leadership is an ideal training and development offering. Programs of this type can incorporate texts concerning advanced leadership techniques as well as leadership biographies of great leaders, emphasizing the lessons to be gleaned from such texts and avoiding clichés. For example, "Lincoln on Leadership" is teeming with leadership tips, including President Lincoln's technique of personally delivering paychecks to his direct supports so that he maintained a steady system of feedback and leadership direction. Organizational culture should also be part of these programs, which should include a study of successful corporate cultures informed with discourse on the participants' specific organizational culture. Leadership communication strategies in the areas of structured employee selection and performance evaluation should also be featured. Issues of cultural communication from an ethnic, economic, and behavioral perspective relative to both the customer-patient community and employees within the organization should also be addressed in such a program, including techniques for making cultural communication a vivid component of daily leadership. In this particular regard, the human resources management department can provide a wealth of information and perspectives. Finally, having participants—with the help of the instructional staff—each compile an individual leadership strategic plan that includes a personal development plan makes this a most useful training module.

SUMMARY

Training is the systematic process by which employees learn the KSAOCs necessary to do their job. It is typically associated with improving the performance, knowledge, or skills of employees in their present position. Career development is viewed as a continuous process consisting of evaluating abilities and interests, establishing career goals, and planning development activities that relate to employees' and the organization's future needs. Organizations must recognize the importance of both training and career development planning and provide career enhancement and development opportunities.

Given the advances in and growing availability of technology, employees and agencies have a greater variety of training methods to select from. E-learning and technology-based training have become more common. For technology-based training to be effective it needs to be designed with good learning principles, match the agency's technology infrastructure, and have the support of top management. Additional factors to consider include the following: What budget and resources will be provided to develop and support the use of new technology? Are trainees geographically dispersed, and are the travel costs of getting to training high? Are trainees comfortable using technology? Do employees have a difficult time attending scheduled training programs? Is there limited time for practice, feedback, and assessment? Such traditional training methods as classroom instruction and behavioral modeling can be delivered to trainees online rather than requiring them to come to a central training location.

It is important that once their career development programs have been developed organizations maintain their programs and revive them with new initiatives. Career development should be linked with other elements of strategic human resources management, such as succession planning, performance evaluations, quality-management initiatives, and new-employee orientation. Managers should be held accountable for developing their individual employees, and one of their main responsibilities should be providing their staff with feedback and coaching.

Agencies that are serious about training and career development should continue to monitor, evaluate, and revise their training and career development programs. To be successful, training and career development programs need to be fully integrated with the organization's strategic focus and strategic human resources management system. Increased skill acquisition will be effective only if agencies accurately identify and predict the types of KSAOCs and positions that will be required. If career paths are identified, then training and development programs must be used to move employees along those paths. New approaches to training need to be considered, and organizational reward structures should encourage individual growth and development that benefits both the employee and the organization.

KEY TERMS

audiovisual methods	needs assessment
career development	programmed instruction
case studies	role playing
community resources	simulators
computer-based training	streaming media
curriculum	training and development
experiential exercises	training objectives
lecture	virtual reality

DISCUSSION QUESTIONS

1. How does the effectiveness of a progressive health care organization's training and development programs support the overall quality of its human resources program?

2. Why is the needs assessment process so critical to the overall success of a health care training and development program?

3. What pieces of strategic human resources management guidance provided in this chapter seem to be the most important to remember when conducting fieldwork in health care training and development?

4. Why do you think training and development are considered to be a "major morale booster" in most successful health care organizations?

5. What type of training and development delivery, in your estimation, is the most effective?

6. Name three to five additional topics for a successful health care training and development program in addition to the nine cited in the last section of this chapter, complete with short descriptions of your proposed program's content.

This chapter was adapted and updated from Pynes, 1997, 2004a, 2009a.

13

Organizational Development Strategies

LEARNING OBJECTIVES

- Articulate the essential objectives of health care organizational development
- Understand how organizational development works in concert with the other essential functions of health care human resources
- Apply the basic strategies of organizational development to a specific health care organization
- Relate the specific illustrations and case exemplars in this chapter to a health care organization of your selection from your studies or professional life
- Select the organizational development strategies that would be most relevant and useful in your academic and professional endeavors

ESSENTIAL OBJECTIVES OF HEALTH CARE ORGANIZATIONAL DEVELOPMENT

Health care organizational development is defined as a comprehensive strategy dedicated to the growth and development of the organization as a total entity, and to the personal and professional growth of each and every employee—and thus is a mainstay accountability of health care human resources management. The human resources team of a progressive health care organization must take a leading role in innovating and implementing a successful organizational development strategy, replete with programs that are realistic, resonant, and results oriented. Figure 13.1 demonstrates essential tenets of health care organizational development.

Given the constant change and escalating challenges health care organizations face, objectives of efficacious organizational development include the following:

Organizational Viability

For a health care organization to survive, it must devote its everyday efforts, overall mission, and operational intentions to the needs of its most important stakeholder—the customer-patient. The provision of stellar health care should be the guiding beacon during times of change and is the charter item of a progressive health care organization, supported by the daily actions of every member of the agency. Organizations that truly embrace this charter

Figure 13.1   Essential Tenets of Health Care Organizational Development

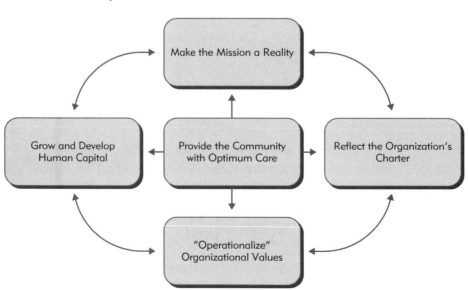

not only survive but also thrive, especially today when the customer-patient discerns the relative quality of care based on personal interactions with staff members. Organizational development, when effective, reflects the overarching values, mission, and charter of the health care organization in meeting the present and future needs of the customer-patient constituency.

Future Readiness

The progressive health care organization must be ready to meet its future needs, insofar as those needs can be predicted at present, as well as emergent trends. When they incorporate thoughtful planning, insightful needs assessment, and capable program development, organizational development efforts enable the organization to adapt to future customer-patient needs.

Community Commitment

Organizational development within a health care facility indicates to its customer-patient community that the organization is truly dedicated to long-term goals, growth, and development in pace with the needs of its customer-patients. Like any credible and respected community-driven organization, the progressive health care organization acknowledges a responsibility to constantly improve services, upgrade the efficacy of its personnel, redefine its operational goals, and maintain a steady commitment to the constituent community. The launch of a purposeful organizational development program in a small rural hospital, for example, can reflect the organization's commitment to its future while reinforcing trust between the community and the organization. The communication of the organizational objectives and major organizational achievements to the customer-patient community during times of change—which can be accomplished with the organizational development process involving time lines demonstrated in Chapter Three of this text—demonstrates a firm commitment to long-term growth and dedication to the community's needs.

Performance Maximization

The well-worn cliché of being "lean and mean" is perhaps the most useful way to define performance maximization. In the progressive health care organization, great performers are given the opportunity to excel, to create new ways to address customer-patient needs and concerns, and to thrive during times of change. These stellar employees, referred to throughout this text as superstars, should also be given the opportunity to help contribute to their organization's growth and development—as well as to their own basic job security during times of turbulence—by contributing fully to the institution and using all of their talents on a daily basis.

For individual members of the organization who are not particularly committed to the health care facility—such as the nonplayers discussed throughout this text—organizational development efforts should provide the opportunity to help them decide, as adults and professionals, whether they want to be long-term members of the organization. For employees at all three levels of performance—the superstars, the steadies, and the nonplayers—organizational development provides an opportunity to grow and develop to escalate expertise, improve performance, and maintain employment (or, in the case of nonplayers, to show who should ultimately be removed from the organization).

Maintaining Fiscal Responsibility

Another positive outcome of organizational development is its potential contribution to organizational fiscal responsibility. Organizational development presents a wonderful opportunity to elicit, garner, and incorporate cost-efficient, quality-conscious solutions to pressing operational, organizational, and patient care quandaries. When done effectively and with focus, organizational development enhances the quality of services provided while realizing measurable cost savings. By maintaining a focus on service, commitment, and selfless compassion as everyday commitments among all members of the progressive health care organization, the human resources team can help set parameters that enable fiscal responsibility and increase the intelligent use of existing staff and available resources.

Organizational Galvanization

Just as rubber and other synthetic compounds must be galvanized—that is, blended together for a tight, cohesive structure—one of the underlying objectives of organizational development is the galvanization of the institution. Put simply, most members of a progressive organization in the competitive health care business arena are usually very appreciative of the basic and realistic fact that they still have a job. As a result, individual commitment to organizational development efforts, such as town hall meetings, performance improvement initiatives, and other approaches discussed throughout this chapter, can be bountiful because most reasonable employees are more than willing to participate in any efforts that might strengthen the organization and, in turn, their job security. Furthermore, organizational development can work as a catalyst in interdepartmental cooperation and coordination through targeted efforts and enlightened needs analysis and programming. "Nobody wins unless everybody plays to win" can be a suitable summation statement as well as a rallying cry for intelligent organizational development efforts.

Opportunity to Redirect Performance and Actions

A progressive health care organization should have a current and relevant organizational chart, a credo, and a known set of organizational objectives, as discussed specifically later in this chapter. During times of change—which in reality is all of the time in American health care—the human resources team, in concert with executive management, has a tremendous opportunity to communicate two critical organizational directions with its organizational development programs. First, given the change, chaos, and challenge omnipresent in health care, the organization must redirect and remodel organizational development efforts to thrive as a business entity. Second, the senior executive team can present new organizational development initiatives, such as a new credo and charter, to trigger some intended renewal and to keep the organization on the right track (or in some cases to get it *back* on the right track through the strength of its human capital). In both cases the promise of a renewed organization has the potential to generate a sense of enthusiasm for the organization's new direction.

Optimization of Resources

Although the phrase *optimization of resources* typically connotes fiscal assets, a progressive health care organization undertakes organizational development to fully use the talents of the individuals—the human resources—doing the majority of the work to meet the demands of the customer-patient community. Organizational development can help empower and encourage the strongest contributors in an organization to practice their craft, and it gives these stellar performers as well as the high-potential steadies the opportunity to grow and develop in their specific areas of expertise while contributing optimally to the organization.

Competitive Edge

A progressive organization can compete more effectively against its rivals in the hypercompetitive health care business arena with a strong organizational development strategy. The health care organization that models itself according to the needs of customer-patients is logically the competitor that will be the preeminent provider of health care services in its particular market. What is more, the organization that embraces the best organizational development strategy is the one that will appear the most "user-friendly" to both its employees—most of whom are probably members of the organization's service community—as well as a critical mass of its larger customer-patient constituency. To this end, organizational development can provide the stellar health care organization with the opportunity to get the jump on its competitors and maintain a critical performance edge.

Social Commitment

A progressive health care organization demonstrates commitment to its community during the upheavals relative to health care that American society faces. The renewed organization attends to the needs that the typical American hospital heretofore did not address, such as critical outpatient services, wellness and health maintenance, and a host of other programs. The progressive health care organization fully and competently prepares its entire workforce to meet the needs of new constituents and the shifting needs of current constituents, who are naturally apprehensive and indeed fearful of health care providers, and who are concerned about the eventual outcomes of their treatment. Through efficacious organizational development the progressive health care organization can maintain the proper array of health care professionals and ensure that the continuity of its professional education facilitates the professional growth necessary to meet the new demands from its customer-patients.

High Organizational Morale and Positive Outlook

Health care employees at every level of progressive health care organizations are currently fearful. They are fearful for their job security, fearful about the future of American health care and the impact of ongoing legislation, fearful of increased and often mendacious scrutiny by the media, and fearful concerning their organization's potential inability to find sufficient resources to provide care while contending with restricted operational and fiscal assets. To combat misdirected apprehension, the organizational development process helps staff members maintain a healthy perspective by not worrying about things they cannot change and concentrating on positive workplace actions that they competently control on a daily basis. That is, the individual staff member can control his or her contribution to the health care organization through communication, staff input, education and personal knowledge, and work performance. The staff member should be encouraged to participate in—rather than to observe or ignore—the organizational development process, which can help relieve the individual staff member's anxiety.

Limitation of Negative Employee Emotionalism

People become fearful when faced with change. Health care organizations today—all of which are facing change in one form or another—have staff members who understandably react poorly to nearly constant nonplayer contention, rampant negativism, and a host of other destructive workplace forces that inhibit the effective delivery of everyday services. Therefore the health care organization that undertakes a renewed, dedicated organizational development initiative is one that will demonstrate a sense of strength by also addressing fear-causing change. The organization can illuminate and resolve negative emotionalism through concentrated and targeted organizational development strategies in organizational sectors in which such canards as "Nothing is done about the people who don't care" and "We've always done it that way, so who cares?" are the rule of the day. Most members of health care organizations are savvy enough to know that no institution is insulated from change and chaos, but that insular thinking can result in the demise of the organization. As employees recognize this from a larger perspective, organizational development that is realistic, resonant, and results oriented can become a major catalyst in shifting organizational emotionalism from negative to positive.

Introduction of a New Era

Given the impression by most members of health care organizations that something "new and different" must be done to meet current and emerging organizational challenges, health care human resources professionals must seek a theme for their organizational development strategy that incorporates the wisdom of individuals as varied as Bill Gates, Thomas Edison, and other great American thinkers. Although this group may at first seem eclectic, all of these individuals, as illustrated in Table 13.1, aptly balanced two themes—taking care of business and taking care of the people depending on them. A progressive health care organization takes into account many business dynamics, new organizational practices, and a spectrum of

Table 13.1   Organizational Development Themes from Great American Innovators

Leader	Mission	Theme
Clara Maass	Modern nursing	Apply skills and technology systematically to healing; self-sacrifice
Thomas Edison	Electrical power for the world	Take risks, learn from mistakes, and always go forward
Abraham Lincoln	Creation of the Veterans Administration system	Care for those who have "borne the battle" and their families (according to Lincoln's charter for establishing veterans' health care)
Bill Gates	Transformative technology	Encourage problem definition, innovate solutions, and lead action
Juliette Low	Founding of the Girl Scouts	Learn through selfless service to the community
Eleanor Roosevelt	Leading the recovery after the Great Depression and World War II	Seek light and goodness after dark times

creative, progressive business approaches. However, a new era of health care organizational development can be created with the reintroduction of basic principles to help return organization members' focus to basic precepts that can spark enthusiasm:

- The customer-patient is at the top of the organizational chart.
- Compassion and dignity are time-honored traditions of our organization.
- Although a business, we are essentially a human service.
- We are the community trust for health care in our area.
- Change is not just made for the sake of change; change takes place to make us better so that we can do our job better.
- Our job is among the most important in our community—taking care of people who need our services in times of desperate need, ill health, and life-or-death situations.

From an individual perspective, a mantra of five factors should be introduced at the forefront of health care organizational development efforts by all members of the organization's leadership:

- Know what you are doing
- Know what you want to do
- Remember that you are doing good work
- Remember how important it is to do good work
- Seek to give everyone around you selflessness, commitment, and fairness

A new era for a progressive health care organization, brought about through organizational development efforts, can indeed be exciting and can help establish new directions for the institution's mission, strategic plan, and focus. This happens only when organizational development is consistently and continually underscored by an allegiance to the basic mission of the health care institution as a community trust.

Sending Appropriate Messages

One of the major benefits of health care organizational development is its conveyance of appropriate, pertinent messages to all constituents, both internal and external. It communicates to customer-patients that their voice has been heard and that efforts are under way to meet their needs more efficiently and effectively. Organizational development also sends a message to employees that participants and individuals who are committed to organizational growth and progress will be rewarded. It further reminds contentious and self-serving individuals that their performance must become more selfless, productive, and effective. It is important to note that stakeholders in a health care organization will interpret organizational development from various perspectives. The organization's leaders must clearly and comprehensively underscore the importance of health care organizational development with a message encompassing these points:

- Organizational development helps to meet the demands of the customer-patient.

- Organizational development positions all of us to meet the demands of the future.

- Organizational development increases the organization's overall efficiency and effectiveness.

- Organizational development increases the stability, progress, and security of our jobs.

- Organizational development challenges and inspires all members of the organization toward peak performance.

In considering these tenets when communicating organizational development—particularly with the launch of new programs and initiatives, such as those delineated throughout this chapter—leaders of the health care organization take a proactive and progressive approach toward getting the right message out to all stakeholders and constituents.

Public Relations and Community Relations Impact

As implied in the previous subsection, the entire customer-patient community of a particular health care organization interprets organizational development through varied personal prisms. Therefore, the cosmetic aspects of organizational development that contribute to how the effort is perceived are as important as organizational development itself, as perception is often as important as reality (a common theme to guide all efforts of health care human resources). For example, health care organizations have adopted a new color scene, a new credo, or a new advertising tagline that not only celebrates the new organizational development efforts but also reinforces the traditions and lore of the particular health care institution. There are several strategies that can be used to realize the full public relations value of health care organizational development. For example, the veteran and customer-patient in West Virginia can feel more confident about the competency of the Huntington VA Medical Center upon review of the Huntington VA Medical Center fact sheet presented later in this chapter, and a resident of the Marshall Islands knows that her national hospital means business and reflects the values of her culture when reviewing the credo statement of the Majuro Medical Center.

ORGANIZATIONAL DEVELOPMENT STRATEGIES FOR BUILDING PRIDE

For health care organizational development to be considered successful, health care employees must feel as though their organization is indeed "playing to win." Most employees are motivated by a sense that their institution is doing all it can to meet the needs of the customer-patient; and providing excellent care is of great importance to the average health care employee.

Even in a successful health care organization employees may be fearful that the organization might soon be unable to provide exemplary care due to a lack of resources and increased confusion in financial reimbursement procedures. The institution must therefore make every effort possible to create a sense of strong affiliation and unity among staff members by taking five action steps concerning organizational development initiatives:

1. Reinforce the basic mission, values, and objectives of the organization

2. Pragmatically describe how organizational development will help enhance the quality of health care services on a daily basis

3. Reinvest in community relations

4. Highlight the successes and "wins" of the renewed progressive health care organization

5. Communicate a strengthened allegiance between the organization and each staff member, which will lead to greater commonality of purpose and, ultimately, to organizational achievement

This section discusses central strategies that enable a human resources team, in concert with managers at all levels, to achieve these five objectives.

Credo

The **credo** is a review of the institution's basic beliefs. Going beyond the basic mission statement, the credo should reflect the core values and restate the organization's commitment to the customer-patient. As per the sample in Figure 13.2 from the Majuro Medical Center in the Marshall Islands—a small, independent country in the Pacific that is also an American protectorate with 250,000 citizens—the credo is a basic set of statements that reflects the beliefs and charter of the organization's nursing corps. As is the case with the Majuro sample, the most well-received credo statements have been those that reflect sentiments commonly held by managers, employees, and members of the service community. In fact, nursing students composed this statement by working with community focus groups that clearly offered valid

---

Figure 13.2   Majuro Medical Center Credo of Nursing

As a community committed to our Nation's education in the strongest traditions of *manit*,*
the Members of the Marshall Islands Nursing Corps:

- Seek always to support a stellar professional educational environment that prepares us to make an optimum contribution to the development of the Marshall Islands Healthcare

- Affirm our desire to become a vanguard Pacific institution of health care by adhering to the highest standards of academic quality, institutional effectiveness, and social responsibility in all regards and in all of our actions

- Dedicate our everyday efforts to being a credible agent of change in preparing the next generation of our Nation's health care leaders in a manner that reflects great credit on our traditions and culture

- Celebrate our rich tradition of cultural wisdom, human diversity, and national aspiration in our everyday actions

- Work together toward consistently providing all with a caring and healing experience enriched with an inspired vision of wellness, selflessness, and honorable action

*This is a Marshallese belief that "an adult never stands taller than when reaching down to help one in need."

input; they garnered even more valuable suggestions by eliciting input from hospital staff and management. Simply by asking staff members, "What is the most important thing to you and your daily responsibilities?" a manager should be able to collect five to ten possible statements for inclusion in the organization's credo—or even for a departmental credo. These efforts can culminate in an overall organizational credo systematically developed by the human resources staff.

Emblazoned with the organization's logo and printed on parchment-style paper in the institution's colors, the credo should be framed and posted at all employee entry points, patient service areas, and other spots where it can be readily observed, as well as on the organization's Web site(s). This is a direct sign to patients and employees alike that the organization is serious about its fundamental community commitment, and that the credo is more than just words—it is a way of doing business on a daily basis.

Organizational Handbook of Values

The credo should be supplemented by a handbook that contains the organization's essential values. In addition to reflecting the organization's core values, the handbook should list performance criteria, which in turn can be used when selecting new employees, when deciding which employees will receive promotions and transfers, and for evaluating organizational performance.

The organizational handbook book of values not only supplements the credo but also attests to how the organization seeks to serve the customer-patient. Put simply, it is a set of guidelines for how the institution pursues its mission of taking care of the customer-patient. As with the credo statement, the handbook should be professionally printed, replete with the organization's logo and color scheme. The most effective handbooks feature photographs of actual staff members conducting their daily work. Pictures of individuals working in the cafeteria line are just as essential to the organizational handbook as photos of individuals working in the emergency room. This type of imagery reinforces the institution's belief that the work of the cafeteria employee is just as necessary to the progressive health care organization's mission as that of the emergency room doctor. Such themes as allegiance, compassion, dignity, respect, and quality should be incorporated in the organizational handbook. Each page should have a value that is clearly defined and that is supplemented by at least five supporting criteria, as depicted in Figure 13.3.

Figure 13.3   Example Criteria Page for an Organizational Handbook of Values

Independent judgment—Capable of ascertaining direction and goals using individual talent and ability; basically self-starting, makes appropriate decisions and executes action without undue reliance on others

Defining Criteria:

Resolves problems with quick, resolute action

Achieves set goals and objectives on time consistently

Gets involved in the resolution of tough problems constructively

Has logical rationales for decision making and performance action

Works well independently without alienating colleagues or other stakeholders

The handbook should be presented to each staff member as soon as it's published and, moreover, to each new employee as an integral part of the orientation process. Many organizations have used a handbook effectively when conducting their new staff orientation program. The presentation of the institution's values and a comprehensive review of how it operates individually and collectively are vital to any health care facility operating under the pressure of constant change. Based on input from across the organization and artfully produced, published, and distributed under the auspices of the human resources management department, the handbook takes a prominent operational role for all well-intentioned managers and employees.

Community-Driven Education

The progressive health care organization uses the credo and handbook both internally and also as the foundation of the community education process. Because many customer-patients truly believe that they are not only stakeholders but also investors in a local health care institution, prevailing apprehension, skepticism, curiosity, and in some cases fear in the community can match that of the institution's employees. Every effort should thus be made to educate the community about the organization. The human resources management department's distribution of the credo and handbook to the community is an effective first step in enlightening customer-patients and assuring them that their health care needs will be met fully and effectively through active, value-driven organizational development.

Community education is not solely the responsibility of the public relations office, the human resources management department, or the organization's leadership. Staff members also become ambassadors to the community and should be charged with the responsibility of educating their friends, neighbors, and family members whenever possible about the organization's daily workings, new initiatives, and strategic plans for meeting emergent needs. Staff members should, for example, prepare presentations for community groups, such as the local Rotary Club, and should also educate others through impromptu, informal conversations at barbecues, picnics, and church events. Supplying such resources as the credo, updates on organizational progress, and facts about the organization's current and new health programs can help enhance both organizational development and community awareness, as these provide education and represent current, relevant communication.

The human resources management department should maintain responsibility for educating staff members on how to communicate with community members relative to the organization's initiatives and strategic plans. Attendance at formal events, such as open houses, can help educate the staff as well as the community. In fact, an open house can become a forum in which to train health care organization members in how to communicate new initiatives to the community. Health fairs can also educate the community while offering various preventive screening services, blood bank operations, and testing procedures. Involving staff members in these activities as well as incorporating training and development that teaches methods on how to educate community members about health care initiatives is a point-specific organizational development approach. In a similar sense, the institution should also support "Career Days" at local schools, not only to spark an interest in health careers among students but also to provide general awareness about their local health care provider.

House Rules

As already discussed, the constant change that affects most community health care organizations necessitates the provision of ever-more-comprehensive health care services to maintain customer-patients' trust. To this end, the human resources team, in concert with appropriate organizational leadership, should produce a set of "house rules" that help reinforce the lessons learned by employees in guest relations programs provided by the organization's training and development cadre. These rules might include commonsense maxims, such as those in the following list of excerpts from the employee manual of the member hospitals of the **Stevens Healthcare Educational Partnership,** a national leader in using government resources to provide free education to health care staff and managers in nonprofit urban hospitals:

- Never say, "I don't know"; immediately find someone who can answer the question at hand.

- Never say, "It's not my job"; find the individual whose job it is.

- Treat the fortieth person you deal with today as well as you treated the first person you treated today.

- Focus on each patient as a source of motivation and inspiration.

- Make certain that your work area is always clean, professional, and safe.

- Extend every small decency necessary and needed at any time.

- Treat your colleagues as well as you treat the patient.

- Remember always that you are our organization, and your conduct is the most prominent personification of our organization.

- Demonstrate compassion, sensitivity, and perceptiveness in everything you do when you are on the medical center campus.

These rules not only represent a set of standards for conduct but supplement the credo, the organizational handbook of values, and other organizational development initiatives. Because most health care professionals practice the standards anyway, they act as only a positive reinforcement for the majority of staff members. However, they do put certain nonplayers on notice relative to the essential truth that *how* a staff member does something is just as important as *what* he or she does on a given day in a progressive health care organization.

Branding and Signage

Some progressive health care organizations give themselves, as well as some internal divisions, new titles to indicate their commitment to a new era in health care. This is a good idea, provided that the new labels do not create confusion or, worse, spread fear throughout the constituent community. For example, if the customer-patient does not recognize the new label and thinks that the organization "has been bought out and is not the same anymore," the label can clearly do more harm than good. New signage and branding have the potential, however, to help the progressive health care organization reestablish its identity with additional strength. For example, if a renewed hospital calls itself a "medical center," the community gets the impression that the organization has actually gotten "bigger and stronger" and can provide more services. In many areas of the Metropolitan East Coast, several community hospitals have formed affiliations and alliances with local teaching universities and have accordingly been branded as "university medical centers," adding panache, gravity, and a sense of an improved identity in the eyes of local community members. In addition, the organization gives itself a wonderful opportunity to garner a renewed commitment from the majority of its staff, provided that the new identity is communicated clearly, cogently, and comprehensively to all staff members. Likewise, if a hospital has acquired an outpatient clinic, or is merged with a home for the aging, it can change its name from "community hospital" to "community health system," again reinforcing the impression that it has become bigger and stronger.

If an organization adopts a new label, its logo and colors should remain the same. This helps maintain consistency for the benefit of customer-patients as well as the organization's staff members, the latter being of particular interest to human resources professionals.

CEO Report

The CEO report can be a strong motivating force in increasing organizational affiliation and pride, and consists of a comprehensive outline of the organization's major achievements for the past year and the major objectives for the coming year. It can be published at three critical opportunities during the organizational development process. First, during any rightsizing or critical change effort it can delineate organizational imperatives as well as the rationale and the need for the change. The second opportunity is during a reconstruction effort, such as when a new organizational structure is introduced and the report is used to highlight the new model's benefits.

The third logical point for introducing a CEO report is during the launch of a new calendar year, at which time the report should contain these six features:

- Expressed appreciation to all staff members for their participation in and support of the organization's progress over the previous year

- A basic review of the organization's progress, complete with positive points, such as financial progress, or other indicators that demonstrate the organization is indeed on the right track

- If applicable, the introduction of the credo, organizational handbook, and new label, in an effort to spark interest in, resonance with, and support for those initiatives

- A review of the institution's current status, including positive indicators of performance

- A brief assessment of the organization's immediate future to help staff comprehend and support new initiatives and significant change dynamics

- A long-range perspective from the CEO on the organization's growth and progress, supported by a time line depiction

The CEO report should be delivered to each employee and augmented whenever possible with comments from each supervisor or manager during monthly meetings and other forums. In addition, the CEO report should be distributed appropriately to community members and presented in conjunction with CEO briefings, town hall meetings, community action nights, and other gatherings at which these six essential messages can be conveyed.

Celebrating the Wins

Every superstar manager in a progressive health care organization must celebrate the "wins," at least at the level and intensity with which he or she reviews and agonizes over the "losses." Because of perfectionist tendencies, health care managers often dwell on "what went wrong and needs to be fixed" rather than "what is going good and needs to be built on." This can be devastating to a progressive organization, as fear and apprehension are already naturally abundant throughout the health care workplace. All leaders therefore need the support, communication acumen, and consultative help of the human resources team to identify wins that can be celebrated to enhance pride and commitment, as such efforts demonstrate the organization's ability to provide excellent services.

Celebrating the wins can take several shapes. For example, by comparing last year's results to this year's—given, of course, that this year's results are positive—a clear analysis can be provided that shows the benefits of embracing organizational development. Comparing the organization's success with the failings of a competing institution that has not pursued organizational development in a relevant and resonant manner is another way to celebrate success. The use of a time line also helps to chart organizational progress and increase team allegiance.

Moreover, organizational leadership's recognition of an individual's strong work contribution goes a long way toward celebrating the wins. This again is the health care leader's responsibility and can be facilitated with the professional support of the human resources management department. Praise from customer-patients, for example, that describes the specific actions of an employee that resulted in better health care is also a win that merits celebration. Perhaps more important, the health care leader who asks employees, "What have we been doing right recently?" is laying the ground-work for a discussion of wins that are clearly recognized, are valid in the eyes of all employees, and reflect the progressive health care organization's success.

"Garment Gimmicks"

Using T-shirts, windbreakers, and other garments bearing the organization's logo, new motto, and other features can seem trivial at first. However, consider how brand-name garments are not only fashionable but a major factor in American society. Certain sportswear companies now manufacture more garments with their own logo than with logos of professional sports teams. In a similar vein, garments that have the logo of the progressive health care organization can be used as inducements and rewards for participation in organizational development efforts. From a broader perspective, they also become a source of advertising as giveaway items at major organizational events both on the medical center campus and across the community—all under the direction and at the discretion of the organization's human resources office.

In other words, using garments that have the organization's logo and other features can be a powerful marketing tool as well as a component of the employee affiliation process. Many progressive health care organizations have used clothing, hats, golf shirts or T-shirts, and other garments not only to demonstrate their logo and name to the community but also to increase employee awareness of new initiatives. Branded items—which could also include coffee cups, golf towels, and related pieces—can be given out meritoriously, for example as an award for assisting as a team leader in an organizational survey process or as part of other recognition strategies, or can simply be distributed to all staff members on the occasion of the organization's Founders' Day. These kinds of giveaways should not be discounted in the overall organizational development scheme, as they have a tremendous impact on staff members and their friends and neighbors throughout the community.

The eight affiliation strategies discussed in this section can help create a sense of allegiance among all staff members and, when used in concert, can help set the pace and raise new expectations for employees as the progressive health care organization moves forward to a promising future while undertaking comprehensive organizational development.

ORGANIZATIONAL DEVELOPMENT STRATEGIES FOR ESCALATING ACCOUNTABILITY

The success of a progressive health care organization rests on its ability to create a sense of renewed accountability among all employees. This individual accountability can be found in the collective belief by most employees that the organization's traditional strength is augmented by its current ability to meet the escalating demands of the health care environment. This section offers practical ways to reinforce accountability though organizational development strategies fostered and implemented by human resources leadership and action.

Human Capital Board Summit

In order to engage all levels of leadership in the organizational development effort, the human resources management department should conduct a board summit as a forum to discuss the organizational development strategy with appropriate members of the **board of directors.** The word *summit* should be used instead of *retreat,* as the organization is moving forward and upward, not retreating from its competitive environment. The board summit should be specifically scheduled to discuss the progressive health care organization's current strategy and strategic plans relative to increasing the quality of its human capital.

The summit, attended by either the entire board or a select committee dedicated to addressing human capital issues, should include a discussion of organizational strategic imperatives. The CEO and the vice president of human resources should take primary responsibility for expressing the institution's specific goals and suggesting ways in which the board can best support the organization relative to organizational development. Although the opinions of all board members are always valued when they are thoughtful, direct, and honest, the specific actions undertaken by board members to support new organizational development are particularly essential. These include efforts in increasing community awareness of the renewed organization and committing available resources (money, time, contacts, or otherwise) toward the organizational development process.

At the summit all board members should understand three critical facts. First, the organization intends to concentrate on the future, not the past. Board members should all commit themselves to the future organizational development efforts; they should not use the past as a basis for understanding or formulating future strategy. Second, "nobody wins unless everybody plays to win"; this means that all board members need to participate as action agents, active players, and proponents of the new system—not as backward-looking, regressive second-guessers. Third, the renewal process is permanent, and change will be a constant factor as the organization moves forward. With these facts as standards, all board members should then be encouraged to participate in shaping the future direction of the progressive health care organization.

The summit's purpose is not only to increase organizational pride but also to enlist board members' support and gain their commitment to future action. The renewal process is a prime opportunity to reconstruct boards, adding new board members or perhaps removing board members who are resistant to change and new challenges.

Volunteer Activation

As discussed in detail in Chapter Six, volunteers are an essential component of any health care organization. They bring their skills as well as continuing commitment to the organization's objectives and mission. Unfortunately, volunteers can often be lost in the shuffle during organizational development, and as a result their accountability in the organization can wane.

Volunteer activation should take two forms. First, the education or human resources management department should provide education to all volunteer groups throughout the organization, particularly during the organizational development process. A clear picture should be presented about the future objectives and mission of the renewed organization. In addition, the particular role of each volunteer—and the role of the entire volunteer corps—should be defined clearly to eliminate any apprehension and fear. Second, each volunteer's abilities should be fully examined in the interest of optimizing his or her potential contribution. For example, if a volunteer has particular marketing skills, he could be asked to create a new logo, signage, and any other marketing details; if another volunteer is a retired teacher, she can be consulted when creating a new day care center. In concert with the suggestions in Chapter Six, the organizational development process offers a natural opportunity not only to reinvest volunteer accountability into the organization but also to reassess and make the most of specific volunteer skills.

Fan Mail Bulletin Board

Investing fifty dollars to erect the bulletin board on which to post "fan mail" to employees and volunteers might be the most intelligent expenditure a human resources management department can make during the organizational development process. Whereas many of us are inundated with e-mails to the extent that we give most online correspondence very little attention, a tangible bulletin board that contains letters from patients, family members, and other stakeholders will be appreciated by all staff members. The bulletin board should be placed in a prominent location, such as the employee cafeteria. Whenever clinical directors receive a letter highlighting individual action—especially when the action occurred at least in part because of the organizational development process—the correspondence should be posted immediately on the fan mail bulletin board.

Likewise, any fan mail received by individual department leaders or unit supervisors should be posted as well. This correspondence is equally important and relevant in the eyes of all staff members. Furthermore, any newspaper articles or positive local press coverage should be posted. The fan mail bulletin board is a simple idea and is extremely effective if well managed. Correspondence should be placed on the bulletin board in a timely manner, with new material added as old correspondence is removed. This is because when an article or letter stays on the board for more than a month, many nonplayers will think—and say—that the organization has done nothing of any good consequence lately. However, certain correspondence that is particularly significant should be placed on the bulletin board, perhaps under a designated "hallmarks of our success" section. The fan mail bulletin board increases staff members' pride in, affiliation with, and respect for the health care organization.

"Big Events"

The progressive health care organization can use "big events" to launch new aspects of the organizational development process and as an educational opportunity to increase the awareness of organizational development programs and strategies. At these events a short speech is mandatory on the part of the organization's CEO, as is the distribution of "garment gimmicks" and other giveaway items. Naturally, food should also be part of the process. Classic examples of big events are employee picnics or holiday parties at which food is provided, creating a relaxed atmosphere for discussing the organization as well as for renewing acquaintances with colleagues and community members.

A benchmark that reflects the lore, legacy, and legend of the organization might be an appropriate occasion for a big event. For example, Founders' Day is typically celebrated by major corporations but not as often by health care facilities. By researching when the community hospital was founded, for example, and celebrating the anniversary date in concert with the launch of new organizational development efforts, the organization can establish a new benchmark that can be used in subsequent years as a new "special day" for staff members and stakeholders to anticipate and enjoy.

Organizational Surveys

The intelligent use of organizational surveys is essential to any health care organization. In a progressive organization in particular, however, the survey results can become a catalytic force in organizational development. For example, a survey that evaluates organizational effectiveness, departmental efficiency, leadership perception, job scope validity, and other critical issues is a useful tool, particularly when participants are asked to make comparisons between the "old organization" and the "new one" (that is, the organization as it existed in recent memory compared to its current status).

With this in mind, it might be useful to conduct a survey immediately after launching an organizational development effort and then, six months later, to take a comparison survey. Regardless of their specific outcomes, surveys of this type can be become clear, direct indicators to leadership concerning the relative efficiency of the organizational development process.

The **Change Readiness Inventory** should also be used. In organizations in which leadership is fearful that the survey results might actually dampen enthusiasm for organizational development efforts—a common reaction even under the best of circumstances, given the fear and apprehension existent in most health care organizations—another approach to garnering employee input might useful. This can be a simple, open-ended questionnaire—a Change Readiness Inventory set of questions—with the following queries:

- What can we be doing during the next six months to get better?

- The three biggest things I've learned over the past six months are _____, _____ and _____.

- In order to be truly successful, we must understand _____ and _____.

- For our organization to be successful, my colleagues and I must always _____.

Using these open-ended questions can generate positive data for pragmatic use by staff members while providing a reflection of prevailing sentiments among staff members across the organization.

Quarterly Reviews

Every three months each department should chart significant quantitative results, which can be posted using numbers that reflect significant gains. Such reports can also reflect percentages—both positive and negative—that have an impact on organizational performance. In addition, time efficiency and cost effectiveness should also be charted each quarter.

These quarterly reviews should be conducted by the line manager and his or her work team. Such reviews can be a tremendous tool for assessing departmental progress, and they can also be rallying points for renewed commitment to departmental objectives. If used artfully throughout the organization, the results of all quarterly reviews can be combined into a comprehensive institutional review; this review can become an integral part of an annual report that contributes to organizational pride and redefined staff commitment.

Time Lines

As mentioned earlier, all managers should use time lines throughout the organizational development process. The time line for the organizational development process might commence on the date a "big event," such as Founders' Day, takes place and continue to the end of the calendar year, the conclusion of the fiscal year, or the first anniversary of the big event. Time lines are straightforward, readily composed, and extremely open to employee input. When time lines are easily recognizable by employees and received as valid reflections of organizational achievement, they become strong organizational motivators. Time line construction can delineate specific details of a certain project or more general improvement initiatives. In any case they can be both a teaching tool and a good work group or organizational performance evaluation tool.

Annual Report

The annual report, which differs from the CEO report in that it focuses on the entire organization relative to its service community, can be an integral part of the organizational development process. As its name suggests, the annual report is a published document developed by senior management in conjunction with the human resources staff responsible for employee relations and communication. If all of the organization's managers have created quarterly reviews and have composed time lines relative to their work in progress, the data collection process for an overall annual report is a natural and efficient one. The annual report should contain progress notes from financial, operational, and personnel standpoints, linking past progress and future plans.

ORGANIZATIONAL DEVELOPMENT STRATEGIES FOR TEAM BUILDING

Trust, accountability, and work satisfaction are the fundamentals of professional motivation. The ability to practice one's craft and apply all of one's powers—mental, physical, and spiritual—to help fellow human beings in pain and need is the essence of professional motivation for any health care professional. This section explores the strategies a health care organization can use as part of an organizational development process to impart a greater sense of satisfaction to each team member.

Job Component Review

Every employee in every health care organization has set job responsibilities and assigned daily tasks. In the progressive health care organization each and every staff member has an opportunity to review his or her individual job role. The job component review must be implemented with clear participation from employees, starting with a self-directed listing of all of their essential job components, with the designation of an approximate time value and weighed performance value to each. The employee can complete this review together with the line manager or supervisor, or independently pending subsequent review, ratification, and approval by the immediate supervisor. Human resources professionals play an essential role in this process as internal consultants to the reviewing manager as well as consulting facilitators to the individual employee. Both managers and staff members should use earlier job descriptions as a foundation for the review, but a previous description should act as no more than a cursory guide to the process. Instead, employees should consider a typical day given the job role in the renewed organization and construct a review accordingly.

Reviewing job components can help establish a performance review that is criteria based and job specific, as described in Chapter Nine. Furthermore, the employee and manager can use the job component review as a guide for action and as a building block for heightening the employee's performance effectiveness.

"Back to the Basics" Program

A "back to the basics" program can help assuage the employee fear that is always present during times of change and refocus the employee on the critical, essential elements of health care delivery. The best way to implement such a program is to apply a patient-focused set of principles that are simple and clear to offset the complexity of the health care business arena.

Here are three examples of patient-focused practices:

- Focus on one patient each day whom you observe as you walk into work and remind yourself that all of your efforts today will help someone like that person or his or her family to get better.

- Recognize that patient care is everyone's job and that all of your daily efforts are directed toward helping that patient and his or her family.

- Any time is a good time to provide a suggestion that helps the patient receive quality care efficiently and effectively, provided that the suggestion is pertinent, practical, progressive, proactive, and patient focused.

These three practices must be articulated and demonstrated throughout the facility and emphasized during all organizational development efforts. At many organizations these precepts have been attached to the back of employee ID badges and printed on posters placed in employee lunch areas and other zones exclusive to staff members. Because most employees find a sense of satisfaction in helping a patient, the focus on patient care cannot only allay fears but also further their sense of satisfaction.

Educational Needs Analysis

Most health care professionals value education as a key component of their work life. Furthermore, as indicated in Chapter Twelve, an ardent effort to conduct a meaningful needs analysis is key to any organizational development initiative, as are efforts in employee education. However, in many instances the education and training budget is the first casualty of financial stress and reimbursement shortfalls. This is ironic given that in times of change, apprehension, and fear education is more necessary than ever for ensuring that individuals are performing as effectively as possible.

In addition to offering educational change management sessions, the health care facility must ensure that basic employee education will not be sacrificed during times of change and chaos. In fact, the organizational development process is a perfect opportunity for the organization to recommit itself to employee education and development. The best way to demonstrate this new commitment is by conducting a training and educational needs analysis.

This analysis uses a simple questionnaire to determine current educational needs and to indicate opportunities for employee development. The needs analysis could also include a section in which individuals are asked to identify subject areas and areas of expertise in which they feel qualified and comfortable to act as instructors or mentors. The data collected from both parts of this needs analysis—the education staff members require and the education that they themselves can provide—should then form the basis for a cohesive training and development program.

Personal Development Plans

After the completion of job component reviews, the organization's managers, with the assistance of human resources professions, can construct personal development plans, which enhance a sense of job satisfaction throughout the organization. These plans highlight each staff member's technical strengths, development needs, promotability, and long-term potential. Personal development plans can be dedicated schematic charts in their own right or can be a simple supplement on organizational charts indicating individual promotability, potential, and performance.

Going beyond promotional opportunities, when determining the specific needs of each employee a basic development strategy should be formulated by all line managers with the consultative assistance of human resources professionals, especially experts in employee education. This discourse should result in a clear development plan for each member of the organization. Implementing a personal development plan not only increases work satisfaction but also inspires and motivates employees in regard to future opportunities in the organization.

Succession Planning

A natural outgrowth from and result of creating enlightened personal development plans is the formulation of a succession plan. Succession planning helps an organization develop "bench strength" with an identified second tier of executive and management talent that will be targeted for growth and development. The identification of backups for all critical positions means that the organization does not have to waste unnecessary resources recruiting management talent or specialists from outside of the organization because it is "growing its own" systematically and purposefully.

Ambassador Programs

Each staff member is in essence an ambassador to the community. As health care organizations undergo rapid change, it is vital that community members do not lose trust in the institution or feel that it is either "too good" or "too bad" for them; community members must consider the organization to be a staple of community life. As health care customer-patients become more aware of health care needs and the quality of health care in their community, ambassador programs become even more important. On the one hand, as an organization begins to specialize consumers with more typical needs might feel that the organization is now "too good" to address them, as was the case with a major university medical center in New England. This organization was able to achieve a number of noteworthy designations as well as establish several cutting-edge programs, but unfortunately it began to develop a reputation for being unable to handle the more pedestrian concerns of its local community. On the other hand, if the institution undergoes a negative change, such as massive downsizing, consumers might feel that it is too poorly equipped to handle their pressing concerns.

As ambassadors to the community at such settings as health care fairs at local schools, employees can present information about health careers as well as the current focus of their employing organization. In more informal settings individuals can "talk up" their health care facility if they are prepared and properly educated concerning the facility's current capacities and capabilities. Moreover, staff members must understand that they are also ambassadors to the community in their everyday actions. This can be underscored during various organizational development training sessions by human resources and education professionals implementing the programs suggested throughout this chapter, and by using employee-generated data when forming strategic plans and other patient-focused initiatives.

Fact Sheets

Fact sheets are simple, one-page communication missives that briefly highlight the institution's accomplishments, its basic capacity for providing health care services, and its unique features. Fact sheets can present information about specialized services as well as more traditional health care offerings, such as maternity and emergency room services, and should reaffirm continuing community commitment. As illustrated in Figure 13.4, fact sheets are easy to construct, and they can be a useful tool in an ambassador program. These documents should be written with employee input and feedback, and indeed can enhance employee satisfaction if each department at every level has the opportunity to construct a fact sheet detailing that department's specific services and capabilities. These fact sheets can be given to all incoming patients and should be distributed to employees on a regular basis as part of an ongoing organizational development effort. Updating fact sheets as well is including interesting "factoids" about the organization are integral parts of this strategy.

Figure 13.4   Huntington VA Medical Center (VAMC) Fact Sheet

- The Huntington VAMC has been serving the area's veteran community since 1920.
- We are affiliated with nearly twenty academic institutions as a teaching medical center.
- Research conducted at the Huntington VAMC contributed to the development of the Cochlear Implant Program.
- We are also the primary care providers for six counties in Kentucky.
- We opened one of the first two centers dedicated to women veteran services this year.

Redefinition Strategies

Undertaking redefinition strategies based on new job components can be useful in organizational development. For example, if the laboratory and radiology components are combined in an organizational development effort, the resulting Department of Diagnostic Services will have streamlined job positions as well as perhaps a new rank structure. Supplemented by an accurate fact sheet, redefinition efforts increase work satisfaction in several ways, not only among department members but also, sometimes, across the entire institution.

First, many health care professionals think they do not receive enough recognition and credit for what they do. Accordingly, if a job component review is conducted and a position is redefined accurately, the staff member will immediately see the benefit of organizational development. In another sense, if the entire department feels it is not getting enough credit for its efforts, a similar redefinition—perhaps with a new title for the department that is more reflective, resonant, and relevant can again demonstrate the immediate positive impact of organizational development as well as the marketing strength of the particular cadre. It is essential to note that redefinition is not the same as renaming or imposing a new title arbitrarily; redefinition involves an actual review of new position components and a redefining of the entire scope of services provided.

General Employee Education

General employee education that deals with tactical issues can also be a contributor to organizational success and individual satisfaction.

Employee education can be broadened to provide staff with the expertise needed for working in the competitive health care business arena. Possible topics for such employee educational sessions include

- Customer service strategies

- Negotiation skills

- Conflict resolution

- Interpersonal support systems

- Communication skills

- Professional etiquette
- Time management
- Stress management
- Customer-patient relations

Management Education

As discussed in Chapter Twelve concerning training and development, management education also contributes to the satisfaction of employees and does not have to be confined to organizational development efforts, change management, or specific technical applications. Many health care organizations have found that educating managers in the following topics is an integral part of the organizational development process:

- Selection and hiring skills
- Performance evaluation
- Motivating employees
- Managing resistance to change
- Resolving nonplayer performance issues
- Managing conflict among employees
- Managed-care strategies
- Increasing pride and trust among staff members
- Anything indicated as a topic of general interest to managers, such as time management, e-mail management, technology management, and stress management

As is the case with employee education, management education can be provided by a capable in-house human resources development expert or by external experts. It either case the education must be practical, relevant, and timely. The trainings session should ideally be short and act in concert with overall progressive organizational development objectives.

SUMMARY

Organizational development not only can act as a foundation for efficacious human resources support to a progressive health care organization but also has the potential to enhance the organization's overall community relations and business growth initiatives. Designed to maximize the contribution and morale of employees by optimizing the organization's overall performance, health care organizational development programs possess a vibrant and critical charter and offer health care human resources professionals opportunities to undertake exciting and rewarding work.

KEY TERMS

board of directors

Change Readiness Inventory

credo

health care organizational
  development

Stevens Healthcare Educational
Partnership

DISCUSSION QUESTIONS

1. Why is organizational development such a critical component of health care human resources management?

2. The value of organizational development is often overlooked in a fast-paced health care organization experiencing considerable change. How would you advocate its importance to a CEO of such an organization?

3. In addition to the strategies delineated in this chapter, what other strategies and organizational initiatives do you think should be part of an effective organizational development program?

4. Considering the content of Table 13.1, compose a thematic overview for an organizational development program for a health care organization of your selection.

5. Revisit the credo statement that you prepared in the discussion questions section of Chapter Five; revise it based on the new learning in this chapter, with an emphasis on organizational development.

6. For a health care organization of your selection, create a fact sheet similar to that of the Huntington VA Medical Center shown in Figure 13.4.

Labor-Management Relations

Collective Bargaining and Progressive Employer Relations

LEARNING OBJECTIVES

- Understand the elements of labor-management relations and collective bargaining and their importance to strategic human resources management in health care

- Describe what a union is and why employees join unions

- Differentiate between collective bargaining rights for federal employees, state and local employees, and nonprofit employees

- Understand the current trends and issues in health care labor-management relations

THERE WAS A time when employees were considered to be the property of their employers. Workers had few rights and little say over their working conditions, wages, or benefits. Labor unions played an important role in fighting for minimum wages, safe working conditions, health insurance, sick leave pay, vacation pay, employer-provided job training and career development opportunities, and retirement pensions. Many of the rights and benefits that health care employees receive today exist because of the voices and activities of union members.

Health care organizations can be found in the private for-profit and nonprofit sectors, as well as under the auspices of federal, state, and local governments. This chapter discusses the collective bargaining laws that govern private, public, and nonprofit health care organizations. Collective bargaining is the process through which a labor union and employer negotiate the scope of the employment relationship.

COLLECTIVE BARGAINING IN THE PRIVATE SECTOR

Private sector labor-management relations were initially governed by the **National Labor Relations Act (NLRA) of 1935.** The NLRA permitted employees to organize and join unions for the purposes of **collective bargaining.** It addressed the rights of employees in the areas of union security agreements, picketing, and striking. Employer unfair labor practices were defined, as were the criteria for an appropriate bargaining unit, the selection of a bargaining representative, and the enforcement of the act. Under this law, employers were required to bargain in good faith with employee unions and could be cited for unfair labor practices if they attempted to interfere with the establishment of such unions. The NLRA established the **National Labor Relations Board (NLRB)** as the administrative agency responsible for enforcing the provisions of the act.

In 1947 Congress amended the NLRA with the passage of the **Labor-Management Relations Act (LMRA),** also known as the Taft-Hartley Act, which articulated union unfair labor practices. In 1959 Congress passed the Labor-Management Reporting and Disclosure Act, also known as the Landrum-Griffin amendments, which established a bill of rights for union members, specifying internal union election procedures and financial reporting disclosure requirements for unions and union officers. It also added restrictions on picketing, prohibited "hot cargo" clauses, and closed certain loopholes in the LMRA. (Hot cargo agreements are contract provisions in which the employer promises not to handle products that the union finds objectionable due to having been produced by nonunion labor or at a plant on strike.) These three acts have been consolidated and are now referred to as the Labor-Management Relations Act, 1947, as amended. Federal and state government agencies are excluded from coverage by the act. Nonprofits became covered in the 1970s.

The NLRB can direct elections and certify results only in the case of employers whose operations affect commerce. The LMRA applies to any employer or union unfair labor practices affecting commerce. The statute therefore has a broad scope, and because the courts have broadly interpreted what "affecting commerce" includes, the NLRB could theoretically exercise its powers to enforce the act for most employers (Feldacker, 1990). However, the board has chosen not to act in all cases. In 1950 it decided to distinguish between businesses in which any dispute would interrupt the flow of interstate commerce and those that are so small that a dispute would probably have no impact on the flow of commerce. It set monetary cutoff points, or standards, that limit the exercise of its power to cases involving employers whose effect on commerce is substantial. The board's requirements for exercising its power or jurisdiction are called **jurisdictional standards** or jurisdictional yardsticks. These standards are based on the yearly amount of business done by the employer or the yearly amount of its sales or purchases. The standards are stated in terms of total volume of business and are different for different kinds of enterprises (Feldacker; National Labor Relations Board, 1997). Table 14.1 presents the board's current jurisdictional standards for social services and health care organizations.

COLLECTIVE BARGAINING IN HEALTH CARE ORGANIZATIONS

Originally the NLRB excluded nonprofit employers from NLRA coverage. In the 1970s, however, the board asserted jurisdiction over nonprofits that had a "massive impact on interstate commerce" or those that met certain financial criteria, such as nursing homes with revenue over $100,000, visiting nurses associations, and similar facilities as applied to profit-making nursing homes (Drexel Homes, 1970).

In August 1974 Congress amended the LMRA to bring nonprofit health care institutions under the law's coverage (commonly referred to as the

---

Table 14.1   **National Labor Relations Board Jurisdictional Standards for Nonprofit Health Care Organizations (in Effect July 1990)**

Organization	*Standard*
Employers that provide social services	$250,000 gross annual revenue
Privately operated health care institutions; defined as hospitals, health maintenance organizations, health clinics, nursing homes, extended care facilities, or other institutions devoted to the care of the sick, infirm, or aged	$250,000 total annual volume of business
Nursing homes, visiting nurses associations, and related facilities	$100,000 total annual volume of business; regarded as a single employer in that annual business of all association members is totaled to determine whether any of the standards apply

Source: Adapted from National Labor Relations Board, 1997, pp. 54–55.

---

health care amendments). At that time Congress added Section 2(14), which defines health care institutions as including hospitals, nursing homes, and other health care facilities regardless of whether they are operated for profit. The health care amendments indicated that Congress had no objection to bringing nonprofit employers under federal labor law. Now, under 29 U.S.C. Section 152(14), the term *health care institution* includes any hospital, convalescent hospital, health maintenance organization, health clinic, nursing home, extended care facility, or other institution devoted to the care of sick, infirm, or aged persons.

The 1974 health care amendments also limited strikes in health care organizations. Two years later in 1976 the NLRB began to treat nonprofit and charitable institutions the same way it treated businesses operated for profit. If a nonprofit employer was sufficiently involved in the interstate flow of money or goods that a labor dispute might disrupt that flow of commerce, the board would take jurisdiction. The board established a jurisdictional standard of $250,000 annual revenue for all social services agencies other than those for which there is another specific standard according to the type of activity in which the organization is engaged. For example, the specific $100,000 standard still applies for a nursing home (Feldacker, 1990).

The NLRB asserts jurisdiction over nonprofit organizations that provide services to or for an exempt government agency, such as Head Start programs, child care services, and medical clinics supported by state or federal funds (Feldacker, 1990). Some of these agencies have argued that they are excluded by the NLRA according to the exemption for government agencies. The board holds that such agencies are covered by the act, even though they are government funded, if they retain independence in labor-management matters, such as by establishing the wages, hours, and working conditions of their employees. The sole standard for taking jurisdiction is whether the contractor has "sufficient control over the employment conditions of its employees to enable it to bargain with a labor organization as its representative." The board looks closely at the nature of the relationship between the government institution and the contractor.

An interesting issue of jurisdiction surfaced in *National Labor Relations Board v. Catholic Bishop of Chicago* (1979). The Supreme Court held that the NLRB cannot assert jurisdiction over church-operated schools because such jurisdiction would violate the First Amendment establishment of freedom of religion and the separation of church and state. The court held that the religious and secular purposes of church-sponsored schools are so intertwined that the board's jurisdiction would unconstitutionally introduce the board into the operations and policies of the church.

The board does, however, assert jurisdiction over church-operated non-profit social agencies, such as nursing homes, hospitals, and child care centers, because they function in essentially the same way as do their secular counterparts: they receive government financial support, they are regulated by the state along with other nonprofit social agencies, and their activities only tangentially relate to the sponsoring organization's religious mission (Feldacker, 1990).

COLLECTIVE BARGAINING IN FEDERAL GOVERNMENT AGENCIES

The **Civil Service Reform Act (CSRA) of 1978** governs labor relations in the federal sector. It covers most employees of the executive agencies of the United States, including the Library of Congress and the Government Printing Office. However, employees working for a number of federal agencies are excluded from coverage. Title VII of the CSRA enacted the provision known as the Federal Service Labor-Management Relations Statute (LMRS), which created the Federal Labor Relations Authority (FLRA) to administer and enforce the CSRA. The FLRA is governed by three bipartisan members who are appointed by the president with the advice and consent of the Senate. The members are appointed for staggered five-year terms.

Dissatisfied parties may appeal rulings made by the FLRA to the U.S. Court of Appeals. The authority of the FLRA is similar to that of the NLRB. It determines appropriate bargaining units, supervises and conducts union elections, conducts hearings and resolves allegations of unfair labor practices, prescribes criteria for and resolves issues relating to determining a compelling need for agency rules or regulations, resolves exceptions to arbitrators' awards, and takes such other actions as are necessary and appropriate to administer the provisions of Title VII of the CSRA.

Federal employees may not bargain over wages and benefits or prohibited political activities. The scope of negotiable issues is more restrictive for federal employees than for employees at other levels of government, at nonprofits, and in the private sector. For example, federal employees may not strike.

In 1991 Congress amended Title 38 to allow Department of Veterans Affairs physicians, nurses, and other medical professionals to engage in collective bargaining because they were not covered by the statute that authorizes bargaining for most federal employees. Under Title 38, employees can negotiate, file grievances, and arbitrate disputes over working conditions, except for matters concerning or arising out of professional conduct or competence, peer review, or compensation. The U.S. Senate and the U.S. House of Representatives have proposed a bill to eliminate these collective bargaining exceptions. The bill has been referred to the respective committees in each chamber, but no further action has been taken at the time of this writing.

COLLECTIVE BARGAINING IN STATE AND LOCAL GOVERNMENT AGENCIES

Many states have passed legislation that grants state and local government employees the right to participate in collective bargaining with their employers. Other states permit public employees only the right to "meet and confer" with a public employer. Still other states lack statutes that permit or recognize the right of public employees to join unions or bargain with public employers. The duty to meet and confer provides unions with the right to discuss with the public employer their proposals establishing the terms and conditions of employment. However, employers are free to ignore the views of the unions and make unilateral decisions as to the terms and conditions of employment.

It is important to note that at this time the collective bargaining rights of public employees are under attack by some governors. In some states the collective bargaining rights of public employees have been revoked; in other states there are proposed restrictions on the topics that can be negotiated, such as wages, benefits, retirement benefits, working conditions, and whether union dues are to be deducted from the employees' paychecks by the employer. What ultimately results could have a profound impact on the labor-management relations of public health care organizations.

Many state statutes are referred to as comprehensive statutes. These statutes are modeled after the Labor-Management Relations Act, 1947, as amended. Like the LMRS they guarantee public employees the right to join or form labor unions or refrain from joining unions. They also establish procedures for the selection of employee representatives, define the scope of bargaining and unfair labor practices, address union security provisions, permit or prohibit strikes, prescribe remedies to resolve contract negotiation impasses, provide mechanisms for resolving contract grievances, and establish an administrative agency to oversee the law. These statutes are referred to as public employee relations acts (PERAs).

CONCEPTS AND PRACTICES OF COLLECTIVE BARGAINING

This section provides explanations of the issues introduced in the preceding overview, along with specific examples to illustrate the concepts of collective bargaining as they are applied in the federal, state, and local governments and in the private sector. For purposes of this discussion, all of the labor-management collective bargaining acts—private or nonprofit (the LMRA), federal (the LMRS), and state (PERAs)—will be referred to generically as labor-management relations acts.

Labor-management relations acts designate or create agencies to provide oversight of the acts and to administer relations among employers, employees, and unions. The NLRB governs private for-profit and nonprofit labor relations, and the FLRA provides oversight on behalf of the federal government. Although the names of these administrative agencies tend to vary across the states (New Jersey's version is the Public Employment Relations Commission, the Illinois version is known as the Illinois State Labor Relations Board, and Florida calls its board the Public Employee Relations Commission), they are often referred to as public employee relations boards.

Unit Determination

The labor-management relations acts generally define the procedures for designating the employees' representative or union. Before a union can represent a group of employees, the constituency of the group must be established in the process of **unit determination.** The group of employees that can potentially be represented by one representative at the bargaining table is called the **appropriate bargaining unit**. The acts contain guidelines and procedures for the determination of the appropriate bargaining unit.

The labor-management relations acts exclude some general categories of employees from a bargaining unit. For example, managerial and confidential employees are excluded as a matter of policy because their interests are more closely aligned with management than with the bargaining unit. Managerial employees are employed by an agency in positions that require or authorize them to formulate, determine, or influence the policies of the agency. Confidential employees are those who assist the individuals who formulate, determine, or execute labor policies. Included in this category are employees who have access to information about labor relations or who participate in deliberations of a labor relations nature and are required to keep that information confidential from the labor organization representing a bargaining unit.

Professional and technical employees, and in some cases supervisors, may also be excluded from an overall bargaining unit, but they are still entitled to representation as their own respective units. A supervisor is an individual who has the authority to, in the interests of the agency, hire, direct, assign, promote, reward, transfer, furlough, lay off, recall, suspend, discipline, or remove employees and to adjust their grievances or recommend such action. However, there is an exception in the case of nurses as supervisors. On October 3, 2006, the NLRB ruled that nurses with full-time responsibility for assigning fellow hospital workers to particular tasks are supervisors under federal labor law and thus not eligible to be represented by unions. In the *Oakwood Healthcare, Inc. and International Union United Automobile, Aerospace and Agricultural Implement Workers of America (UAW), AFL-CIO* (2006) decision, the board changed course and now interprets Section 2(11) in a way that makes it easier for health care employers to argue that charge nurses are statutory supervisors who should not be included in a bargaining unit of registered nurses. The *Oakwood* decision focused primarily on three of the Section 2(11) factors: assign, responsibly direct, and exercise independent judgment. This decision may have broad applications to supervisory employees in all private industries that fall under the Labor-Management Relations Act, 1947, as amended.

Professional employees perform work of a predominantly intellectual, nonstandardized nature. The work must require the use of discretion and independent judgment as well as knowledge that is customarily acquired through college or university attendance. Technical employees perform work of a technical nature that requires the use of independent discretion and special training. They may have acquired their expertise in college, in technical schools, or through on-the-job training.

Bargaining units for acute care hospitals are regulated under the Code of Federal Regulations. 29 C.F.R. Section 103.30, appropriated bargaining units in the health care industry, permits eight units:

1. All registered nurses

2. All physicians

3. All professionals except for registered nurses and physicians

4. All technical employees

5. All skilled maintenance employees

6. All business office clerical employees

7. All guards

8. All nonprofessional employees except for technical employees, skilled maintenance employees, business office clerical employees, and guards.

The NLRB has the discretion to determine appropriate units in other health care facilities and, under extraordinary circumstances, to do so by adjudication.

Selection of a Bargaining Representative

The labor-management relations acts also contain specific procedures for selecting an exclusive **bargaining representative. Exclusive recognition** is the term applied when one union has the right and responsibility to speak on behalf of all employees in the bargaining unit. Voluntary recognition by the employer is the easiest way of designating a union. It is available only if the union can demonstrate support by a majority of employees in the unit, usually achieved by having employees sign recognition cards authorizing the union to represent them in collective bargaining.

If voluntary recognition is not achieved or is challenged by a claim of majority representation by another representative organization, a secret ballot election may be held to select the exclusive bargaining representative. The administrative agencies have the authority to regulate these representation elections, which are also subject to judicial review. Some states insist that a secret ballot election be held to determine employee representation. A union that has been voluntarily recognized by the employer as the exclusive representative possesses the same rights as a union that has been certified through a formal certification election.

The procedures for a certification election are similar across the for-profit, nonprofit, federal, and state sectors. The union must request that employees in the proposed unit sign recognition cards authorizing the union to represent them. The union must obtain a "show of interest" by the unit members, which is not less than 30 percent for nonprofits, the federal government, and the majority of states. However, if the employer chooses not to voluntarily recognize a union, an election will be held. If the union receives 51 percent of the votes, it will be recognized as the exclusive representative.

Union Security

Labor-management relations acts contain provisions for union security devices that address the degree to which unions can compel union membership or mandate the payment of dues to support their activities. Most contracts contain some kind of union security provision, and union security provisions are articulated in each state's public employee relations act. Federal employees are free not to join unions. The different types of union security provisions are explained in the following paragraphs.

Closed Shop

Under a **closed shop** agreement, an employer was not permitted to hire anyone who was not already a member of the union. Closed shop arrangements became illegal in the private sector under Section 8(a)(3) of the Labor-Management Relations Act, 1947, as amended. These arrangements have always been prohibited in the public sector because they infringe on the employer's prerogative in determining employment standards, as well as restrict the selection of new employees.

Union Shop

Under a **union shop** provision, all unit employees are required to join the exclusive bargaining representative after being hired. An employer operating under this agreement may hire employees who are not members of the union. However, the nonunion employees must join the union within the period specified in the agreement, which is usually thirty days, and must remain members of the union as a condition of continued employment. Compulsory membership by a certain date after employment prevents free riders: employees who are not union members but benefit from union negotiations without paying their share of the union's operating expenses. Free riders are a particular problem in the federal government, where union shops are prohibited.

Agency Shop

Under an **agency shop** agreement, all unit employees, whether or not they are union members, are required to pay a service fee to the exclusive bargaining representative. The service fee is designed to make nonmembers pay their share of the expense of representing all of the unit employees.

Fair Share

The **fair share** provision resembles the agency shop provision in that employees must pay a proportion of regular union dues to cover the exclusive representative's costs for collective bargaining. However, unlike agency shops, nonbargaining activities are not funded by nonunion members.

Maintenance of Membership

Under **maintenance of membership** provisions, employees are not required to become union members. However, those who join a union must remain members and pay membership dues to the union until the contract expires.

Dues Checkoff

Because unions depend on the fees collected from employees for their support, they must have a reliable and continuous system for collecting membership dues. A **dues checkoff** mechanism permits unions to collect fees from employers, who withhold the union dues from the employees' paychecks and forward the funds to the union. This is a more efficient process than collecting fees from individual members. Dues checkoff is typically combined with one of the other union security provisions.

Right-to-Work States

The following states are known as **right-to-work states:** Alabama, Arizona, Arkansas, Florida, Georgia, Idaho, Iowa, Kansas, Louisiana, Mississippi, Nebraska, North and South Carolina, North and South Dakota, Tennessee, Texas, Utah, Virginia, and Wyoming. According to right-to-work laws, individuals cannot be forced to join or pay dues to a labor union. Furthermore, no worker need be a union member to acquire or retain employment. In the private sectors, Section 14(b) of the LMRA permits states to outlaw various forms of union security provisions:

> Nothing in this Act shall be construed as authorizing the execution or application of agreements requiring membership in a labor organization as a condition of employment in any State or Territory in which such execution or application is prohibited by State or Territorial law.

This provision means that an employer can reject a union's demand for the recognition of union security arrangements that are illegal under state law.

Unfair Labor Practices

Labor-management relations acts enumerate specific unfair labor practices that may be committed by the employer, the union, or both. Unfair labor practices are actions by either the employer or the union that interfere with employees' ability to exercise their statutory rights. The administrative agencies generally have exclusive jurisdiction to hear unfair labor practice suits filed by an employee, the employer, or the union, which is subject to limited judicial review.

Provisions to address unfair labor practices are intended to protect the rights of employees, unions, and employers by prohibiting discrimination, interference, and coercion by both employers and unions. For unions, unlawful activities would constitute interference with the employer's management duties and rights. Charges of employer discrimination, interference, and coercion often pertain to the rights of employees to engage in union activity and the rights of unions to represent their members.

The Scope of Collective Bargaining

The scope of collective bargaining constitutes which subjects are negotiable. Specific topics have generally been classified on a case-by-case basis into three types: mandatory, permissive, and illegal or prohibited.

Mandatory Topics

Mandatory topics of bargaining are issues that the laws (whether private, nonprofit, federal, or state) require management and labor to bargain over. Either side can bargain to an impasse on a mandatory topic if the parties can demonstrate that they made a good-faith effort to reach agreement on it. Mandatory topics in both the nonprofit and for-profit sectors typically include wages, salaries, fringe benefits, and working conditions. Mandatory topics for federal employers and employees are restricted to conditions of employment that affect working conditions, including personnel policies, practices, and other matters, whether established by rule, by regulation, or otherwise. Federal employees may not bargain over wages or fringe benefits.

The statutes that permit collective bargaining by public employees vary in what they consider to be mandatory topics of bargaining.

Permissive Topics

Permissive topics are matters related to optional policy issues that may be bargained over if there is mutual agreement between labor and management. Neither management nor labor may unilaterally insist on such bargaining, and neither has to bargain over permissive topics. In many states permissive topics of bargaining include insurance benefits, retirement benefits, productivity bargaining, and grievance and discipline procedures. Permissive topics in the federal sector include, at the election of the agency, work projects, tours of duty, or the technology, methods, and means of performing work. Education benefits could be considered a permissive topic. Because these benefits are not wages, hours, or working conditions, they would not be considered mandatory topics, but the employer and union could elect to negotiate them.

Deciding whether an issue is mandatory or permissive has generally been accomplished on a case-by-case basis. Administrative agencies and the courts have devised varying and flexible tests rather than establishing fixed rules. The decision is difficult because many issues affect the terms and conditions of both employment and management policymaking. Examples of this dilemma surface frequently in teaching and social work. Teachers want to negotiate such issues as class size, curriculum, teaching loads, and nonteaching duties and responsibilities. Social workers want to bargain over caseload, treatment alternatives, or the process of deciding what services are appropriate for clients. These issues address working conditions, but they are also dimensions of management policy.

Illegal or Prohibited Topics

Illegal or prohibited topics cannot be bargained, and any agreement to bargain with respect to illegal topics will be void and unenforceable. Instead, illegal topics typically must be resolved through the legislative process. Examples of illegal or prohibited topics of bargaining at the federal and state levels are the negotiation of the organization's objectives, how the objectives should be implemented, the agency's organizational structure, and employment standards. Issues concerning retirement, job qualifications, selection, placement, promotion criteria, and the functions of the organization's civil service commission or merit system are often excluded from bargaining in the public sector. Some states, such as Iowa, specifically exclude the public retirement system from the scope of mandatory bargaining. Other states exclude the merit system. Illegal topics for private organizations could include a closed shop union security provision or contract terms in violation of state or federal laws. For example, contract clauses that permit unions to discriminate against persons of color or against members of certain religious groups would be illegal because they violate Title VII of the Civil Rights Act of 1964 and many state fair employment practice acts.

Management Rights

The missions of public sector organizations are decided by legislative bodies. The managers responsible for the performance of these functions are accountable to those legislative bodies and ultimately to the people. Major decisions made in bargaining with public employees are inescapably political because they involve critical policy choices. The matters debated at the bargaining table are not simply questions of wages, hours, and vacations. Directly at issue are questions of the size and allocation of the budget, tax rates, the level of public services, and the long-term obligation of the government. These decisions are political in the sense that they are to be made by elected officials who are politically responsible to the voters. They are generally considered legislative decisions and not subject to delegation to nonelected persons (Edwards, Clark, & Craver, 1979). Therefore, public sector employers tend to have more discretion than private employers in exercising their management rights.

Impasse Resolution

When management and labor are unable to agree to contract terms, an impasse occurs. Third-party intervention often becomes necessary to help resolve their differences. Three procedures are commonly used to resolve impasses: mediation, fact finding, and interest arbitration.

Mediation

When a bargaining impasse occurs, either one or both of the parties may request **mediation:** the introduction of a neutral third party into the negotiation process to assist the bargaining parties in resolving their differences. Mediators often meet with the parties individually at first to discover the conflict. They then encourage the parties to resume bargaining. Mediators may suggest compromise positions that bridge the gap in negotiations, or they may act as intermediaries to persuade the parties that their proposals are unrealistic. Mediators assume only an advisory role. They have no power to compel the settlement of disputes. Mediation findings are not binding unless approved by both parties in the dispute.

Fact Finding

Fact finding involves holding an adversarial hearing at which each side presents its position on the issues in dispute. The fact-finding body studies the evidence presented at the hearing and then makes recommendations for a final settlement.

The fact finder's recommendations are not binding on the parties. However, these recommendations are often made public, and the threat of unfavorable publicity can make both sides more willing to reach a negotiated settlement. Fact finding is grounded in the belief that public opinion will encourage the parties to accept the fact finder's report so as not to appear unreasonable.

Interest Arbitration

Interest arbitration is the procedure used when mediation and fact finding have not resolved bargaining impasses. An arbitrator will hold an adversarial hearing and, based on the evidence presented, determine the terms of the final agreement. Arbitration resolves conflicts without the use of a strike. State and local governments typically use arbitration as a substitute for permitting the right to strike. Only statutes may compel the use of arbitration to conciliate contract disputes. The courts lack jurisdiction to compel arbitration in the absence of statutory authority. To discourage routine reliance on arbitration, many statutes impose the cost of arbitration on the parties.

Interest arbitration has been criticized for intruding on the sovereignty of government entities. The third party is unaccountable to the voters or elected officials, yet makes decisions that affect the employer-employee relationship. To avoid this concern, many statutes require that arbitration decisions be approved by a majority of the appropriate legislative body.

Public sector arbitration varies across the states, and there are several forms. Compulsory binding arbitration requires that any dispute not settled during negotiations must end in arbitration. Arbitrators are free to make awards based on the evidence presented. The arbitrator may take any reasonable position and is usually inclined to make a decision that accommodates the positions of both parties to create a realistic and effective agreement.

Final-offer arbitration permits each party to submit proposals, or final offers, to arbitration. There are two types of final-offer arbitration: final offer by issue and final offer by package. In final-offer-by-package arbitration the arbitrator must select either the union's or the employer's final offer on all of the disputed issues. The arbitrator may not modify the proposals or compromise on the two offers. This procedure assumes that each side will make reasonable offers to prevent the arbitrator from selecting the other party's final package. In final-offer-by-issue arbitration the arbitrator selects either side's final offer on an issue-by-issue basis. The arbitrator is free to select the most reasonable position on each issue. The arbitrator's decision may reflect a combination of employer and union offers. Arbitration by issue gives the arbitrator more flexibility in developing an agreement because the award may incorporate proposals from both sides. This method has been criticized for possibly producing compromise awards that eliminate some of the risk by going to arbitration.

An arbitrator's decision tends to be final and is limited to issues within the permissible scope of collective bargaining. The determination of an issue outside the scope of bargaining will be viewed as a decision made beyond the jurisdiction of the arbitrator and will therefore be reversed. All mandatory topics of bargaining are considered to be within the scope of compulsory arbitration. Nonmandatory topics of bargaining generally are not considered to be within the scope of arbitration unless both parties agree to submit the topic. Most arbitration statutes contain specific criteria that arbitrators must consider in making their decisions. In addition to guiding arbitrators, these criteria facilitate judicial review.

Strikes

For-profit and nonprofit employees are permitted to strike; however, most public employees do not have a legally protected right to strike. Federal employees are prohibited from striking, and currently a number of states have laws that permit some public employees to strike; however, there is little consistency across the states in which employees are covered and in the conditions that permit them to strike.

Among states that permit strikes by public employees, a clear delineation is made between employees who are permitted to strike and those prohibited from striking. Most states limit permission to employees who are not responsible for the public's welfare. The state of Alaska, for example, divides its employees into three classes. Employees who are prohibited by law from striking must go to arbitration to resolve a negotiation impasse. Employees prohibited from striking are those whose services may not be lost for even the shortest time; police, fire, and hospital employees are in this class. In the second class are employees who are permitted to strike until there is a threat to public safety and welfare, at which point a court may enjoin the strike and order arbitration. In the final class are all other employees who may strike after a majority vote. Other employees may engage in a strike if there has first been an attempt at mediation with the employer and if a majority of employees in the unit vote by secret ballot to authorize the strike.

In most states that permit public employee strikes, the union and its members must adhere to a set of stipulations before a strike is considered allowable. For example, Hawaii state statutes permit strikes for nonessential employees in a bargaining unit if the unit has no process for binding arbitration. Before these employees may strike, they must comply with impasse procedures, sixty days must be allowed to elapse after the fact-finding board publishes its recommendations, and the unit must give a ten-day notice of intent to strike. Still, the Hawaii Labor Relations Board retains the right to set requirements to avoid danger to public health or safety.

Nurses in public health care facilities in Montana are permitted to strike only if written notice is given thirty days in advance and no other health care facility within a 150-mile radius intends to strike or is engaged in a strike. These limitations to strike permit the public employer to take action to prevent the strike or prepare for the absence of public workers. If the restrictions concerning strikes are not adhered to, public employers have the right to certain disciplinary actions toward the union and the striking employees.

Even where strikes are permitted, many state statutes grant courts the authority to issue injunctions or restraining orders if the strike presents a danger to public health or safety. If a strike is enjoined by the courts, violation of the court order could result in civil contempt penalties for the union and employees.

As noted earlier in this chapter, the 1974 health care amendments limited strikes in health care organizations. The union must give a ten-day notice to the health care facility, and the Federal Mediation and Conciliation Service must be advised of the union's intent to strike.

Grievance Arbitration

Grievance arbitration occurs when labor believes that management has violated the terms of a labor contract and files a grievance. In grievance arbitration a neutral third party is asked to resolve the disagreement that could not be settled by the involved parties. A hearing is held that enables the parties to present evidence and testimony that support their respective positions on the case. After reviewing all of the evidence presented, the arbitrator renders a decision based on the merits of the case. The decision tends to be final and legally binding on both parties.

The scope of an arbitrator's authority is usually negotiated and stated in the collective bargaining agreement. A commonly negotiated clause authorizes the arbitrator to resolve all disputes concerning the application or interpretation of the contract, but it prohibits the arbitrator from adding to or subtracting from the express terms of the agreement in formulating an award.

Grievance arbitration is undertaken as the last resort in settling disputes because it is expensive. Direct costs involve the expenses associated with preparing the case and the arbitrator's fee. Indirect costs involve all the time spent away from work by the grievant, supervisor, union representative, witnesses, and other associated employees. The contract usually specifies which party will be responsible for paying the arbitrator's fee. It is common for labor and management to equally share the cost of an arbitration proceeding. Because sharing the costs makes it less expensive for the union to extend the grievance and appeal process until arbitration, some agreements require that the losing party pay all of the fees associated with arbitration. Holding the losing party responsible for all of the costs should provide the party whose grievance is weak with an incentive to settle at a lower level in the proceedings, and it should encourage the union to screen cases carefully.

Grievance arbitration is expressly authorized by statute for the private sectors. The LMRA requires that all contracts contain a grievance resolution procedure. This requirement is also found in Section 7121 of the Federal Service Labor-Management Relations Statute and in most state statutes.

The *Semi-Annual Labor Activity in Health Care Report,* prepared by the American Society for Healthcare Human Resources Administration and IRI Consultants (2009), found the issues important in health care organizing to include pay, staffing levels, benefits, having input in decisions, job security, leadership interpersonal skills, leadership management practices, the quality of patient care, workload and distribution of work, safety and security, and situational staffing coverage.

The impact of competition and organizational restructuring has become an issue in health care organizations. Contracts have called for employers to notify employees of impending layoffs and offer voluntary leaves of absence to employees before reducing their hours. In other circumstances, unions have been called on to defend professional autonomy and improve working conditions. Collective bargaining has expanded the scope of labor negotiations to include such issues as agency-level policymaking, agency missions, standards of service, and professional judgment. Other negotiated topics have been coverage for malpractice and professional liability insurance, legal representation of workers, workload issues, the provision of in-service training, financial assistance for licensing examinations, and remuneration for enhanced education. Professional employees are joining unions due to changes brought about with privatization and the shift toward managed care, not only in the health care field but also in the provision of social services.

SUMMARY

Union contracts with health care organizations recognize that new issues have emerged that make labor-management understanding and cooperation more important than ever. The uncertainty inherent in numerous workplace changes has shaken the confidence of many employees that their job is secure and their wages will remain competitive. Uncertain economic times, a decrease in health care benefits for many workers, an increase in the temporary workforce, and reduced or lost pensions have contributed to growing insecurity in the labor market. Changes in the labor market coupled with ineffective and sometimes arbitrary and unfair management often lead employees to unionize when they feel threatened.

The future of the labor movement will hinge on its ability to reach out to new constituencies and collectively develop a new agenda for political action. Women, people of color, and new immigrants typically work in the service sector and might benefit by joining a union. The California Nurses Association (CAN), National Nurses Organizing Committee (NNOC), Service Employees International Union (SEIU), and American Federation of State, County and Municipal Employees (AFSCME), among others, have reframed their respective platforms to emphasize such issues as wage stagnation, employment insecurity, and the growing economic inequality between workers and owners. They are talking about corporate responsibility, democracy in the workplace, and worker rights. Other important issues being discussed are universal health care, continuing education and retraining, and making child care available to low-wage earners. Unions have begun to emphasize the need for greater racial, gender, and class equality and for improving the political and economic status of workers and their community. Moving beyond the traditional topics of collective bargaining, such as wages, hours, and working conditions, these new issues focus attention on the need for affordable and safe day care, maternal leave benefits, an increased ability to work flexible hours, eliminating sexual harassment and discrimination in the workplace, and ending the exploitation of immigrant workers.

Unions have sought to expand the scope of bargaining to include such issues as agency-level policymaking, agency missions, standards of service, coverage for malpractice and professional liability insurance, legal representation of workers, workload issues, the provision of in-service training, financial assistance for licensing examinations, and remuneration for enhanced education. New employee benefits, including the introduction of labor-management committees; mental health and substance abuse benefits; child care benefits; employee development plans; incentive awards; counseling for tests; alternative work schedules; safety precautions, such as guidelines covering the use of video display terminals; and tax-sheltered annuities are also finding their way into collective bargaining agreements.

When employees choose to join a union, increased compensation and benefits are not their only reasons. Often there are concerns about effective management and the quality of the workplace climate. For example, market-based health care reforms are having a negative impact on the environment in which registered nurses work. They have been replaced with less qualified and less expensive personnel, such as licensed practical nurses and technicians. Patient-to-staff ratios have also been increased. Many nurses feel that some of the reforms threaten the quality of patient care, and many believe that joining a union will help them gain greater control over patient care. Collective bargaining affords professionals the ability to demand that the standards of their profession be respected and enforced. For registered nurses, the threat of losing control over their environment is a factor in the decision to vote for union representation (www.uannurse.org). Nurses with a negative perception of their work climate are more likely to vote for a union in a representative election than nurses who have a positive perception of the climate (Clark, Clark, Day, & Shea, 2000).

For health care organizations that are not yet unionized, it is important to have a progressive human resources management system in place that respects employees. Examinations, performance appraisals, promotions, and merit pay systems must be administered in an equitable and consistent manner. Jobs must be enriched to eliminate tasks that are routine and boring, and career development opportunities must be provided. Employees must feel that their job is important and that they are contributing to the mission of the agency. Whether or not workers join unions depends on their perceptions of the work environment and their desire to have a say in decisions that affect them or to influence employment conditions. Organizations that provide employees with the opportunity to participate in the decision-making process are less likely to be the targets of unionization.

KEY TERMS

agency shop	fact finding
appropriate bargaining unit	fair share
bargaining representative	illegal or prohibited topics
Civil Service Reform Act (CSRA) of 1978	interest arbitration
	jurisdictional standards
closed shop	Labor-Management Relations Act (LMRA)
collective bargaining	
dues checkoff	labor-management relations acts
exclusive recognition	maintenance of membership

mandatory topics

mediation

National Labor Relations Act
(NLRA) of 1935

National Labor Relations Board
(NLRB)

permissive topics

right-to-work states

union shop

unit determination

DISCUSSION QUESTIONS

1. Define collective bargaining.

2. What did the National Labor Relations Act (NLRA) of 1935 permit?

3. When were health care organizations covered under the NLRA?

4. Define exclusive recognition.

5. Describe the following union security provisions: closed shop, union shop, agency shop, fair share, maintenance of membership, dues checkoff, and right-to-work states.

6. What are mandatory topics? What do mandatory topics typically include?

7. Discuss the three procedures commonly used to resolve impasses: mediation, fact finding, and interest arbitration.

8. When does grievance arbitration occur?

This chapter was adapted and updated from Pynes, 1997, 2004a, 2009a.

15

Strategic Health Care Human Resources Technology

LEARNING OBJECTIVES

- Understand the importance of technology to strategic human resources management

- Discuss what a human resources information system (HRIS) is

- Explain how an HRIS is useful when undertaking HR planning

- Recognize how technology is promoting changes in organizational structures and job design

TECHNOLOGY IS MAKING health care more portable. In a *Wall Street Journal* article titled "Medicine on the Move," Stephanie Simon (2011) writes that Vscan, a portable ultrasound device that is approximately the size of a cell phone, allows cardiologists and their patients to look directly into the heart to check out the muscle, valves, rhythm, and blood flow. Other technology tools allow health care providers to monitor vital signs, note changes in activity levels, and verify that medications have been taken without seeing a patient. The Regenstrief Institute and Wishard Health Services in Indianapolis, Indiana, established the nation's first ambulance-based information system, which allows paramedics and emergency personnel immediate access to the statewide electronic health records (EHRs) of patients. Its purpose is to help the medics provide more effective emergency care by giving them real-time access to a digital record of the patient's preexisting medical conditions, previous treatments, allergies, current medications, and other information. Some ambulances have computer applications on board that can identify whether a patient has been transported before and the reasons for the transport, and supply some medical facts about the patient. These data are provided on the way to the accident or incident scene so that care at the scene can begin immediately. When a medical emergency is reported to 911, the dispatch center automatically picks up a name and location, and then based on this information accesses the relevant EHRs and transmits them to ambulances (Lipowicz, 2009).

When we think of a health care organization, we think of a hierarchical, centralized structure of specialists that typically rely on a fixed set of standard operating procedures. That model is no longer always the case. Many agencies have become flatter and decentralized. These new organizational structures rely on networks of teams and individuals to ensure the effective delivery of services. Advances in information technology have assisted in making this possible. In a knowledge- and information-based economy, information systems technology takes on greater importance. Computers and information technology are being used to design and manage health care programs. Information technology is being used not only to automate routine tasks but also increasingly to restructure and integrate procedures and programs for delivering services.

Information systems optimize the flow of information and knowledge within the organization and help management maximize knowledge resources. Because the productivity of employees will depend on the quality of systems serving them, management decisions about information technology are important determinants of the effectiveness of a health care organization.

INFORMATION SYSTEMS TECHNOLOGY

To understand information systems requires understanding the problems they are designed to solve, their architectural and design elements, and the organizational processes that are needed to accomplish the required tasks.

To be able to use an information system, a manager must understand the organization, management, and technology dimensions of the system and how they can be used to provide information leading to effective solutions. Computer-based information systems rely on computer hardware and software technology to process and disseminate information, although computers are only part of an information system.

Information systems incorporate computer hardware and software, storage, and telecommunication technology. Computer hardware is the physical equipment used for input, processing, and output activities in an information system. The software consists of the detailed, preprogrammed instructions that control and coordinate the computer hardware in an information system. Storage technology includes media for storing data, such as magnetic or optical disc, or tape. Telecommunication technology consists of physical devices and software that link the various pieces of hardware and transfer data from one physical location to another. Computers and communication equipment can be connected in networks for sharing voice, data, images, sound, and video. A network links two or more computers to shared data and resources, such as a printer.

The capabilities of information technology (IT) can help organizations in a variety of ways (Davenport & Short, 1990, p. 17):

- *Transactional capability:* IT can transform unstructured processes into routine transactions.

- *Geographical capability:* IT can transfer information with rapidity and ease across large distances, making processes independent of geography.

- *Automational capability:* IT can replace or reduce human labor in a process.

- *Analytical capability:* IT can bring complex analytical methods to bear on a process.

- *Informational capability:* IT can bring vast amounts of detailed information into a process.

- *Sequential capability:* IT can enable changes in the sequence of tasks in a process, often allowing multiple tasks to be worked on simultaneously.

- *Knowledge management capability:* IT allows the capture and dissemination of knowledge and expertise to improve the process.

- *Tracking capability:* IT allows the detailed tracking of task status, inputs, and outputs.

- *Disintermediation capability:* IT can be used to connect two parties within a process who would otherwise communicate through an intermediary (internal or external).

ORGANIZATIONAL CHANGE

Information technology can promote various degrees of organizational change. The most common change is the automation or mechanization of routine tasks. However, IT can also be used for more sophisticated tasks, such as reengineering and redesigning business processes, whereby business and work processes are analyzed, simplified, and reconstructed. Processes have two important characteristics: they have defined business outcomes, and the outcomes have recipients (the customers). Customers can be internal or external to the organization. Processes can also occur across or between organizational units. Davenport and Short (1990) provide the following examples of processes: investigating and paying an insurance claim, writing a proposal for a contract, creating a marketing plan, developing a new product or service, and ordering goods from a supplier. There are typically five steps in organizational process redesign:

1. Developing a business vision and process objectives to prioritize objectives and set targets

2. Identifying the processes to be redesigned to identify critical or bottleneck processes

3. Understanding and measuring existing processes to identify problems and set baseline performance expectations

4. Identifying IT levers to brainstorm new process approaches

5. Designing and building a prototype of the process to implement organizational and technical aspects

The most likely objectives related to process redesign are reducing costs, reducing the time for tasks to be completed, increasing or improving the quality of output, and empowering individuals and providing them with more control over their output (Davenport & Short, 1990).

Improved work flow management has enabled many agencies to reduce costs and improve customer service at the same time. Information systems can make organizations more efficient, and information technology can be used to redesign and reshape organizations, transforming their structure, scope of operation, reporting and control mechanisms, work practices, work flows, products, and services. Flatter organizations have fewer levels of management; lower-level employees are given greater decision-making authority, and employees may work away from a manager. Information systems make information available to line workers so they can adhere to decisions that managers previously made. Networks of computers have made it possible for employees to work together as a team. E-mail, the Internet, and videoconferencing, among other forms of information technology, allow employees to work from different locations. For example, employees can work remotely from their home or car and can collaborate while miles away from the office or other structures, thus vastly expanding organizational boundaries.

TYPES OF INFORMATION SYSTEMS

There are five main types of information systems, each serving a different organizational level: operational-level systems, knowledge-level systems, expert-based systems, management-level systems, and strategic-level systems.

Operational-Level Systems

Operational-level systems support operational managers by helping keep track of the elementary activities and transactions of the organization, such as the clinical and administrative health care information related to patient encounters (Wager, Lee, & Glaser, 2009). Examples of patient-specific clinical information are patient records, including such items as medication records, progress notes, consultations, physicians' orders, imaging and X-ray results, lab results, and diagnoses codes. Examples of administrative information include such items as consents for procedures, authorizations, scheduling data, admission registration, insurance eligibility, and billing, diagnoses, and procedure codes (Wager, Lee, & Glaser, 2009).

To fight medication errors, hospitals have adopted bar code and scanner technology. Having bar codes on medications and on patients' armbands will automate the routines nurses perform before administering medicine. This is consistent with the movement toward electronic medical networks and the national e-record network (Adams, 2009; "Work Begins," 2009).

The principal purpose of information systems at this level is to answer routine questions and track the flow of transactions through the organization.

Knowledge-Level Systems

Knowledge-level systems support the knowledge and data workers in an organization. The purpose of these systems is to help the organization integrate new knowledge into the agency and control the flow of paperwork. Reporting systems support knowledge-level systems. Generating reports is a basic function of most information systems. For example, demographic data could be used to complete required government forms, or a system for tracking time and attendance data could be used to generate reports on sick time, which different departments could then examine to identify those with high absenteeism. In the case of a health care organization receiving public funds, the hours of services delivered can be reported to receive reimbursement. This would allow for future planning and budgeting.

Expert-Based Systems

Expert-based information is generally collected by experts outside of the health care organization as part of **expert-based systems.** Health care providers and executives use this information for clinical and administrative decision making, and they rely on it to stay abreast of changes in their discipline, to remain professionally competent, and to discover the latest techniques and procedures in their field. Regional and national databases and informational Web sites related to health care management, as well as online and print professional journals, are examples of sources of expert knowledge (Wager, Lee, & Glaser, 2009, pp. 8, 37).

Management-Level Systems

Management-level systems are designed to serve the monitoring, controlling, decision-making, and administrative activities of middle managers. Decision-support systems support management-level systems. They go beyond simply reporting information, typically incorporating rules, formulas, or specialized displays that are designed to help end users make decisions. Scheduling and staffing are areas in which decision support can be useful. A routine question in scheduling is how many people should be scheduled for a given time period or a particular event. If there are changes in workload or seasonal variations due to an increasing or decreasing need for services or attendance at events, it may be helpful to have a model that recommends the number of people in each job category who should be scheduled. Similar questions emerge over the longer term with respect to recruitment and staffing. If middle managers are expecting increasing retirements, what are the knowledge, skills, abilities, and other characteristics (KSAOCs) of people they need to hire, and how many people should they hire? Other human resources management (HRM) topics, such as benefits planning and analysis, are good candidates for receiving decision support.

Strategic-Level Systems

Strategic-level systems help senior managers address strategic issues and long-term trends in both the agency and the external environment. Executive-support systems support strategic-level systems. Whereas traditional decision-support systems are directed at well-defined, narrowly focused problems, executive-support systems bring together data from diverse sources to help senior managers assess broader strategic questions. Strategic human resources management figures into these decisions. When a health care organization considers a merger, for example, labor costs, including pensions and benefits, are usually significant concerns. Having access to timely and accurate information can provide the necessary perspective.

Health care organizations and each department need to be aware of their revenue and expenditures. All organizations have an accounting function that is responsible for maintaining and managing the agency's financial records, receipts, disbursements, and payroll expenditures. An accounting information system enables a manager to keep track of the financial assets and flow of funds. It provides a record of transactions for disbursements, receipts, and other expenditures.

Most health care organizations, regardless of size, also have an accounts receivable system to keep track of money. For example, health care organizations must keep track of the grants they receive from public and private sources, as well as their cash and noncash donations, gifts, and contributions. They need to monitor their fees for services and have a system in place for billing and collections. The information system keeps track of the outstanding bills and can produce a variety of reports. The system supplies information to the general ledger system, which tracks the agency's total cash flow. Senior managers can use the financial reports gleaned from the accounting information system to make immediate and strategic decisions.

HUMAN RESOURCES INFORMATION SYSTEMS

The HRM function is responsible for attracting, developing, and maintaining the agency's workforce. Human resources identifies potential employees, maintains complete records on existing employees, and creates programs to develop employees' talents and skills.

Strategic-level human resources information systems identify the personnel requirements, such as the skills; educational levels; types of positions; number of positions; and costs of recruiting, advertising, benefits, promotions and so on, for meeting the agency's strategic plans. At the management level, a **human resources information system (HRIS)** helps managers monitor and analyze the recruitment, allocation, and compensation of employees. HR knowledge-level systems support analysis activities related to job design, training, and the modeling of employee career paths and reporting relationships. HR operational-level systems track the recruitment and placement of the agency's employees.

Technological advances not only have changed how organizations are structured and work is performed but also have begun to change the tasks of HRM specialists. Computers are used to perform many of the functions for which employees were once responsible.

A typical HRIS for employee record keeping maintains basic data, such as each employee's name, age, sex, marital status, address, educational background, salary, job title, date of hire, and date of termination. The system can produce a variety of reports, such as lists of newly hired employees, terminated employees, employees on a leave of absence, employees classified by job type or educational level, or employees grouped by job performance level. Such systems are typically designed to provide data necessary for federal and state record-keeping requirements.

Compensation and Benefits

At a higher level of the HRIS is the integration of payroll operations with the HRIS and benefits unit in HR. Government regulations and the complexity of benefits in many organizations warrant HRM expertise. Interfacing or integrating payroll and HR systems within the HRIS enhances efficiency because data entry and maintenance tasks are reduced.

When payroll operations are moved to the HRM department, HR specialists, with their benefits and compensation expertise, make certain that benefits plans remain qualified under government regulations; ensure the accuracy of payroll deductions for HR-managed plans; and have the opportunity to answer employees' questions about pay and benefits, in person or through interactive HRIS technology.

When organizations offer flexible benefits plans to employees, the HRIS can be used to communicate information to the employees that can have an impact on the costs associated with benefits and their administration. Employees can obtain information about the benefits available and make changes in their plan by enrolling in a new benefits plan, adding or changing dependents, changing the amount of monthly savings deducted from paychecks, making a cash withdrawal, taking out a loan, or withdrawing from a plan altogether. In some systems these decisions are supported by a simple "what-if?" analysis that shows the employee choices in regard to available plans, pension projections, how much would be saved after five years at a certain rate of deduction, and so on.

Giving employees direct access to benefits plans and the ability to self-enroll in or change benefits plans reduces staffing requirements in the benefits department, eliminates paperwork, and otherwise improves the administration of benefits. New employees who want to know when they are eligible to enroll in a certain plan can find this information without going to the benefits department, a change in dependents covered by health insurance can be made without paperwork, and retirement benefits at different ages can be projected.

Career Planning and Staffing Systems

Employees and employers can use the HRIS to access career planning and staffing systems. At the simplest level electronic bulletin boards list basic job information, and at a more complex level they include online position descriptions; job advertisements when openings arise; résumés of all covered employees; knowledge-based assessment modules; and systematic procedures that link qualified candidates and open positions, providing managers with the backgrounds and résumés of employees and applicants who meet the position requirements.

Career planning and staffing systems that are accessible to employees permit employees' direct involvement in their own career development or movement in the organization. A career development system that is accessible to employees can provide information about positions at the next level; job descriptions; information about steps in career paths leading to certain positions; training and development activities that may be required; and information about trends in workforce movement, surpluses and shortages, and other career-relevant areas. In some systems the employee can select a training class or another development activity or create an entirely new career plan, subject to authorization, which also can be handled electronically. Most career development is essentially self-development and requires personal motivation, commitment, and clear linkages between individual efforts and career results. Extending information through an HRIS gets the employees involved.

Communicating Policies and Procedures

Distributing agency policies and procedures using technology is less expensive than printing hard copies and handing them out to employees. Employees and employers can make changes and communicate them in an expedited manner. Information systems permit automatic communication that provides uniformity and consistency in implementing some policies and procedures yet allows for flexible and audience-specific variations in implementing others. For example, regional pay levels may influence hourly rates, different labor contracts may be in effect in different locations, and paid holidays may vary. However, other policies with respect to nondiscrimination, privacy, and federal legislation, such as the Fair Labor Standards Act, may apply to all employees, requiring record keeping and in some cases overtime pay.

Organizations are using technology to offer quick online access to company policies. By entering the organization's online system, managers and employees can examine company policy with respect to time off, vacations, holiday pay, or infractions leading to discipline. Merit pay guidelines, performance appraisal instructions, training programs, and instructions on how to transfer or hire an individual can also be made available online.

Employee Participation

Employees' access to the HRIS also permits employees to make their views and ideas known to management in a timely, cost-efficient manner. When employee attitudes are important to the organization, the timeliness, accuracy, and identification of different attitudes and perceptions among different types or categories of employees is important. Online employee surveys can eliminate the administration of paper-and-pencil surveys and automatically summarize data and trends, such as changes in attitudes that may deserve prompt management intervention. Linked to the HRIS, an automated attitude survey can produce summaries of employee responses by such groupings as management level, job function, location, or demographic characteristics without requiring manual analysis.

Training and Performance Support

In a complex HRIS, job analysis data, productivity data, skills and competencies information, performance ratings, applicant qualifications, test results, and other types of information relevant to training can be integrated:

- HRIS demographic data can be analyzed to develop audience-specific curricula and training formats that are tailored for different groups.

- Job requirements can be linked to training. This could include competency-based training and assessment.

- The HRIS can provide online training courses or provide links to approved vendor-supplied training courses.

- The HRIS can analyze the relationships among training and performance ratings, turnover, compensation, and other variables to establish cost-benefit data on specific types of training.

- The HRIS can develop new recruitment practices, preemployment tests, and other employment process tools based on analysis of training data and the requirements of positions.

Integrating Work and Technology

Integrating employees and technology can be a complex, multifaceted function. For information systems to work, many factors need to be considered: conducting job and work flow analyses, recruiting and selecting qualified people, and providing training and retraining so that employees are knowledgeable about and comfortable with technology.

The implementation of an HRIS can also lead to the outsourcing of the HRM function. Many small health care organizations lack the organizational capacity to develop and administer HRM programs and find it less expensive to outsource HRM functions than to hire new employees with expertise and invest in technology. However, outsourcing must be done with caution. A vendor hired by the California Department of Health Care Services mailed letters to 49,352 Medi-Cal beneficiaries that included each patient's Social Security number on the address label. The department followed up with notification letters alerting patients to the security breach and instructing them on how to protect themselves from identity theft by contacting credit agencies and putting fraud alerts on the files (McIntosh, 2010).

Electronic Human Resources Management

Electronic human resources management is used to enhance such human resources processes as job analysis, recruitment, selection, training, performance management, and compensation. Data can be collected for job analysis from employees and supervisors using online questionnaires. Data can be summarized and job descriptions can be created. Some of the systems can transfer the data to a job evaluation form and create job evaluation point scores for use in compensation systems. Many agencies now use Web-based portal systems to post job openings and screen résumés. E-recruiting systems can be used to track applicants and provide them with virtual job previews. Some organizations are using e-selection systems to assess job applicants' KSAOCs, manage applicant flow, and evaluate the effectiveness of selection processes. Some agencies use technology to conduct interviews, personality assessments, and background checks online and use computerized testing to examine candidates' cognitive abilities.

E-learning is used for a variety of education and training programs. Web-based systems, CD-ROMs, and audio- or videoconferencing can be used at remote locations. Electronic performance management systems are used to facilitate the writing of performance appraisals. Agencies can also use technology to track unit performance, absenteeism, grievance rates, and turnover levels over time. E-compensation mechanisms are used to help agencies administer compensation, benefits, and payroll systems. Technology can also provide managers with comparable labor market data and with tools to design and model the costs of compensation systems, provide employees with information about benefits as well as self-service systems to select or change benefits, and enable agencies to comply with laws and union contracts.

Strategic Human Resources Management

Human resources information systems applications must go beyond payroll and benefits administration and tracking employee records. They must connect to the strategic objectives of the agency to facilitate more effective recruitment and selection, training and development, communication, manpower planning, and other core HR processes. Managers and workers can use data assembled and gleaned from an HRIS to analyze problems and make informed decisions.

Ashbaugh and Miranda (2002) identify the following strategic applications of HRIS:

- *Align HRIS to organizational performance issues*. Use technology to evaluate organizational performance.

- *Improve core business processes*.

- *Develop a human capital inventory*. Organizations can combine information for education and skills tracking and matching, career planning, succession planning, and performance evaluations.

- *Link position control to budgeting*. By integrating HR with the financial planning process, organizations can develop a compensation management program that includes automated position control to serve as a check that a department will not exceed its salary budget and the ability to develop projections or forecasts based on hours, actual expenditures, or staff totals. They can link HR, benefits, and payroll data to the budget planning process that includes the ability to develop "what-if?" analyses.

- *Facilitate labor-management relations*. To be knowledgeable about the ramifications of decisions made between employers and employees, both unions and management need accurate information for tracking seniority, disciplinary actions, and the number of grievances filed. Data can also be provided for labor negotiations such as pension changes, trend analysis for employee absences and use of sick time, analysis of the costs for overtime, and comprehensive employee benefit costs.

Other strategic applications include having employees update address changes, enroll in training courses, change benefits plans, and disseminate policies. Business intelligence can also be increased by using new technology. Advanced analytical tools, such as online analytical processing, data mining, and executive-support systems, provide insight into trends and patterns and can be used to improve the organization's decision-making capability. In a strategic human resources management context, those tools can be used to support HRM decisions.

SUMMARY

The changing dynamics in technology have brought about changes in the way health care organizations are organized and how services are delivered. Many health care organizations now use technology designed specifically to schedule patients, to code insurance forms, and to keep records for insurance claims and bill collections. Using electronic health records, clinicians, such as doctors, nurses, and physical therapists, can record a patient's medical history, including vital signs and diagnoses. It is not just the direct service providers and clinicians that are using technology, however; human resources information systems have brought about changes in human resources management functions. The new health care law has created a Center for Medicare and Medicaid Innovation to identify, test, and disseminate new ways of delivering and paying for health care (Landro, 2011). As health care organizations confront these challenges, strategic human resources management will become even more important. Innovative strategies will be necessary to assist organizations in preparing for changing missions, priorities, and programs.

KEY TERMS

expert-based systems

human resources information
    system (HRIS)

knowledge-level systems

management-level systems

operational-level systems

strategic-level systems

DISCUSSION QUESTIONS

1. Describe at least six types of information technology capabilities.

2. What are the five steps in organizational process redesign?

3. Briefly discuss the five types of information systems.

4. What factors should be considered in information systems design?

5. How is electronic human resources management used to enhance human resources processes?

This chapter was adapted and updated from Pynes, 2004a, 2009a.

BIBLIOGRAPHY

Accrediting Commission on Education for Health Services Administration. (1997). *Self-study guide for graduate programs in health services administration.* Washington DC: Author.

Adams, J. S. (1965). Inequity in social exchange. In L. R. Berkowitz (Ed.), *Advances in experimental social psychology* (Vol. 2), pp. 267–299. New York: Academic Press.

Adams, R. W. (2009, October 24). Polk hospitals using bar codes to improve safety. *The Ledger,* p. B1.

Affara, F. (2009). *ICN framework of competencies for the nurse specialist.* Geneva, Switzerland: International Council of Nurses.

Agochiya, D. (2002). *Every trainer's handbook.* New Delhi: Sage.

Albert, S. (2000). *Hiring the chief executive: A practical guide to the search and selection process* (Rev. ed.). Washington DC: National Center for Nonprofit Boards.

Alderfer, C. P. (1972). *Existence, relatedness, and growth: Human needs in organizational settings.* New York: Free Press.

American Society for Healthcare Human Resources Administration & IRI Consultants. (2009). *Semi-annual labor activity in health care report.* Detroit, MI: IRI Consultants. www.iriconsultants.com.

Arline v. School Board of Nassau County. (1987). 479 U.S. 8937.

Arvey, R. D., Nutting, S. M., & Landon, T. E. (1992). Validation strategies for physical ability testing in police and fire settings. *Public Personnel Management, 21,* 301–312.

Ashbaugh, S., & Miranda, R. (2002). Technology for human resources management: Seven questions and answers. *Public Personnel Management, 31,* 7–20.

Barr, S. (2008, April 21). Election e-mails can end your term in office. *Washington Post,* p. D01.

Bartram, D. (2005). The great eight competencies: A criterion-centric approach to validation. *Journal of Applied Psychology, 90,* 1185–1203.

Board of Trustees of the University of Alabama v. Garrett. (2001). 531 U.S. 356.

Borman, W. C., & Motowidlo, S. M. (1993). Expanding the criterion domain to include elements of contextual performance. In N. Schmitt & W. C. Borman (Eds.), *Personnel Selection* (pp. 71–98). San Francisco: Jossey-Bass.

Borzo, J. (2004, May 24). Almost human. *Wall Street Journal,* pp. R1, R10.

Bramley, P. (1996). *Evaluating training effectiveness* (2nd ed.). London: McGraw-Hill.

Branti v. Finkel. (1980). 445 U.S. 506.

California Federal Savings & Loan Association v. Guerra. (1987). 479 U.S. 272.

Calvert, C. T. (2010). *Family responsibilities discrimination: Litigation update 2010.* Center for Worklife Law: The University of California Hasting College of the Law. www.worklifelaw.org/pubs/FRDupdate.pdf.

Cascio, W. F. (1991). *Applied psychology in personnel management* (4th ed.). Upper Saddle River, NJ: Prentice Hall.

Cayer, N. J. (2003). Public employee benefits and the changing nature of the workforce. In S. W. Hays & R. C. Kearney (Eds.), *Public personnel administration: Problems and prospects* (4th ed.), pp. 167–179. Upper Saddle River, NJ: Prentice Hall.

Cayer, N. J., & Roach, C.M.L. (2008). Work-life benefits. In C. G. Reddick & J. D. Coggburn (Eds.), *Handbook of employee benefits and administration* (pp. 309–334). Boca Raton, FL: CRC Press.

Champion-Hughes, R. (2001). Totally integrated employee benefits. *Public Personnel Management, 30,* 287–302.

Clark, D., Clark, P., Day, D., & Shea, D. (2000). The relationship between health care reform and nurses' interest in union representation: The role of workplace climate. *Journal of Professional Nursing, 16*(2), 92–97.

Coggburn, J. D. (2007). Outsourcing human resources: The case of the Texas Health and Human Services Commission. *Review of Public Personnel Administration, 27*(4), 315–335.

Coggburn, J. D., & Reddick, C. G. (2007). Public pension management: Issues and trends. *International Journal of Public Administration, 30,* 995–1020.

Collins, S. K., & Collins, K. S. (2007, January-February). Succession planning and leadership development: Critical business strategies for healthcare organizations. *Radiology,* pp. 16–21.

Commerce Clearing House Business Law Editors. (1992). *Workers' compensation manual: For managers and supervisors*. Chicago: Commerce Clearing House.

Connick v. Myers. (1983). 461 U.S. 138.

Cook v. State of Rhode Island, Department of Mental Health, Retardation, and Hospitals. (1993). 10 F.3d 17, 1st Cir.

Corporation of the Bishop of the Church of Jesus Christ of Latter Day Saints v. Amos. (1987). 483 U.S. 327.

Costa, P. T., McCrae, R. R., & Kay, G. G. (1995). Persons, places and personality: Career assessment using the revised NEO Personality Inventory. *Journal of Career Assessment, 3,* 123–139.

Council for Adult and Experiential Learning. 2004. *The promise and practice of employer educational assistance programs: 2004 state of the field strategies and trends.* www.cael.org/PDF/CAEL_Tuition_Survey.pdf.

Daley, D. (1998). An overview of benefits for the public sector: Not on the fringe anymore. *Review of Public Personnel Administration, 19*(3), 5–22.

Daley, D. (2008). Strategic benefits in human resources management. In C. G. Reddick & J. D. Coggburn (Eds.), *Handbook of employee benefits and administration* (pp. 15–27). Boca Raton, FL: CRC Press.

Davenport, T. H., & Short, J. E. (1990, Summer). The new industrial engineering: Information technology and business process redesign. *Sloan Management Review,* pp. 11–27.

DeNavas-Walt, C. C., Proctor, B. D., & Smith, J. C. (2010). *Income, poverty, and health insurance coverage in the United States: 2009* (Current Population Reports P60–238). U.S. Census Bureau. Washington DC: U.S. Government Printing Office.

Dorschner, J. (2010, February 23). Jackson health system to cut 900 jobs. *Miami Herald.* www.miamiherald.com.

Dothard v. Rawlinson. (1977). 433 U.S. 321.

Drexel Homes, Inc. (1970). 182 NLRB, No. 151.

Dubois, C.-A., & Singh, D. (2009). From staff-mix and beyond: Towards a systemic approach to health workforce management. *Human Resources for Health, 7*(89), 1–19.

Durst, S. (1999). Assessing the effect of family friendly programs on public organizations. *Review of Public Personnel Administration, 19*(3), 19–33.

Edwards, H. T., Clark, R. T., Jr., & Craver, C. B. (Eds.). (1979) *Labor relations law in the public sector* (3rd ed.). Riverside, NJ: Bobbs-Merrill.

Elrod v. Burns. (1976). 427 U.S. 347.

Evercare and National Alliance for Caregiving. (2007, November). *Evercare study of family caregivers: What they spend, what they sacrifice: Findings from a national survey.* www.caregiving.org/data/Evercare_NAC _CaregiverCostStudyFINAL20111907.pdf.

Feldacker, B. (1990). *Labor guide to labor law* (3rd ed.). Upper Saddle River, NJ: Prentice Hall.

Feuer, D. (1987). Paying for knowledge. *Training, 24,* 57–66.

Fitz-enz, J. (1996). *How to measure human resources management* (2nd ed.). New York: McGraw-Hill.

Fitz-enz, J. (2000). *The ROI of human performance: Measuring the economic value of employee performance.* New York: AMACOM.

Fitzgerald, W. (1992). Training versus development. *Training and Development Journal, 5,* 81–84.

Flynn, J. P. (2006, May). Designing a practical succession planning program. *PA Times,* 4, 6.

Gael, S. (1988). *The job analysis handbook for business, industry, and government* (Vols. 1–2). Hoboken, NJ: Wiley.

Garcetti v. Ceballos. (2006). 547 U.S. 410.

Garcia v. San Antonio Metropolitan Transit Authority. (1985). 488 U.S. 889.

Garrett, B., Buettgens, M., Doan, L., Headen, I., & Holahan, J. (2010, March). *The cost of failure to enact health reform 2010–2020.* Washington DC: Urban Institute & Robert Wood Johnson Foundation. www.rwjf.org/files/research/57449.pdf.

Garry, P. M. (2007, Fall). Constitutional relevance of the employer-sovereign relationship: Examining the due process rights of government employees in light of the public employee speech doctrine. *St. John's Law Review.* http://findarticles.com/p/articles/mi_qa3735/is_200710/ai_n21100611/print.

Goldberg, L. R. (1999). A broad-bandwidth, public-domain, personality inventory measuring the lower-level facets of several five-factor models. In I. Mervielde, I. Deary, F. De Fruyt, & F. Ostendorf (Eds.), *Personality psychology in Europe* (Vol. 7, pp. 1–28). Tilburg, The Netherlands: Tilburg University Press.

Gossett, C. W., & Ng, E.S.W. (2008). Domestic partnership benefits. In C. G. Reddick & J. D. Coggburn (Eds.), *Handbook of employee benefits and administration* (pp. 379–397). Boca Raton, FL: CRC Press.

Gottfredson, G. D., & Holland, J. L. (1994). *Position Classification Inventory.* Odessa, FL: Psychological Assessment Resources.

Greenberg, J. (1986). Determinants of perceived fairness of performance evaluations. *Journal of Applied Psychology, 71*, 340–342.

Greenberg, J. (1996). *The quest for justice on the job: Essays and experiments.* Thousand Oaks, CA: Sage.

Guion, R. M., & Highhouse, S. (2006). *Essentials of personnel assessment and selection.* New York: Lawrence Erlbaum.

Guion, R. M., Highhouse, S., Reeve, C., & Zickar, M. J. (2005). *The Self-Descriptive Index.* Bowling Green, OH: Sequential Employment Testing.

Gupta, N. (1997). Rewarding skills in the public sector. In H. Risher, C. Fay, & Associates (Eds.). *New strategies for public pay: Rethinking government compensation programs.* San Francisco: Jossey-Bass.

Gupta, N., Jenkins, G. D., Jr., & Curington, W. P. (1986). Paying for knowledge: Myths and realities. *National Productivity Review, 5,* 107–123.

Harshbarger, S., & Crafts, A. (2007). The whistle-blower: Policy challenges for nonprofits. *Nonprofit Quarterly, 14*(4), 36–44.

Healy, B., & Southard, G. D. (April, 1994). *Pay for performance, administrative policy manual, policy no. 30–19.* City of Claremont.

Healey v. Southwood Psychiatric Hospital. (1996). Cal. 3, 70 FEP 439.

Henderson, R. I. (2000). *Compensation management in a knowledge based world* (8th ed.). Upper Saddle River, NJ: Prentice Hall.

Heneman, R. D. (1992). *Merit pay: Linking pay increases to performance ratings.* Reading, MA: Addison-Wesley.

Herzberg, F. (1964, January-February). The motivation-hygiene concept. *Personnel Administration,* pp. 3–7.

Herzberg, F. (1968). One more time: How do you motivate employees? *Harvard Business Review, 46,* 36–44.

Hoff, J. (2006, May 1). My virtual life. *BusinessWeek,* 72–78.

HRO Today 2010 resource guide. (2009, October). *HRO Today, 8*(8), 24–72.

Hudson, D. L., Jr. (2008, January). The Garcetti effect: Government employees fear high court case undermines retaliation protections. *ABA Journal,* pp. 16–17.

Hughes, M. A., Ratliff, R. A., Purswell, J. L., & Hadwiger, J. (1989). A content validation methodology for job related physical performance tests. *Public Personnel Management, 18,* 487–504.

Hyland, S. L. (1990, September). Helping employees with family care. *Monthly Labor Review,* pp. 22–26.

Illinois Department of Central Management Services. (n.d.). Upward mobility program. www.state.il.us/cms/2_servicese_edu/umprgm.htm.

Issenberg, S. B., McGaghie, W. C., Hart, I. R., Mayer, J. W., Felner, J. M., Petrusa, E. R., . . . Ewy, G. A. (1999). Simulation technology for health care professional skills training and assessment. *Journal of the American Medical Association, 282,* 861–866.

Johnson, R. E. (1988). Flexible benefit plans. In John Matzer Jr. (Ed.), *Pay and Benefits: New Ideas for Local Government*. Washington DC: ICMA.

Kaiser Family Foundation. (2010, September). Employer health benefits 2010 annual survey. http://ehbs.kff.org/.

Kaplan, R. S., & Norton, D. (1996). Using the balanced scorecard as a strategic management system. *Harvard Business Review, 70*(1), 71–79.

Kellough, J. E., & Lu, H. (1993). The paradox of merit pay in the public sector. *Review of Public Personnel Administration, 13,* 45–64.

Kellough, J. E., & Nigro, L. G. (2002). Pay for performance in Georgia state government: Employee perspectives on GeorgiaGain after 5 years. *Review of Public Personnel Administration, 22*(2), 146–166.

Khatri, N., Wells, J., McKune, J., & Brewer, M. (2006). Strategic human resource management issues in hospitals: A study of a university and a community hospital. *Hospital Topics, 84*(4), 9–20.

Kimmel v. Florida Board of Regents. (2000). 528 U.S. 62.

Kirkpatrick, D. L. (1994). *Evaluating training programs: The four levels.* San Francisco: Berrett Koehler.

Kirkpatrick, D. L. (1998). *Evaluating training programs: The four levels* (2nd ed.). San Francisco: Berrett-Koehler.

Kolb, D. A. (1984). *Experiential learning: Experience as a source of learning and development*. Upper Saddle River, NJ: Prentice Hall.

Kossek, E. E., DeMarr, B. J., Backman, K., & Kolar, M. (1993). Assessing employees' emerging elder care needs and reactions to dependent care benefits. *Public Personnel Management, 22*, 617–638.

Landro, L. (2011, March 28). The time to innovate is now. *Wall Street Journal*, p. D1.

Lavarreda, S. A., Brown, E. R., Cabezas, L., & Roby, D. H. (2010, March). *Number of uninsured jumped to more than eight million from 2007 to 2009*. UCLA Center for Health Policy Research. www.healthpolicy.ucla.edu/pubs/files/Uninsured_8-Million_PB_%200310.pdf.

Lawler, E. (1989). Pay for performance: A strategic analysis. In L. R. Gomez-Mejia (Ed.), *Compensation and benefits* (pp. 136–181). Washington DC: Bureau of National Affairs.

Lawler, E. (2000). *Rewarding excellence: Pay strategies for the new economy*. San Francisco: Jossey-Bass.

Lipowicz, A. (2009, October 21). Wireless medical records system comes to Indianapolis. *Federal Computer Week*. http://few.com/Articles/2009/10/21/Indianpolis-ambulance-accessing-wireless-EHR-syst.

Locke, E. A. (1968). Towards a theory of task motivation and incentives. *Organizational Behavior and Human Performance, 3*, 157–189.

Lombardi, D. N. (1988a). *Handbook of personnel selection and performance evaluation in healthcare*. San Francisco: Jossey-Bass.

Lombardi, D. N. (1988b). Mind trust: Dimensions of healthcare leadership. *Administrative Radiology, 9*, 25–29.

Lombardi, D. N. (1988c). Performance evaluation techniques. *Administrative Radiology, 5*, 35–39.

Lombardi, D. N. (1990a). Eliminating future tense. *Administrative Radiology, 9*, 14–19.

Lombardi, D. N. (1990b). Ethics, healthcare and the 1990's: Part 1. *Clinical Laboratory Management, 6*, 416–425.

Lombardi, D. N. (1990c). Ethics of the heart and mind. *Administrative Radiology, 10*, 17–22.

Lombardi, D. N. (1990d). Intrapreneurial constituency management: A success profile for the 1990's. *Hospital Material Management Quarterly, 11,* 26–31.

Lombardi, D. N. (1990e). *Progressive leadership with values: Progressive strategies for healthcare management.* Chicago: ACHE.

Lombardi, D. N. (1990f). *Stress and the healthcare environment.* Ann Arbor: Health Administration Press.

Lombardi, D. N. (1990g). Urban healthcare in crisis. *Administrative Radiology, 2,* 14–22.

Lombardi, D. N. (1991a). Ethics and the organizational human resources strategy. *Clinical Laboratory Management, 1,* 31–39.

Lombardi, D. N. (1991b). The new pyramid: Laying the groundwork with motivational power. *Administrative Radiology, 6,* 45–50.

Lombardi, D. N. (1992a). Healthcare and the new union movement. *Materials Administrative Radiology, 4,* 16–21.

Lombardi, D. N. (1992b). *Progressive healthcare management strategies.* Chicago: American Hospital.

Lombardi, D. N. (1993a). *Handbook for the new healthcare manager.* Chicago: American Hospital.

Lombardi, D. N. (1993b). Human resource management in the health care setting. *Hospital and Health Services Administration, 3,* 298–299.

Lombardi, D. N. (1994a). *The healthcare organizational survey system.* Chicago: American Hospital Publishing.

Lombardi, D. N. (1994b). How to diagnose and treat conflict in your department. *Materials Management in Healthcare, 1.*

Lombardi, D. N. (1994c). The last public trust. *Administrative Radiology, 1.*

Lombardi, D. N. (1994d). The pyramid organization: Maximizing performance strategies. *Healthcare Executive.*

Lombardi, D. N. (1996). *Thriving in an age of change: Practical strategies for health care leaders.* Chicago: Health Administration Press.

Lombardi, D. N. (1997). *Reorganization and renewal: Strategies for healthcare leaders.* Chicago: Health Administration Press.

Lombardi, D. N. (2002). *Handbook for the new healthcare manager* (2nd ed.). Hoboken, NJ: Wiley.

Lombardi, D. N. (2005). Preparing for the future: Leadership and management strategies. *Healthcare Executive, 11,* 8–14.

Lombardi, D. N. (2006). *Health care management.* Hoboken, NJ: Wiley.

Manzo, P. (2004, Winter). The real salary scandal: It isn't that some nonprofit CEOs make big bucks. It's that most nonprofit employees are paid too little. *Stanford Social Innovation Review,* pp. 65–66.

Maslow, A. H. (1954). *Motivations and personality.* New York: HarperCollins.

McClelland, D. C. (1961). *The achieving society.* New York: Free Press.

McCrae, R. R. (2002). NEO-PI-R data from 36 cultures: Further intercultural comparisons. In R. R. McCrae & J. Alik (Eds.), *The five-factor model of personality across cultures* (pp. 105–125). New York: Kluwer Academic.

McCrae, R. R., & Costa, P. T. (2004, February). A contemplated revision of the NEO five-factor inventory. *Personality and Individual Differences, 36,* 587–596.

McCurdy, A. H., Newman, M. A., & Lovrich, N. P. (2002). Family-friendly workplace policy adoption in general and special purpose local governments: Learning from the Washington State experience. *Review of Public Personnel Administration, 22*(1), 27–51.

McDonnell Douglas v. Green. (1973). 401 U.S. 424.

McIntosh, A. (2010, February 9). Health care department breaches privacy. *Sacramento Bee,* p. 3A.

McKay, J. (2007, June). Mind reader. *Government Technology, 20*(6), 38, 40.

McPherson v. Rankin. (1987). 483 U.S. 378.

Meacham v. Knolls Atomic Power Laboratory. (2008). No. 06-1505.

Mount Healthy City School District Board of Education v. Doyle. (1977). 429 U.S. 274.

Nason, J. W. (1993). *Board assessment of the chief executive: A responsibility essential to good governance* (4th ed.). Washington DC: National Center for Nonprofit Boards.

National Labor Relations Board. (1997). *A guide to basic law and procedures under the NLRA* (Rev. ed.). Washington DC: U.S. Government Printing Office.

National Labor Relations Board v. Catholic Bishop of Chicago. (1979). 440 U.S. 490.

National Treasury Employees Union v. Von Raab. (1989). 489 U.S. 656.

Nelson-Horchler, J. (1989). Elder care comes of age. *Industry Week, 238,* 54–56.

Nevada Department of Human Resources v. Hibbs. (2003). 538 U.S. 721.

Newlin, J. G., & Meng, G. J. (1991). The public sector pays for performance. *Personnel Journal, 70,* 110–114.

Oakwood Healthcare, Inc. and International Union, United Automobile, Aerospace and Agricultural Implement Workers of America (UAW), AFL-CIO. (2006). 348 NLRB, No. 37.

Oblinger, D. (2003, July-August). Boomers, Gen-Xers Millennials: Understanding the new students. *EDCAUSE,* pp. 37–47.

O'Connor v. Consolidated Coin Caters Corporation. (1996). 517 U.S. 308.

Office of National Drug Control Policy. (2004). *The economic costs of drug abuse in the United States, 1992–2002.* Washington DC: Author.

Perry, J. L. (1995). Compensation, merit pay, and motivation. In S. W. Hays & R. C. Kearney (Eds.), *Public personnel administration: Problems and prospects* (3rd ed.), pp. 121–317. Upper Saddle River, NJ: Prentice Hall.

Perry, J. L. (2000). Bringing society in: Toward a theory of public service motivation. *Journal of Public Administration Research and Theory, 10*(2), 471–488.

Phillips, J. J., & Stone, R. D. (2002). *How to measure training results.* New York: McGraw-Hill.

Phillips, P. P., & Phillips, J. J. (2002). The public sector challenge: Developing a credible ROI process. In P. P. Phillips (Ed.), *Measuring ROI in the public sector* (pp. 1–32). Alexandria, VA: ASTD.

Pickering v. Board of Education. (1968). 391 U.S. 563, 568.

Pierson, J., & Mintz, J. (1995). *Assessment of the chief executive: A tool for governing boards and chief executives of nonprofit organizations.* Washington DC: National Center for Nonprofit Boards.

Pillay, R. (2008). Managerial competencies of hospital managers in South Africa: A survey of managers in the public and private sectors. *Human Resources for Health, 6*(4), 1–7.

Primoff, E. S. (1975, June). *How to prepare and conduct job-element examinations.* Washington DC: U.S. Civil Service Commission, Personnel Research and Development Center.

Primoff, E. S., & Eyde, L. D. (1988). Job element analysis. In S. Gael (Ed.), *The job analysis handbook for business, industry, and government* (Vol. 2), pp. 807–825. Hoboken, NJ: Wiley.

Pynes, J. E. (1997). *Human resources management for public and nonprofit organizations.* San Francisco: Jossey-Bass.

Pynes, J. E. (2003a). Pay for performance and merit pay. In J. Rabin (Ed.), *Encyclopedia of public administration and public policy* (pp. 885–889). New York: Marcel Dekker.

Pynes, J. E. (2003b). Strategic human resources management. In S. Hays & R. Kearney (Eds.), *Public personnel administration: Problems and prospects* (4th ed.), pp. 93–105. Upper Saddle River, NJ: Prentice Hall.

Pynes, J. E. (2003c). Training and development. In J. Rabin (Ed.), *Encyclopedia of public administration and public policy* (pp. 1219–1225). New York: Marcel Dekker.

Pynes, J. E. (2004a). *Human resources management for public and nonprofit organizations* (2nd ed.). San Francisco: Jossey-Bass.

Pynes, J. E. (2004b). The implementation of workforce and succession planning in the public sector. *Public Personnel Management, 33*(4), 389–404.

Pynes, J. E. (2007a). Pay for performance and merit pay. In E. M. Berman & J. Rabin (Eds.), *Encyclopedia of public administration and public policy* (2nd ed.), pp. 1423–1427. New York: Taylor & Francis.

Pynes, J. E. (2007b). Training and development. In E. M. Berman & J. Rabin (Eds.), *Encyclopedia of public administration and public policy* (2nd ed.), pp. 1942–1948. New York: Taylor & Francis.

Pynes, J. E. (2009a). *Human resources management for public and nonprofit organizations: A strategic approach* (3rd ed.). San Francisco: Jossey-Bass.

Pynes, J. E. (2009b). Strategic human resources management. In S. Hays, R. Kearney, & J. Coggburn (Eds.), *Public personnel administration: Problems and prospects* (5th ed.), pp. 95–106. Upper Saddle River, NJ: Prentice Hall.

Rainey, H. G. (2003). *Understanding and managing public organizations* (3rd ed.). San Francisco: Jossey-Bass.

Raymark, P. H., Schmit, M. J., & Guion, R. M. (1997). Identifying potentially useful personality constructs for employee selection. *Personnel Psychology, 50,* 723–736.

Reddick, C. G., & Coggburn, J. D. (2007). State government employee health benefits in the United States: Choices and effectiveness. *Review of Public Personnel Administration, 27*(5), 5–20.

Risher, H. (2002). Pay-for-performance: The keys to making it work. *Public Personnel Management, 31,* 317–332.

Risher, H., Fay, C. H., & Perry, J. L. (1997). Merit pay: Motivating and rewarding individual performance. In H. Risher & C. H. Fay (Eds.), *New strategies for public pay: Rethinking government compensation programs* (pp. 253–271). San Francisco: Jossey-Bass.

Roberts, G. E. (2000). An inventory of family-friendly benefit practices in small New Jersey local governments. *Review of Public Personnel Administration, 20*(2), 50–62.

Roberts, G. E. (2002). Municipal government part-time employee benefit practices. *Public Personnel Management, 33,* 1–22.

Roberts, G. E. (2004). Mental health benefits in New Jersey state and local government. *Public Personnel Management, 31,* 211–224.

Rutan v. Republican Party of Illinois. (1990). 497 U.S. 62.

Shareef, R. (1994). Skill-based pay in the public sector. *Review of Public Personnel Administration, 14*(3), 60–74.

Shareef, R. (1998). A midterm case study of skill-based pay in the Virginia Department of Transportation. *Review of Public Personnel Administration, 18*(1), 5–22.

Shareef, R. (2002). The sad demise of skill-based pay in the Virginia Department of Transportation. *Review of Public Personnel Administration, 22*(3), 233–240.

Simon, S. (2011, March 28). Medicine on the move. *Wall Street Journal.* http://online.wsj.com/article/SB10001424052748703559604576174842490398186.html.

Sims, R. R. (1998). *Reinventing training and development.* Westport, CT: Quorum.

Skipp, C. (2010, March 5). Miami board looks to close two hospitals. *New York Times,* p. A13.

Smith v. City of Jackson. (2005). 544 U.S. 228.

Society for Human Resources Management. (2010). *What senior HR leaders need to know: Perspectives from the United States, Canada, India, the Middle East and North Africa.* Arlington, VA: Author.

Society for Industrial and Organizational Psychology. (2003). *Principles for the validation and use of personnel selection procedures* (4th ed.). www.siop.org/_Principles/principles.pdf.

St. Mary's Honor Center v. Hicks. (1993). 509 U.S. 502.

Tanner, A. (2002). Professional staff education: Quantifying costs and outcomes. *Journal of Nursing Education, 32*(2), 91–97.

Thompson, J. R. (2007). *Designing and implementing performance-oriented payband systems.* Washington DC: IBM Center for the Business of Government. www.businessofgovernment.org.

Thompson, J. R., & Lehew, C. W. (2000). Skill-based pay as on organizational innovation. *Review of Public Personnel Administration, 20*(1), 20–40.

Towers Perrin. (1992). *Why did we adopt skill-based pay?* New York: Author.

Trans World Airlines, Inc. v. Hardison. (1977). 432 U.S. 63.

Uniform guidelines on employee selection procedures. (1978, August 25). *Federal Register, 43*(166), 38290–38315.

United Automobile Workers v. Johnson Controls. (1991). 499 U.S. 187.

U.S. Merit Systems Protection Board. (2006). *Designing an effective pay for performance compensation system.* Washington DC: U.S. Government Printing Office.

U.S. Merit Systems Protection Board. (2008). *Attracting the next generation: A look at federal entry-level hires.* Washington DC: U.S. Government Printing Office.

U.S. Office of Personnel Management. (2005). *OPM's workforce planning model.* www.opm.gov/hcaaf_resource_center/assets/Sa_tool4.pdf.

U.S. Office of Personnel Management. (2006). *Career patterns: A 21st century approach to attracting talent.* Washington DC: Author.

U.S. Office of Personnel Management. (2010). Salary table 2010-GS. www.opm.gov/oca/10tables/html/gs.asp.

Vroom, V. H. (1964). *Work and motivation.* Hoboken, NJ: Wiley.

Wager, K. A., Lee, F. W., & Glaser, J. P. (2009). *Health care information systems: A practical approach for health care management* (2nd ed.). San Francisco: Jossey-Bass.

Wallace, M. J., Jr., & Fay, C. H. (1988). *Compensation theory and practice* (2nd ed.). Boston: PWS-Kent.

Washington counties create training video on pandemic flu preparation. (2008, February 6). Government Technology. www.govtech.com/gt/print_article.php?id=261382.

Watson v. Fort Worth Bank and Trust. (1988). 487 U.S. 977.

West, D. J., Jr. (2002). Healthcare management competencies for physician leaders in clinical settings in CEE/NEE countries. *Journal of Health Sciences Management and Public Health, 3*(2), 105–112.

Wexley, K. N., & Latham, G. P. (1991). *Developing and training human resources in organizations* (2nd ed.). Upper Saddle River, NJ: Prentice Hall.

White, G. (2007, July 22). Resuscitating Grady: Buyouts leave hospital with large talent drain. *Atlanta Journal Constitution*, pp. D1, D10–D11.

Work begins on national e-health record network. (2009, September 30). *Associated Press.*

INDEX

Page references followed by *fig* indicate an illustrated figure; followed by *t* indicate a table.

A

Accountability: action versus discussion, 59–61; backstage versus onstage, 62–63; closure versus "revisiting," 61–62; customer focus versus nonplayer focus, 59; deniability versus, 59; encouragement versus empowerment, 65; "how" versus "if," 62; known versus unknown, 63–64; leaders versus leaners, 64–65; PACT Formula component of, 55*fig*, 58–59, 61–65; performance management focus of, 210; positions versus postures, 65; practical versus conceptual, 61; strategies for escalating, 338–344; written versus verbal, 63

Accountability strategies: annual report, 343–344; "big events," 341–342; fan mail bulletin board, 340–341; human resources board summit, 338–339; organizational surveys, 342; quarterly reviews, 343; time lines, 343; volunteer activation, 340

Accrediting Commission on Education for Health Services Administration, 169

Achievement tests, 189

Action agents/superstars, 50–52

Action orientation, 78–79

Acumen of volunteers, 137*fig*, 139–141

ADA Amendments Act (2008), 90–93

Administrative services organizations (ASOs), 36

"Administrator's Interpretation Letter" (DOL), 96

Administrivia, 313–314

Advertising: external recruitment using, 196–197; media used for recruitment, 185

Advocates/steadies, 51*t*, 52–53

Affirmative action: description of, 98–99; Executive Orders 11246 and 11375 on, 99–101; Rehabilitation Act (1973) on, 101–102; SHRM planning focus on, 112; Uniformed Services Employment and Reemployment Rights Act (USERA) [1994], 102; Vietnam Era Veterans' Readjustment Act (1974), 102

Age Discrimination in Employment Act (ADEA) [1967], 89–90, 103*t*

Agencies (search), 184–185

Agency shop agreement, 363–364

Agitators/nonplayers, 51*t*, 53, 311

AIDS/HIV status of employees, 91, 92, 283, 293

Air Training Command, 172

Alderfer, Clayton P., 249

All My Children (TV soap opera), 19

Ambassador programs, 347–348

Ambulance-based information system, 378

American innovators, 326*t*

American Society for Healthcare Human Resources Administration, 372

Americans with Disabilities Act (1990), 90–93, 94, 103*t*, 158, 197

Amos, Corporation of the Bishop of the Church of Jesus Christ of Latter Day Saints v., 88

Annual reports, 343–344

Appraisal discussion format: step 1: opening overview, 231–232; step 2: key goal attainment, 232; step 3: work personality assessment, 232–233; step 4: developmental direction, 233; step 5: constructive consensus, 233

Appropriate bargaining unit, 360

Arbitration: grievance, 371–372; interest, 368–369

Arline v. School Board of Nassau County, 101

Assessment: executive performance use of, 223–224; of job candidate KSAOCs, 187–192; work personality, 232–233. *See also* Evaluation; Performance evaluation

Audiovisual methods, 297–298

B

"Back to the basics" program, 345

Balanced scorecard approach, 219–220

Baptist Hospital (Louisville), 126

Bargaining representative, 362–363

Barnabas Health, 5, 6, 8

Behavior-common cultures, 127–128

behavioral observation scales (BOS), 213, 217*fig*

Behaviorally anchored rating scales (BARS), 214–215, 216*fig*

Belief-centered cultures, 126

Benchmark positions, 255

Benchmarking: accountability encouraged through, 341–342; human resources (HR), 43–44

Benefits: description of, 271–272; discretionary, 276–282, 277*t*; domestic partnership, 283; employee assistance program (EAP), 283–284; flexible, 282–283; flexible job environment, 284–285; government required, 272–276, 277*t*; human resources information

systems (HRIS) employees, 385; outplacement assistance, 284. *See also* Compensation

Benefits consulting services, 35

The Beth Blog, 128

The Beth (NBIMC), 5–6, 128

"Big events," 341–342

Blood drives, 147

Board of directors, 339

Board of Education, Pickering v., 105

Board of Trustees of the University of Alabama v. Garrett, 93

Bon Secours Health System, 126

Bona fide occupational qualification (BFOQ), 85–87

Branding, 334–335

Branti v. Finkel, 106

Broadbonding (or paybanding), 261

Budget Reconciliation Act (1986), 273

Business Not As Usual: Preparing for Pandemic Flu (Public Health Seattle and King County), 297

Business operations: health care training and development to manage, 310–311; volunteer role in, 146–147

Business orientation, 75

C

"C Factors," 76, 121–122

California Department of Health Care Services, 388

California Federal Savings & Loan Association v. Guerra, 89

California Psychological Inventory, 189

Cancellation of employees, 244–245

Career development: description and benefits of, 306–307; human resources information systems (HRIS), 385–386; job analysis used to design, 156. *See also* Health care training and development; Training and development

Case studies, 296

Catholic Bishop of Chicago, National Labor Relations Board v., 357

CD-ROM software, 301, 388

Ceballos, Garcetti v., 106

Celebrating the wins, 336–337

Centers for Disease Control and Prevention, 196

CEO report, 335–336

Change Readiness Inventory, 342

Change. *See* Organizational change

Chicago Hope (TV show), 19

Chief executive officer (CEO): annual report issued by, 335–336; "big events" role of, 341;

human resources board summit role of, 339; of progressive health care organizations, 22, 24; volunteer summit participation by, 148

Chief financial officer (CFO), 25–26

Chief information officer (CIO), 26

Chief operating officer (COO), 24

Children's Hospital of New Jersey, 6

Children's Hospital (Philadelphia), 141

City of Jackson, Smith v., 90

Civil Rights Act (1964): description of the, 103*t*; involuntary affirmative action permitted under, 100; Sections 702 and 703, 87–88; Title VII, 84–87, 94, 367

Civil Rights Act (CRA) [1991], 93–94, 104*t*

Civil Rights Acts (1866 and 1871), 84, 94, 103*t*, 104–105

Civil Rights Attorney's Fee Awards Act (1976), 94

Civil Rights Division (Department of Justice), 158

Civil Service Reform Act (CSRA) [1978], 358–359

Clara Maass Medical Center (CMMC), 6–7

Clarity, 76, 122

Classification Act (1923), 254

Classification Act (1949), 255

Clock management, 76

Closed shop agreement, 363

Closure, 76, 122

Cognitive ability and aptitude tests, 189

Collective bargaining: in federal government agencies, 358–359; grievance arbitration, 371–372; in health care organizations, 355–357; impasse resolution, 367–369; management rights, 367; in the private sector, 354–355; scope of, 365–367; selecting bargaining representative, 362–363; in state and local government agencies, 359; strikes, 369–371; unfair labor practices, 365; union security, 363–365; unit determination, 360–362

Commitment: contribution versus criticism, 69–70; fact versus fiction, 69; majority commitment versus 100 percent consensus, 67; need versus want, 67; outcomes versus opinions, 69; PACT Formula component of, 55*fig*, 66–70; participants versus spectators, 68–69; perspective versus perception, 68; solution formulation versus problem reiteration, 67–68; specific versus general, 68; taking a stand versus having a committee, 70; telling versus selling, 70

Communication: five "C Factors" of, 76, 121–122; health care training and development for strategic, 315–316, 320*t*, 328–329; HR professionals' skill for direct, 76; human resources information systems (HRIS) policies and procedures, 386; interest-motivated cultures and medical lexicon, 128; psychographics of, 129–132; responsive, 76; unique vernacular of health care organizations, 121; volunteer with skills related to, 142–143

Community: health care organizational development focus on, 320*fig*, 321; health care volunteers and the, 147; training resources form within the, 298; volunteer summit agenda on local, 149

Community resources for training, 298

Community-based recruitment, 186–187

Community-driven education, 332–333

Compassion, 76, 122

Compensation: Equal Pay Act of 1963 governing, 268–269; executive benefits and, 265–267; Fair Labor Standards Act (FLSA) governing, 42, 267–268; human resources information systems (HRIS) employees, 385; job analysis to development systems of, 156; pay differentials, 260–261; unemployment, 274; workers,' 274–275. *See also* Benefits

Compensation systems: employee equity used for, 258, 260265; external equity used for, 253–254; General Schedule (GS), 255, 258, 259*t*; internal equity used for, 254–255, 258; typical compensable factors considered in, 256*t*–257*t*

Competencies: description of, 168; eight managerial positions, 168–169; executive performance evaluation of, 224–225; for health care organization positions, 169–170; International Council of Nurses identification for nurse specialist, 170

Competency modeling, 168–170

Competitive edge, 324

Comprehensive communication, 76, 122

Comprehensive Occupation Data Analysis Program, 172

Computer-based training, 298

Conciliation agreement, 100

Confluent skills, 139

Connick v. Myers, 105

Consent decree, 100

Consolidated Coin Caters Corporation, O'Connor v.,
      90

Consolidated Omnibus Budget Reconciliation Act
      (COBRA), 279

Constitutional rights: due process rights, 108–109;
      expressive rights, 105–106; freedom of
      association, 106–107; limits on political
      participation, 107–108; overview of, 102,
      104–105; privacy rights, 108. *See also* U.S.
      Constitution

Content theories of motivation: ERG theory, 249;
      hierarchy of needs, 248–249;
      motivator-hygiene theory, 250–251; theory of
      needs, 249–250

Contextual performance analysis, 173–174

Continuous quality improvement (CQI) craze, 65,
      70

*Cook v. State of Rhode Island, Department of Mental
      Health, Retardation, and Hospitals,* 102

Coordination, 76, 122

*Corporation of the Bishop of the Church of Jesus Christ
      of Latter Day Saints v. Amos,* 88

Council for Adult and Experiential Learning, 281

Credo: community-driven education use of,
      332–333; definition of, 330; Majuro Medical
      Center Credo of Nursing, 330*fig*; strategies for
      building, 330–331

Crisis Intervention Team (CIT) [Memphis], 300

Critical incident reports, 214*fig*

Critical incident technique, 162

Cultural composition foundations, 122–123*fig*

Cultural factors: behavior-common cultures,
      127–128; belief-centered cultures, 126;
      cultural composition foundations
      determining, 122–123*fig*; experience-based
      cultures, 124–125; HR (human resources)
      and relevance of, 122–128; interest-motivated
      cultures, 128; objective-driven cultures, 125;
      psychographics for charting, 129–132;
      regionally founded cultures, 127. *See also*
      Organizational culture

Curriculum. *See* Training curriculum

Customer-patients: declining public trust in health
      care by, 19–21; escalating expectations of,
      15–16; factual perception of, 13, 14;
      "life-or-death" perception collectively
      prevalent in, 14–15; new era of focus on, 327;
      sending appropriate messages to, 327–328;
      "tender loving care" (TLC) provided to, 117,
      121. *See also* Patient care

D

Decency value, 66*fig*

Decision making: criteria and process of, 77*fig*;
      decisive approach to, 76–77

Decisiveness, 76–77

Defined-benefit pension plans, 276–277

Defined-contribution pension plans, 277–278

Department of Justice, 98, 158

Department of Labor, 96, 98, 99

Department of Labor Procedure and Functional
      Job Analysis, 171

Department of Labor's Employment and Training
      Service, 276

Department of Veterans Affairs (VA) Health Care
      System: employee pay scale for employees of,
      258; experienced-based culture of, 124–125;
      external recruitment requirements of, 196;
      time line system used at, 58, 60*fig*

Development: career, 156, 306–307, 385–386;
      organizational themes from great American
      innovators, 326*t*; strategies for health care
      organization, 319–351. *See also* Training and
      development

"Difficult personality" employees, 311

Direct communication, 76

Disability insurance, 280

Discretionary benefits: description of, 276;
      disability insurance, 280; education programs,
      281–282; health insurance, 278–280; paid
      time away from work, 280–281; pensions,
      276–278; summary of, 277*t*

Discrimination: age, 89–90; disparate impact,
      97–98; disparate treatment, 96–97;
      individuals with disabilities and, 90–93;
      pregnancy, 89; religious, 87–88

Disparate impact, 97–98

Disparate treatment, 96–97

Distributive justice, 263

Documentation: performance evaluation form,
      226–231; performance evaluation program,
      220–221

Domestic partnership benefits, 283

Dothard v. Rawlinson, 86

*Doyle, Mount Healthy City School District Board of
      Education v.,* 105

Drug addiction, 283–284

Drug testing, 191

Drug-related problems, 283–284

Due process rights, 108–109

Dues checkoff mechanism, 364

E

E-learning training: simulators, 299–300; streaming media, 299; virtual reality, 300–301

E-mail management, 313–314

Edison, Thomas, 326*t*

Education programs, 281–282

Educational needs analysis, 345–346

Edwards Personal Preference Schedule, 189

800-number help lines, 13

Electronic health records (EHRs), 378

Electronic human resources management, 388–389

Employee assistance program (EAP), 283–284

Employee equity: broadbonding or paybanding, 261; description of, 258; gainsharing, 264–265; General Schedule (GS) for federal employees, 258, 259*t*; longevity pay, 261; merit pay or pay for performance, 262–264; pay differentials, 260–261; skill-based pay or pay for knowledge, 261–262

Employee Polygraph Protection Act (1988), 192

Employee referral system, 184

Employees: "Administrator's Interpretation Letter" (DOL) on gay and lesbian, 96; affirmative action and, 98–102; benefits for, 271–284, 385; cancellation of, 244–245; collective bargaining by, 354–369; compensation of, 42, 156, 260–269, 274–275, 385; constitutional rights of, 102–109; "difficult personalities," 311; discrimination against, 87–93, 96–98; employment at will doctrine and, 110–111; fan mail bulletin board made available to, 340–341; federal equal employment opportunity protections of, 84–96; grievance arbitration and, 371–372; H-IB visas for temporary foreign workers, 197–198; HIV/AIDS status of, 91, 92, 283, 293; human resources information systems (HRIS) access by, 387; independent contractors compared to, 275; integrating HRIS technology and, 387–388; limiting negative emotionalism of, 325–326; morale and positive outlook of, 325; recruitment and selection of, 155–156, 181–206, 385–386; strategies for halting the retirement of productive, 42; strikes by, 369–371; suspension of, 243–244; whistle-blower protection of, 109–110. *See also* Health care workforce; Human capital; Performance evaluation

Employment at will doctrine, 110–111

Employment Retirement Income Security Act, 42

Employment Verification (I-9) Form, 93

Enterprise human resources outsourcing services, 36

Equal Employment Opportunities Commission (EEOC), 85, 91, 93, 98, 158, 187

Equal Employment Opportunity Act, 42

Equal employment opportunity laws: addressing religious discrimination, 87–88; Age Discrimination in Employment Act (ADEA) [1967], 89–90, 103*t*; Americans with Disabilities Act and ADA Amendments Act, 90–93, 94, 103*t*; bona fide occupational qualification (BFOQ), 85–87; Civil Rights Act (CRA) of 1991, 93–94, 104*t*; Civil Rights Acts (1866 and 1871), 84, 94, 103*t*; Family and Medical Leave Act (FMLA) [1993], 42, 94–96, 104*t*; Immigration Reform and Control Act (IRCA) [1986], 93; Pregnancy Discrimination Act (1978), 89, 103*t*; SHRM planning focus on, 112; summary of the, 103*t*–104*t*; Title VII of the Civil Rights Act (1964), 84–87, 94, 103*t*; Uniformed Services Employment and Reemployment Rights Act (USERA) [1994], 102, 104*t*

Equal Pay Act of 1963, 268–269

Equity theory, 252–253

ER (TV show), 19

ERG theory, 249

Essay for performance evaluation, 212–213

Evaluation: of candidate interviews, 204–206; of candidate résumés, 194*fig*; Kirkpatrick's four level model for, 303–305; of SHRM effectiveness, 42–44; 360-degree, 215–217, 218*fig*; of training and development, 303–306. *See also* Assessment; Performance evaluation

Exclusive recognition, 362

Executive compensation and benefits, 265–267

Executive Order 11246 (1965), 99–101

Executive Order 13198 (2001), 88

Executive Order 13199 (2001), 88

Executive Order 13279 (2002), 88

Executive Order 13280 (2002), 88

Executive performance evaluation: competencies evaluated as part of, 224–225; conducting a, 222–225; four methods of assessment used for, 223–224

Expectancy theory, 251–252

Experience and training rating, 190

Experience-based cultures, 124–125

Experiential exercises, 297
Expert-based systems, 382
Expressive rights, 105–106
External equity, 253–254
External recruitment: advertising and legal issues of, 196–197; description of, 195–196; technology used for, 196

F

Facilitating employees, 242–243
Fact finding, 368
Fact sheets, 348*fig*
Factual perception: on customer-patients, 13, 14; on Internet health information, 13–14
Fair dealing exception, 111
Fair Labor Standards Act (FLSA), 42, 267–268, 386
Fair share provision, 364
Family and Medical Leave Act (FMLA) [1993], 42, 94–96, 104*t*
Family Responsibilities Discrimination: Litigation Update 2010, 283
Fan mail bulletin board, 340–341
Federal Insurance Contributions Act (FICA), 273
Federal laws: collective bargaining, 354–372; equal employment opportunity, 42, 87–104*t*; governing compensation, 267–269; government required benefits, 272–276. *See also* Legislation; U.S. Constitution
Federal Service Labor-Management Relations Statute (LMRS), 358, 371
Fifth Amendment, 109
Finkel, Branti v., 106
First Amendment, 105–106
Fiscal responsibility, 322
Five "C Factors," 76
Flexible benefits, 282–283
Flexible job environment, 284–285
Florida Board of Regents, Kimmel v., 90, 93
The Florida Hospitals, 142
Ford Motor Company, 291
Forecasting: description of, 38; SHRM use of, 38–42
Fort Worth Bank and Trust, Watson v., 98
Fortitude value, 66*fig*
Founders' Day, 341–342
Fourteenth Amendment, 109
Fourth Amendment, 108
Franciscan Health System, 126
Freedom of association, 106–107

G

Gainsharing: compensation bonus program, 264–265; as performance evaluation technique, 219–220
Garcetti v. Ceballos, 106
Garcia v. San Antonio Metropolitan Transit Authority, 267–268
"Garment gimmicks," 337–338
Garrett, Board of Trustees of the University of Alabama v., 93
Gates, Bill, 326*t*
Gay employees, 96
General employee education, 349–350
General Schedule (GS) system: Classification Act (1949) establishment of, 255; criticisms of, 255, 258; for federal employees, 258, 259*t*
Glass Ceiling Act (1991), 94
Goal-setting book, 253
Goalsharing plan, 219, 220
Good faith exception, 111
Government Accountability Office, 44
Government Employee Rights Act (1991), 94
Government required benefits: description of, 272; Medicare, 273; military leave, 276; Social Security, 272–273; summary of, 277*t*; unemployment compensation, 274; workers' compensation, 274–275
Grady Memorial Hospital (Atlanta), 41–42
Green, McDonnell Douglas v., 97
Grievance arbitration, 371–372
Guerra, California Federal Savings & Loan Association v., 89

H

H-IB visas, 197–198
"Halo Effect," 205
Hardison, Trans World Airlines, Inc. v., 87
Hatch Act, 107–108
Hawaii Labor Relations Board, 370
Head Start programs, 147
Healey v. Southwood Psychiatric Hospital, 86–87
Health benefits services, 35
Health care: demands for nontraditional services as part of, 9; escalating expectations of, 15–16; five change dynamics of modern, 12–21; as media target, 16–19; unique models of health care in the, 3–4
Health care change dynamics: escalating expectations, 15–16; health care as a media target, 16–19; life-or-death outcomes, 14–15;

overview of, 12–14; "people intensity," 21; public trust, 19–21

Health care leaders: accountability characteristic of, 55*fig*, 58–59, 61–65; celebrating the wins, 336–337; commitment characteristic of, 55*fig*, 66–70; defined values of progressive, 66*fig*; pride characteristic of, 55*fig*, 56–58, 60*fig*; training and development specifically for, 308*fig*–316; trust characteristic of, 55*fig*, 71–74. *See also* PACT Formula

Health care organizational development: community commitment/public relations objective of, 320*fig*, 321, 328–329; competitive edge objective of, 324; definition of, 319–320; essential tenets of, 320*fig*; fiscal responsibility objective of, 322; future readiness objective of, 321; for introduction of a new era, 326–327; morale and positive outlook objective of, 325; optimization of resources objective of, 323–324; organizational galvanization objective of, 322–323; organizational viability objective of, 320–321; performance maximization objective of, 321–322; redirecting performance and action objective of, 323; on sending appropriate messages, 327–328; social commitment objective of, 324. *See also* Organizational change; Strategic human resources management (SHRM)

Health care organizational strategies: for building pride, 329–338; for escalating accountability, 338–344; for team building, 344–350

Health care organizations: collective bargaining, 355–357; current perceptions of, 7–9; importance of volunteers in, 135–151; organizational culture standards for HR of, 49–80; unique models of U.S., 3–4; unique vernacular of, 121. *See also* Human resources (HR); Progressive health care organizations

Health care professionals: "difficult personalities" among, 311; organizational chronology of a, 25*fig*; strategies for halting the retirement of productive, 42; unique characteristics of, 115–122

Health care training and development: critical dimensions of, 308*fig*–310; efficiency of, 308*fig*, 309–310; for encouraging workplace innovation and creativity, 313; for essential management and leadership strategies, 311; immediate usefulness of, 308*fig*, 309; for

leading through change, crisis, and conflict, 311–312; limiting negative employee emotionalism objective of, 325–326; to manage changes in today's business environment, 310–311; on presentation skills, 314–315; relevance of, 308*fig*–309, 310–316; resonance of, 308*fig*, 309, 310–316; for strategic analysis and planning, 312–313; for strategic communication and leadership, 315–316; on stress management, 313–314; for team building, 312. *See also* Career development

Health care workforce: collective bargaining by, 355–357; cultural factors relevant to HR (human resources), 122–128; "difficult personalities" among, 311; limitations to strikes by, 369–371; nonplayers/agitators among, 51*t*, 53, 311; steadies/advocates among, 51*t*, 52–53; superstars/action agents among, 50–52, 311; unique characteristics of, 115–122. *See also* Employees; Human capital

Health insurance: COBRA legislation on, 279; costs and types of, 278–279; importance as benefit, 278; Mental Health Parity Act (1996) impact on, 279–280

Health Insurance Portability and Accountability Act (HIPAA), 279

Health maintenance organization (HMO) plans, 278

Health Research and Educational Trust, 272

Health savings accounts (HSAs), 279

HEALTHeCAREERS network, 196

Herzberg, Frederick, 250–251

Hibbs, Nevada Department of Human Resources v., 95

Hicks, St. Mary's Honor Center v., 97

Hierarchy of needs, 248–249

High visibility, 74–75

High-deductible health plans (HDHPs), 278, 279

HIV/AIDS status of employees, 91, 92, 283, 293

Hoboken Gen X crew: compared to New Jersey Retirees, 131*t*–132; psychographics of, 129, 130*t*

Hoboken University Medical Center (HUMC), 5

Honesty and integrity tests, 192

Hope Credit, 281

Hospital Jobs Online, 196

The Hospital for Special Care (Connecticut), 141

"Hot cargo" clauses, 354

House rules, 333–334

How to Measure Training Results (Phillips and Stone), 306

HRO Today (2009), 35

Human capital: effective strategic management of, 47; health care organizational development focus on, 320*fig*; Performance Matrix used to enhance, 50–54, 311; recruitment and selection for increasing, 155–156, 178–207. *See also* Employees; Health care workforce

Human resources board summit, 338–339

Human resources (HR): compensation and benefits manager of, 28; cultural factors relevant to, 122–128; director of employee relations of, 29; health care organization role of, 11–12; human resources generalist of, 28; job analysis for planning, 156; organizational chart of health care organization, 27*fig*; organizational culture standards for, 49–80; outsourcing, 35–36; recruiting manager of the, 28; SHRM approach to planning, 36–38; training and development specialists of, 28–29. *See also* Health care organizations

Human resources information systems (HRIS): applications to SHRM, 389–390; career planning and staffing systems, 385–386; caution with outsourcing, 388; communicating policies and procedures, 386; compensation and benefits, 385; costs and factors to consider for developing, 40; description of, 35, 384; employee access to, 387; forecasting workforce needs using computerized, 39–40; integrating employees and technology through, 387–388; outsourcing, 35; training and performance support of, 387. *See also* Information technology services; Technology

Human resources management (HRM): changing role of, 32–34; electronic, 388–389; human resources outsourcing by, 35–36; for improving organizational effectiveness, 155; job analyses providing foundation for, 155–164; recruitment using contacts of, 183; strategic requirements for, 74–79; understanding long-term implications of, 32. *See also* Strategic human resources management (SHRM)

Human resources management (HRM) requirements: action orientation, 78–79; business orientation, 75; decisiveness, 76–77*fig*; direct communication, 76; high visibility, 74–75; knowledgeability, 77–78; pragmatism, 79; responsiveness, 76; strength, 79; user-friendliness, 75

Human resources planning model, 37–38

Huntington VA Medical Center (VAMC), 329

Huntington VA Medical Center (VAMC) fact sheet, 348*fig*

I

"I" formula, 313, 314*fig*

I-9 (Employment Verification) Form, 93

IBM, 291

Identity theft, 388

Illegal Immigration Reform and Immigrant Responsibility Act (1996), 197

Illegal or prohibited topic of bargaining, 366–367

Illinois Department of Central Management Services, 307

Immigration Reform and Control Act (IRCA) [1986], 93, 103*t*, 197

Impasse resolution: definition of, 367; fact finding for, 368; interest arbitration for, 368–369; mediation for, 367–368

Implied contract exception, 110–111

In-basket exercises, 190–191

Incentive services, 36

Independent contractors, 275

Industry value, 66*fig*

Informal staff referrals, 185

Information technology services: ambulance-based, 378; description of, 36, 378–379; electronic health records (EHRs), 378; expert-based systems, 382; health care capabilities of, 379–380; knowledge-level systems, 382; management-level systems, 382–383; operational-level systems, 381–382; organizational change facilitated by, 380–381; outsourcing, 36; strategic-level systems, 383–384. *See also* Human resources information systems (HRIS); Technology

Integrity value, 66*fig*

Interest arbitration, 368–369

Interest inventories, 190

Interest-motivated cultures, 128

Intergenerational day care, 141

Internal equity: description of, 254–255, 258; typical compensable factors considered for, 256*t*–257*t*

Internal job candidates, 185–186

Internal recruitment, 185–186

Internal Revenue Service (IRS), 275
International Council of Nurses, 170
International Personality Item Pool, 174
Interviewing. *See* Job candidate interviews
IRI Consultants, 372

J
Jackson Health System (Miami), 45
Job analyses: developing compensation systems, 156; HR planning, career development, and training, 156; information gathered for, 158–163; job design using, 157; KSAOCs identified through, 155–156, 292–293; legal significance of, 157–158; performance evaluation using, 156; personality-based, 173–174; recruitment and selection component of, 155–156; risk management using, 156–157; Structured Checklist, 161*fig*; team-based, 174; techniques for, 170–174
Job analysis program: considerations for, 163; designing a, 163–164
Job Analysis Questionnaire, 160*fig*
Job analysis techniques: Comprehensive Occupation Data Analysis Program, 172; contextual performance analysis, 173–174; Department of Labor Procedure and Functional Job Analysis, 171; job element method, 172–173; Occupational Information Network, 173; Position Analysis Questionnaire (PAQ), 171
Job candidate interviews: conducting the, 199–204; dyad dynamics of, 202*fig*–203; evaluating the, 204–206; preparing and planning for, 198–199; reviewing résumés and setting slate for, 193–195
Job candidates: interviewing, 193–195, 198–206; likeability of, 204–205; recruitment of, 155–156, 181–187, 195–197; reviewing résumés, 193–195; selection of, 155–156, 178–195, 198–206; undertaking applications and screening, 187–193
Job component review, 344–345
Job description: definition of, 157–158; example of a, 166*fig*–167*fig*; overview of, 164–165, 167–168; performance evaluation form on, 227; preselection process of reviewing the, 181
Job design, 157
Job element method, 172–173
Job fairs, 183
Job family, 157

Job rotation, 285
Job specifications list, 164–165
Johnson Controls, United Automobile Workers v., 85–86
The Joint Commission. *See* TJC (The Joint Commission)
Jurisdictional standards, 355

K
Kaiser Family Foundation, 272
Kimmel v. Florida Board of Regents, 90, 93
Kirkpatrick's evaluation model, 303–305
Knolls Atomic Power Laboratory, Meachan v., 90
Knowledge, skills, abilities, and other characteristics (KSAOCs): developing training objectives for, 293–294; as employee equity compensation factor, 260; job analysis information on, 158–163; job analysis program designed around, 164; job analysis to identify, 155–156, 292–293; job description including required, 164–168, 182–183; job element method consideration of, 172–173; management-level systems to identify, 383; performance evaluation of, 210; presentation skills, 314–315; screening job candidates for, 187–192; tracting for recruitment, 185–186; training curriculum that imparts, 294, 295–296, 301, 304
Knowledge-level systems, 382
Knowledgeability: as human resource management requirement, 77–78; as leadership value, 66*fig*

L
Labor-management relations: collective bargaining in federal government agencies, 358–359; collective bargaining in health care organizations, 355–357; collective bargaining in the private sector, 354–355; collective bargaining in state and local government agencies, 359; grievance arbitration, 371–372; impasse resolution, 367–369; management rights, 367; scope of collective bargaining, 365–367; selecting bargaining representative, 362–365; strikes, 369–371; unfair labor practices, 365; unit determination, 360–362
Labor-Management Relations Act (LMRA) [Taft-Hartley Act]: grievance arbitration requirements by, 371; *Oakwood* decision impacting, 361; provisions for the private sector, 354–355; Section 2(14) provisions for

Labor-Management Relations Act (LMRA)
  [Taft-Hartley Act]: (*Continued*)
  health care organizations, 355–357; Section
  14(b) on union security provisions, 364–365;
  state statutes modeled after the, 359
Labor-Management Reporting and Disclosure Act
  (Landrum-Griffin amendments), 354
Leaders. *See* Health care leaders
Lecture format, 296
Legal cases: *Arline v. School Board of Nassau County,*
  101; *Board of Trustees of the University of
  Alabama v. Garrett,* 93; *Branti v. Finkel,* 106;
  *California Federal Savings & Loan Association
  v. Guerra,* 89; *Connick v. Myers,* 105; *Cook v.
  State of Rhode Island, Department of Mental
  Health, Retardation, and Hospitals,* 102;
  *Corporation of the Bishop of the Church of Jesus
  Christ of Latter Day Saints v. Amos,* 88;
  Dothard v. Rawlinson, 86; *Garcetti v. Ceballos,*
  106; *Garcia v. San Antonio Metropolitan
  Transit Authority,* 267–268; *Healey v.
  Southwood Psychiatric Hospital,* 86–87;
  Kimmel v. Florida Board of Regents, 90, 93;
  McDonnell Douglas v. Green, 97; *McPherson v.
  Rankin,* 105; *Meachan v. Knolls Atomic Power
  Laboratory,* 90; *Mount Healthy City School
  District Board of Education v. Doyle,* 105;
  *National Labor Relations Board v. Catholic
  Bishop of Chicago,* 357; *National Treasury
  Employees Union v. Won Raab,* 108; *Nevada
  Department of Human Resources v. Hibbs,* 95;
  *Oakwood Healthcare, Inc. and International
  Union United Automobile, Aerospace and
  Agricultural Implement Workers of America
  (UAW), AFL-CIO* decision, 361; *O'Connor v.
  Consolidated Coin Caters Corporation,* 90;
  Pickering v. Board of Education, 105; *Rutan v.
  Republic Party of Illinois,* 106; *St. Mary's Honor
  Center v. Hicks,* 97; *Smith v. City of Jackson,*
  90; *Trans World Airlines, Inc. v. Hardison,* 87;
  United Automobile Workers v. Johnson Controls,
  85–86; *Watson v. Fort Worth Bank and Trust,*
  98
Legislation: Age Discrimination in Employment
  Act (ADEA) [1967], 89–90, 103*t*; Americans
  with Disabilities Act and ADA Amendments
  Act, 90–93, 94, 103*t*, 158, 197; Budget
  Reconciliation Act (1986), 273; Civil Rights
  Act (1964), 84–88, 94, 100, 103*t*, 367; Civil
  Rights Act (CRA) of 1991, 93–94, 104*t*;

Civil Rights Acts (1866 and 1871), 84, 103*t*,
  104–105; Civil Rights Attorney's Fee Awards
  Act (1976), 94; Civil Service Reform Act
  (CSRA) [1978], 358–359; Classification Act
  (1923), 254; Classification Act (1949), 255;
  Consolidated Omnibus Budget Reconciliation
  Act (COBRA), 279; Employee Polygraph
  Protection Act (1988), 192; Employment
  Retirement Income Security Act, 42; Equal
  Employment Opportunity Act, 42; Equal Pay
  Act of 1963, 268–269; Fair Labor Standards
  Act (FLSA), 42, 267–268, 386; Family and
  Medical Leave Act (FMLA) [1993], 42,
  94–96, 104*t*; Family and Medical Leave
  National Defense Authorization Act for FY
  2010 Amendments, 95–96; Federal Insurance
  Contributions Act (FICA), 273; Federal
  Service Labor-Management Relations Statute
  (LMRS), 358, 371; Glass Ceiling Act (1991),
  94; Government Employee Rights Act (1991),
  94; Hatch Act, 107–108; Health Insurance
  Portability and Accountability Act (HIPAA),
  279; Illegal Immigration Reform and
  Immigrant Responsibility Act (1996), 197;
  Immigration Reform and Control Act (IRCA)
  [1986], 93, 197; Labor-Management
  Relations Act (LMRA) [Taft-Hartley Act],
  354–357, 359, 361, 364–365, 371;
  Labor-Management Reporting and Disclosure
  Act (Landrum-Griffin amendments), 354;
  Mental Health Parity Act (1996), 279–280;
  National Defense Authorization Act (NDAA)
  [2008], 95–96; National Labor Relations Act
  (NLRA) [1935], 354; Occupational Safety
  and Health Act, 42; Paul Wellstone and Pete
  Domenici Mental Health Parity and
  Addiction Equity Act (2008), 280; Political
  Activities Act (1939), 107; Pregnancy
  Discrimination Act (1978), 89, 103*t*; Public
  Accounting Reform and Investor Protection
  Act (2002) [Sarbanes-Oxley Act], 110; public
  employee relations acts (PERAs), 359, 360;
  Rehabilitation Act (1973), 91, 101–102,
  103*t*; Section 501 (Rehabilitation Act), 91;
  Section 503 (Rehabilitation Act), 91; Section
  504 (Rehabilitation Act), 102; Section 1981A
  (Title 42 of the U.S. Code), 94; Social
  Security Act (1935), 273, 274; Social Security
  Amendments (1983), 273; Tax Reform Act
  (1986), 277; Title 38 (Civil Service Reform

Act), 358–359; Title VII of the Civil Rights Act (1964), 84–87, 94, 103t, 367; Title VII (Civil Service Reform Act), 358; Uniformed Services Employment and Reemployment Rights Act (USERA) [1994], 102, 104t, 276; Vietnam Era Veterans' Readjustment Act (1974), 102; Whistleblower Protection Act (1989), 110. *See also* Federal laws

Lesbian employees, 96

Lie detector exams, 191–192

Life-or-death outcomes: evidence of public perception of, 14–15; as health care change dynamic, 14–15

Lifetime Learning Credit, 281–282

Limits on political participation, 107–108

Lincoln, Abraham, 326t

"Lincoln on Leadership," 315

"Little Hatch Acts," 107–108

Local government agency collective bargaining, 359

Logos: branding and signage through, 335; credo reflected by, 331; "garment gimmicks" using, 337–338

Long Island Jewish Hospital, 126

Longevity pay, 261

Low, Juliette, 326t

M

Maass, Clara, 326t

McClelland, David, 249

McDonnell Douglas v. Green, 97

McPherson v. Rankin, 105

Maintenance of membership, 364

Majuro Medical Center Credo of Nursing, 330fig

Management by objectives, 213

Management education, 350

Management-level systems, 382–383

Mandatory topic of collective bargaining, 365–366

Marriott, 198

Maslow, Abraham, 248

Mayo Clinics, 17, 142

Meachan v. Knolls Atomic Power Laboratory, 90

Media: doctor icons of television, 18–19; e-learning, 299–301; health care as target of the, 16–19; recruitment through advertising, 185

Mediation, 367–368

"Medicine on the Move" (*Wall Street Journal*), 377

Mental Health Parity Act (1996), 279–280

Mercy Hospital System (Oklahoma), 144

Merit pay (or pay for performance), 262–264

Metropolitan East Coast, 335

Midcareer breaks (or sabbaticals), 285

Military leave, 276

Minnesota Multiphasic Personality Inventory, 189

Mission: of great American innovators, 326t; health care organizational development focus on, 320fig; organizational development strategies to reinforce, 329. *See also* Values

Monster.com, 196

Morale, 325

Motivation: content theories of, 248–251; definition of, 247–248; process theories of, 251–253; words used to describe, 248

Motivator-hygiene theory, 250–251

Mount Healthy City School District Board of Education v. Doyle, 105

Myers, Connick v., 105

N

National Alliance for Caregiving and Evercare, 283

National Defense Authorization Act (NDAA) [2008], 95–96

National Labor Relations Act (NLRA) [1935], 354

National Labor Relations Board (NLRB), 354, 356t–357, 360, 362

National Labor Relations Board v. Catholic Bishop of Chicago, 357

National Treasury Employees Union v. Won Raab, 108

Needs assessment, 291–293

NEO Job Personality Inventory, 174

NEO PI-R Job Profiler, 174

Nevada Department of Human Resources v. Hibbs, 95

New Jersey Retirees: compared to Hoboken Gen X crew, 130t, 132; psychographics of, 129, 131t

Newark Beth Israel Medical Center (NBIMC), 5–6, 128

Newsweek magazine, 17–18

Nonplayers/agitators, 51t, 53, 311

Nontraditional service demands, 9

O

Oakwood Healthcare, Inc. and International Union United Automobile, Aerospace and Agricultural Implement Workers of America (UAW), AFL-CIO decision, 361

Objective-driven cultures, 125

Occupational Information Network, 173

Occupational Safety and Health Act, 42

O'Connor v. Consolidated Coin Caters Corporation, 90

Office of Federal Contract Compliance Programs (OFCCP), 99–100

Office of Personnel Management, 37, 172, 183, 258, 259*t*

Office of Special Counsel (OSC), 107

Operational-level systems, 381–382

Optimization of resources, 323–324

Organizational change: Change Readiness Inventory, 342; five dynamics of health care, 12–21; how information technology can facilitate, 380–381; leading through, 311–312; managing in today's business environment, 310–311. *See also* Health care organizational development

Organizational culture: HR professionals as stewards of, 49–50; PACT Formula as hallmark of, 54–74; Performance Matrix used to enhance human capital, 50–54, 311; strategic communication and leadership training on, 315–316; strategic requirements for HR management department, 74–79. *See also* Cultural factors

Organizational handbook of values, 331–332*fig*

Organizational surveys, 342

Outplacement assistance, 284

Outsourcing: caution on HRIS, 388; HRM services that can be included in, 35–36; *HRO Today* (2009) report on, 35

P

Pacification of employees, 241–242

PACT Formula: accountability component of, 55*fig*, 58–59, 61–65; commitment component of, 55*fig*, 66–70; overview of the, 54–55*fig*; pride component of, 55*fig*, 56–58, 60*fig*; trust component of, 55*fig*, 71–74. *See also* Health care leaders

Paid time away from work: Family and Medical Leave Act (FMLA) [1993] on, 42, 94–96, 104*t*; type of, 280–281

Patient care: progressive placement of volunteers for, 146; volunteer role in, 145–146. *See also* Customer-patients

Paul Wellstone and Pete Domenici Mental Health Parity and Addiction Equity Act (2008), 280

Pay differentials, 260–261

Pay for knowledge (or skill-based pay), 261–262

Pay for performance (or merit pay), 262–264

Paybanding (or broadbonding), 261

Payroll software and services: description of, 35; outsourcing, 35

Pensions: defined-benefit pension plans, 276–277; defined-contribution pension plans, 277–278; description of, 276

"People intensity," 21

Perceptual reality, 14

Performance evaluation: components of an effective form, 226–231; as critical component of SHRM, 210; defusers to employee reactions to, 241–245; format for an appraisal discussion, 231–233; fundamental elements of a sound, 225–226; job analysis for, 156; KSAOCs assessed as part of, 210; managing potential employee reactions to, 233–241; Performance Matrix used for, 53–54, 311. *See also* Assessment; Employees; Evaluation

Performance evaluation employee defusers: cancellation, 244–245; facilitation, 242–243; pacification, 241–242; suspension, 243–244

Performance evaluation employee reactions: charge of personal bias, 237–238; complacency, 239; complete surprise, 234–235; contradiction, 240; expected praise, 235–236; immediate blame, 236–237; misunderstanding of objectives, 235; strong nonverbal reaction, 238–239; strong verbal reaction, 238; taken initiative, 240–241

Performance evaluation form: administrative data section of, 226–227; development plan section of, 229; employee comments section of, 229–230; job description section of, 227; objectives and expectations adjustment section of, 228–229; overall rating section of, 230; review of past year's expectations and objectives section of, 227–228; signatures section of, 230–231; work characteristic ratings section of, 228

Performance evaluation programs: development of, 210–211; documentation used in, 220–221; evaluation review component of, 221–222; executive evaluation component of, 222–225; individual performance appraisal techniques used in, 211–217*fig*; rater training for, 222; team-based performance appraisal techniques used in, 217–220

Performance evaluation review: conducting a, 221–222; defusers to employee reactions during, 241–245; format for an appraisal discussion, 231–233; managing potential employee reactions during, 233–241; performance evaluation form used for, 226–231

Performance evaluation techniques: balanced scorecard approach, 219–220; behavioral observation scales (BOS), 213, 216*fig*, 217*fig*; behaviorally anchored rating scales (BARS), 214–215; critical incident reports, 214*fig*; essays, 212–213; gainsharing plan, 219, 220; goalsharing plan, 219, 220; individual-based, 211–217*fig*; management by objectives, 213; personnel data, 215; productivity data or work standards, 213; team-based, 217–220; 360-degree evaluations, 215–217, 218*fig*; trait rating scales, 212, 213*fig*

Performance management: accountability focus on, 210; health care organizational development strategies for, 321–322, 323; human resources information systems (HRIS), 387; motivation component of, 247–253

Performance Matrix: description of, 12, 50; human capital enhanced through use of, 50–54; nonplayers/agitators category of, 51*t*, 53; performance evaluation systems application of, 53–54; steadies/advocates category of, 51*t*, 52–53; superstars/action agents category of, 50–52; training in order to best use, 311

Permissive topics of collective bargaining, 366

Personal development plans, 346

Personality inventories, 189

Personality-based job analysis, 173–174

Personnel data evaluation, 213

PG Chambers School, 116

Physical ability tests, 192

Physician network listings, 13

Physicians Employment, 196

Pickering v. Board of Education, 105

Point of service (POS) plans, 278

Political Activities Act (1939), 107

Political participation limitations, 107–108

Position Analysis Questionnaire (PAQ), 171

Position Classification Inventory, 174

Pragmatism, 79

Preferred provider organization (PPO) plans, 278, 279

Pregnancy Discrimination Act (1978), 89, 103*t*

Preselection process: compiling a list of expectations, 180–181; compiling a wish list, 179–180; overview of, 178–179; reviewing the job description, 181; reviewing

recruitment tactics, 181–187; reviewing résumés and setting interviewing slate, 193–195; undertaking application and screening procedures, 187–192

Presentation skills, 314–315

Pride: affecting versus annoying, 56–57; majority versus minority, 56; PACT Formula component of, 55*fig*, 56–58; progress versus status quo, 57; VA time lines, 58, 60*fig*; wins versus losses, 57–58

Privacy rights, 108

Procedural justice, 263

Process theories of motivation: equity theory, 252–253; expectancy theory, 251–252; goal-setting theory, 253

Productivity data, 213

Professional contacts, 184

Professional employer organizations (PEOs), 36

Programmed instruction, 298

Progressive health care organizations: composition of HR management department of, 27*fig*–29; defined leadership values of, 66*fig*; defining elements of, 4–7; organizational chart of a midsize community hospital, 23*fig*; profile of a, 22–27; strategies for organizational development of, 319–351; volunteer placement by, 146*t*. *See also* Health care organizations

Psychographics: comparing Hoboken Gen X crew and New Jersey retirees, 129–132; definition of, 129

Psychological examinations, 192

Public Accounting Reform and Investor Protection Act (2002), 110

Public employee relations acts (PERAs), 359, 360

Public policy exception, 110

Public relations impact, 328–329

Public trust, health care and declining, 19–21

Q

Quality of life: employee assistance program (EAP) impacting, 283–284; flexible benefits impacting, 282–283; flexible job environment impacting, 284–285; outplacement assistance impacting, 284

Quality of work: employee assistance program (EAP) impacting, 283–284; flexible benefits impacting, 282–283; flexible job environment impacting, 284–285; outplacement assistance impacting, 284

Quarterly reviews, 343
Queens (New York City), 123–124

R
Rankin, McPherson v., 105
Rawlinson, Dothard v., 86
Recruiting, staffing, and search services: description
    of, 35; outsourcing, 35; search agencies,
    184–185
Recruitment: definition of, 181–182; external,
    195–197; human resources information
    systems (HRIS) professionals, 385–386; job
    analysis used for, 155–156; reviewing tactics
    for, 181–187; sources for, 182*fig. See also*
    Selection
Redefinition strategies, 349
Regenstrief Institute, 378
Regionally founded cultures, 127
Rehabilitation Act (1973): affirmative action
    provision of, 101–102; description of the,
    103*t*; Section 504 on individuals with
    disabilities, 102; Sections 501 and 503 on
    individuals with disabilities, 91, 101
Religious discrimination laws, 87–88
Relocation services: description of, 35; outsourcing,
    35
Republic Party of Illinois, Rutan v., 106
Respondeat superior ("let the master answer"), 105
Responsiveness, 76
Résumés: bridging the interview and review of,
    198–206; reviewing job candidate, 193–195;
    sorting by criteria, 193
Retirement: halting for productive employees, 42;
    pension benefits during, 276–278
Return on investment (ROI) analysis, 43–44
Return to Objectivity formula: cancellation,
    244–245; facilitation, 242–243; pacification,
    241–242; suspension, 243–244
Right-to-work states, 364–365
Risk management, 156–157
Robert Wood Johnson Foundation, 278
Role playing, 296
Roosevelt, Eleanor, 326*t*
Rutan v. Republic Party of Illinois, 106

S
Sabbaticals, 285
St. Mary's Honor Center v. Hicks, 97
*San Antonio Metropolitan Transit Authority, Garcia
    v.,* 267–268

Sarbanes-Oxley Act (2002), 110
School Board of Nassau County, Arline v., 101
School liaison programs, 183–184
Screening services, 35
Search agencies, 184–185
Section 501 (Rehabilitation Act), 91
Section 503 (Rehabilitation Act), 91
Section 504 (Rehabilitation Act), 102
Section 1981A (Title 42 of the U.S. Code), 94
Security: HRIS outsourcing and breach of, 388;
    union, 363–365; workplace, 35
Selection: definition of, 181–182; human resources
    information systems (HRIS) professionals,
    385–386; interviewing for, 193–195,
    198–206; job analysis used for, 155–156;
    preselection process, 178–195; reviewing
    résumés, 193–195; undertaking application
    and screening procedures, 187–192. *See also*
    Recruitment
Self-Descriptive Index, 174
Semi-Annual Labor Activity in Health Care Report
    (2009), 372
Signage, 334–335
Simulators, 299–300
Skill sets of volunteers, 137*fig*, 141–143
Skill-based pay (or pay for knowledge), 261–262
Sloan Kettering Cancer Services, 17
Smith v. City of Jackson, 90
Social commitment, 324
Social Security Act (1935), 273, 274
Social Security Amendments (1983), 273
Social Security benefits, 272–273
Southwood Psychiatric Hospital, Healey v., 86–87
Spheres of Influence Model: description of, 9–12;
    illustrated diagram of, 10*fig*
Standard operating practice (SOP), 139
Start On Success (SOS) Program [NBIMC], 6
State government agency collective bargaining, 359
*State of Rhode Island, Department of Mental Health,
    Retardation, and Hospitals, Cook v.,* 102
Steadies/advocates, 51*t*, 52–53
Stevens Healthcare Educational Partnership, 334
Strategic analysis and planning, 312–313
Strategic human resources management (SHRM):
    basic beliefs and purpose of, 31–32;
    benchmarking and ROI analysis of, 43–44;
    equal employment opportunity and
    affirmative action focus of, 112; forecasting
    by, 38–42; Grady Memorial Hospital as
    example of poor, 41–42; HRIS applications

to, 389–390; HRM audit to assess effectiveness of, 42–43; human resources planning by, 36–38; performance evaluation as critical component of, 210; problems and implications of, 44–45; strategic job analyses as integral to, 155–175. *See also* Health care organizational development; Human resources management (HRM)

Strategic human resources technology, 377–378

Strategic job analysis, 165–166

Strategic-level systems, 383–384

Streaming media, 299

Strength attribute, 79

Stress management, 313–314

Strikes, 369–371

Structured Checklist, 159, 161*fig*

Structured oral exams, 190

Subject matter experts (SMEs): job analysis program designed by, 164; job element method role of, 172; structured checklist developed by, 159, 161*fig*

Succession planning, 347

Superstars/action agents, 50–52, 311

Suspension of employees, 243–244

T

Taft-Hartley Act. *See* Labor-Management Relations Act (LMRA) [Taft-Hartley Act]

Tax Reform Act (1986), 277

Team building: organizational development strategies for, 344–350; training and development for, 312

Team building strategies: ambassador programs, 347–348; "back to the basics" program, 345; educational needs analysis, 345–346; fact sheets, 348*fig*; general employee education, 349–350; job component review, 344–345; management education, 350; personal development plans, 346; redefinition strategies, 349; succession planning, 347

Team-based job analysis, 174

Technical training: human resources information systems (HRIS), 387; importance to health care operations, 24

Technology: assessing job candidate's skills with, 205–206; e-learning, 299–301; integrating employees and HRIS, 387–388; recruitment using, 196. *See also* Human resources information systems (HRIS); Information technology services

Temporary foreign workers, 197–198

"Tender loving care" (TLC), 117, 121

Tennis elbow, 128

Theory of needs, 249–250

Thirteenth Amendment, 84

360-degree evaluations, 215–217, 218*fig*

Time lines: as accountability strategy, 343; VA Health Care System use of, 58, 60*fig*; volunteer summit agenda on, 148

Time magazine, 17–18

Title 38 (Civil Service Reform Act), 358–359

Title VII (Civil Rights Act of 1964), 84–87, 94, 367

Title VII (Civil Service Reform Act), 358

TJC (The Joint Commission), 117, 121, 227

Training curriculum: audiovisual methods used for, 297–298; case studies used for, 296; community resources used for, 298; e-learning and technology used for, 299; experiential exercises used for, 297; issues to consider when developing, 294–296; KSAOCs imparted by, 294, 295–296, 301, 304; lecture format for, 296; programmed instruction and computer-based training, 298; role playing format for, 296

Training delivery, 302–303

Training and development: delivering the, 302–303; description and benefits of, 289–291; developing the curriculum for, 294–301; developing training objectives, 293–294; evaluating, 303–306; experience and training rating, 190; health care, 308*fig*–316; HR job analyses, 156; HR specialists in development and, 28–29; human resources information systems (HRIS), 387; job analysis used to design, 156; needs assessment for, 291–293; performance evaluation rater, 222. *See also* Career development; Development

Training objectives, 293–294

Trait rating scales, 212, 213*fig*

Trans World Airlines, Inc. v. Hardison, 87

Trust: assurance versus apprehension, 73–74; clarity versus complexity, 73; community versus family, 72; PACT Formula component of, 55*fig*, 71–74; patient-driven versus ego-driven, 72; proactive versus reactive, 72–73; running toward versus running from, 73; we versus they, 71

U

Unemployment compensation, 274

Unfair labor practices, 365

Uniform Guidelines on Employee Selection Procedures, 98, 157

Uniformed Services Employment and Reemployment Rights Act (USERA) [1994], 102, 104*t*, 276

Union security: agency shop agreement on, 363–364; closed shop agreement on, 363; description of, 363; dues checkoff mechanism of, 364; fair share provision on, 364; maintenance of membership provision on, 364; right-to-work states, 364–365; union shop provision on, 363

Union shop, 363

Unit determination, 360–362

United Automobile Workers v. Johnson Controls, 85–86

United States Marine Corps, 291

UnitedHealth Group, 283

Upward Mobility Program (state of Illinois), 307

Urban Institute, 278

U.S. Air Force, 172

U.S. Citizenship and Immigration Services, 197

U.S. Civil Service Commission, 98

U.S. Constitution: Fifth Amendment, 109; First Amendment, 105–106; Fourteenth Amendment, 109; Fourth Amendment, 108; Thirteenth Amendment, 84. *See also* Constitutional rights; Federal laws

U.S. Department of Justice, 98, 158

U.S. Department of Labor, 96, 98, 99, 171, 276

U.S. Department of Veterans Affairs. *See* Department of Veterans Affairs (VA) Health Care System

U.S. Equal Employment Opportunities Commission (EEOC), 85, 91, 93, 98

U.S. Merit Systems Protection Board, 196, 262

U.S. Office of Federal Contract Compliance Programs (OFCCP), 99–100

U.S. Office of Personnel Management, 37, 172, 183, 258, 259*t*

U.S. Office of Special Counsel (OSC), 107

USA Today, 17

USAJOBS, 196

User-friendliness, 75

V

Values: community-driven education based on, 332–333; credo reflecting, 330–331,

332–333; house rules reflecting, 333–334; organizational handbook of, 331–332*fig. See also* Mission

Vesting, 276–277

Vietnam Era Veterans' Readjustment Act (1974), 102, 103*t*

Virtual Leaders program (Lowes Hotels), 300–301

Virtual reality, 300–301

Visiting Nurse Association (VNA) Health Group, 116

Volunteer summits: agenda topics for, 148–151; benefits of holding, 148

Volunteers: accountability by activating, 340; acumen of, 137*fig*, 139–141; business operations role of, 146–147; community relations and, 147; confluent skills of, 139; fan mail bulletin board made available to, 340–341; identifying background strengths of, 137*fig*; importance of, 135–136; organizational support of, 143–145; patient care by, 145–146; professional experience of, 136–139; progressive placement of, 146*t*; skill sets of, 137*fig*, 141–1434; ten essential rules for placement of, 150–151

Vroom, Victor H., 251

Vscan technology, 377

W

Wall Street Journal, 377

Watson v. Fort Worth Bank and Trust, 98

Web-based services: description of, 35; outsourcing, 35

WebMD, 13

What Senior HR Leaders Need to Know: Perspectives from the United States, Canada, India, the Middle East and North Africa (SHRM), 33–34

Whistle-blower protection, 109–110

Whistleblower Protection Act (1989), 110

Wishard Health Services (Indianapolis), 378

Won Raab, National Treasury Employees Union v., 108

Work sample or performance tests, 190

Work standards evaluation, 231

Workers' compensation, 274–275

Workforce. *See* Health care workforce

Workplace innovation and creativity, 313

Workplace security services, 35

Y

Youth liaison programs, 147